W0227615

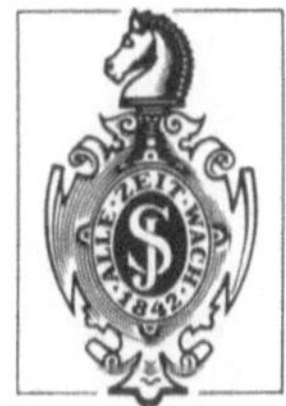
ALLE ZEIT WACH
1842

J. Koscielny F. Jung
H. Kiesewetter A. Haaß (Eds.)

# *Hemodilution*

With 91 illustrations and 79 tables

With contributions by

B. Angelkort, R. Bach, G. Berg, B. Bertram, L. Bette, A. Birk, J. Blume, H. Böhme, I. Bulik, I. Decker, J. Dyckmans, S. Erlenwein, H. Förster, M. Gerhards, A. Haaß, G. Hamann, L. Heilmann, T. Holbach, R. Hubertus, F. Jung, U. Kässer, H. Kiesewetter, W. Kolepke, J. Koscielny, G. Leipnitz, C. Mrowietz, M. Reim, H. Schieffer, W. Schimetta, J. Schwab, J. Simon, S. Spitzer, M. Stoll, T. Tormann, J. Treib, W. Vogel, P. Waldhausen, E. Wenzel, H.-J. Wilhelm and S. Wolf

Springer-Verlag Berlin Heidelberg GmbH

Dr. med. J. Koscielny

Prof. Dr. med., Dr.-Ing. H. Kiesewetter

Priv.-Doz., Dr.-Ing. F. Jung

Abteilung für Klinische
Hämostaseologie und Transfusionsmedizin
Universitätskliniken
W-6650 Homburg/Saar

Prof. Dr. med. A. Haaß

Universitätsnervenklinik – Neurologie
Universitätskliniken
W-6650 Homburg/Saar

ISBN 978-3-540-55352-6 ISBN 978-3-662-07748-1 (eBook)
DOI 10.1007/978-3-662-07748-1

Library of Congress Cataloging Cataloging-in-Publication Data

Hemodilution / J. Koscielny ... [et al.].
Includes bibliographical references and index.
ISBN 978-3-540-55352-6
1. Hemodilution. I. Koscielny, J. (Jürgen)
[DNLM: 1. Blood Circulation – Physiology. 2. Hemodilution.
WG 166 H489] RC671.5.H4546 1992 616.1'06-dc20 DNLM/DLC for
Library of Congress


Originally published by Springer-Verlag Berlin Heidelberg New York in 1992



27/3145/5 4 3 2 1 0 – Printed on acid-free paper

## Acknowledgment

We are especially grateful to Fresenius AG, Bad Homburg, for supporting this research. Special tribute must also be extended to Dr. Elder Granger, Chief, Department of Medicine, Landstuhl Army Regional Medical Center, who kindly reviewed the English version of this book.

# Contents

# List of Contributors

Angelkort, B., Prof. Dr. med.
Medizinische Klinik Nord im Klinikzentrum Nord der Städtischen Kliniken Dortmund, Münster Str. 240, 4600 Dortmund

Bach, R., Dr. med.
Medizinische Klinik und Poliklinik, Innere Medizin III, Universitätsklinik des Saarlandes, 6650 Homburg/Saar

Berg, G., Dr. med.
Medizinische Klinik und Poliklinik, Innere Medizin III, Universitätsklinik des Saarlandes, 6650 Homburg/Saar

Bertram, B., Dr. med.
Augenklinik der Medizinischen Fakultät RWTH Aachen, Pauwelsstraße, 5100 Aachen

Bette, L., Prof. Dr. med. (†)
Medizinische Klinik und Poliklinik, Innere Medizin III, Universitätsklinik des Saarlandes, 6650 Homburg/Saar

Birk, A., Dr. med.
Zentrum für Gefäß- und Kreislauferkrankungen, 5100 Aachen

Blume, J., Dr. med.
Gemeinschaftspraxis für Angiologie, Katschof 3, 5100 Aachen

Böhme, H., Prof. Dr. med.
Institut für Gefäßerkrankungen, Zentralkrankenhaus Gauting, Unterbrunner Str. 85, 8035 Gauting/München

Bulik, I., Dr. med.
Institut für Gefäßerkrankungen, Zentralkrankenhaus Gauting, Unterbrunner Str. 85, 8035 Gauting/München

Decker, I., Dr. med.
Universitätsnervenklinik – Neurologie, Universitätsklinik des Saarlandes, 6650 Homburg/Saar

Dyckmans, J., Dr. med.
Medizinische Klinik und Poliklinik, Innere Medizin III, Universitätsklinik des Saarlandes, 6650 Homburg/Saar

Erlenwein, S.,
Abteilung für Klinische Hämostaseologie und Transfusionsmedizin, Universitätsklinik des Saarlandes, 6650 Homburg/Saar

Förster, H., Prof. Dr. med.
Zentrum für Anaesthesiologie und Wiederbelebung, Klinikum der Johann Wolfgang Goethe-Universität, 6000 Frankfurt am Main 70

Gerhards, M., Dipl.-Ing.
Zentrum für Gefäß- und Kreislauferkrankungen, 5100 Aachen

Haaß, A., Prof. Dr. med.
Universitätsnervenklinik – Neurologie, Universitätsklinik des Saarlandes, 6650 Homburg/Saar

Hamann, G., Dr. med.
Universitätsnervenklinik – Neurologie, Universitätsklinik des Saarlandes, 6650 Homburg/Saar

Heilmann, L., Prof. Dr. med.
Stadtkrankenhaus Rüsselsheim, Abteilung für Gynäkologie und Geburtshilfe, August-Bebel-Str. 59, 6090 Rüsselsheim

Holbach, T., Dr. med.
Abteilung für Chirurgie, St. Elisabeth-Krankenhaus, 6648 Wadern/Saar

Hubertus, R.,
Abteilung für Klinische Hämostaseologie und Transfusionsmedizin, Universitätsklinik des Saarlandes, 6650 Homburg/Saar

Jung, F., Priv.-Doz., Dr.-Ing.
Abteilung für Klinische Hämostaseologie und Transfusionsmedizin, Universitätsklinik des Saarlandes, 6650 Homburg/Saar

Kässer, U., Dr. med.
Abteilung für Kardiologie, Robert-Bosch-Krankenhaus, 7000 Stuttgart 50

Kiesewetter, H., Prof. Dr. med., Dr.-Ing.
Abteilung für Klinische Hämostaseologie und Transfusionsmedizin, Universitätsklinik des Saarlandes, 6650 Homburg/Saar

Kolepke, W., Dr. med.
Abteilung für Klinische Hämostaseologie und Transfusionsmedizin, Universitätsklinik des Saarlandes, 6650 Homburg/Saar

Koscielny, J., Dr. med.
Abteilung für Klinische Hämostaseologie und Transfusionsmedizin, Universitätsklinik des Saarlandes, 6650 Homburg/Saar

Leipnitz, G., Dr. med.
Abteilung für Klinische Hämostaseologie und Transfusionsmedizin, Universitätsklinik des Saarlandes, 6650 Homburg/Saar

Mrowietz, C., Dipl.-Ing.
Abteilung für Klinische Hämostaseologie und Transfusionsmedizin, Universitätsklinik des Saarlandes, 6650 Homburg/Saar

Reim, M., Prof. Dr. med.
Augenklinik der Medizinischen Fakultät RWTH Aachen, Pauwelsstraße, 5100 Aachen

Schieffer, H., Prof. Dr. med.
Medizinische Klinik und Poliklinik, Innere Medizin III, Universitätsklinik des Saarlandes, 6650 Homburg/Saar

Schimetta, W., Dr. rer. nat.
Abteilung für „Infusionen und klinische Ernährung", Laevosan Gesellschaft m. b. H., Estermannstr. 17, A-4020 Linz

Schwab, J., Dr. med.
Abteilung für Geriartrie, Jakobi Krankenhaus, 4440 Rheine

Simon, J., Dr. med.
Fachabteilung für Anästhesie, Caritas-Krankenhaus Dillingen, 6638 Dillingen/Saar

Spitzer, S., Dr. med.
Medizinische Klinik und Poliklinik, Innere Medizin III, Universitätsklinik des Saarlandes, 6650 Homburg/Saar

Stoll, M., Dr. med.
Universitätsnervenklinik – Neurologie, Universitätsklinik des Saarlandes, 6650 Homburg/Saar

Tormann, T., Dr. med.
Institut für Anästhesie, Universitätsklinik des Saarlandes, 6650 Homburg/Saar

Treib, J.,
Universitätsnervenklinik – Neurologie, Universitätsklinik des Saarlandes, 6650 Homburg/Saar

Vogel, W., Dr. med.
Medizinische Klinik und Poliklinik, Innere Medizin III, Universitätsklinik des Saarlandes, 6650 Homburg/Saar

Waldhausen, P., Dr. med.
Abteilung für Klinische Hämostaseologie und Transfusionsmedizin, Universitätsklinik des Saarlandes, 6650 Homburg/Saar

Wenzel, E., Prof. Dr. med.
Abteilung für Klinische Hämostaseologie und Transfusionsmedizin, Universitätsklinik des Saarlandes, 6650 Homburg/Saar

Wilhelm, H.-J., Dr. med.
Klinik und Poliklinik für Hals-Nasen-Ohren-Kranke, Universitätsklinik des Saarlandes, 6650 Homburg/Saar

Wolf, S., Dr. med. Dr.-Ing.
Augenklinik der Medizinischen Fakultät RWTH Aachen, Pauwelsstraße, 5100 Aachen

# Abbreviations Used

| | |
|---|---|
| $\alpha$ | Bunsen's solubility coefficient |
| $\alpha$-amyl | $\alpha$-amylase activity |
| ABO | arterial branch occlusion |
| ADP | adenosine diphosphate |
| Albumin | albumin concentration in serum |
| ART | arm retina time (time) |
| ASA | acetylsalicylic acid |
| ATP | adenosine triphosphate |
| AV | atrioventricular |
| AVP | arteriovenous passage time |
| BF | mean blood flow |
| BFcca | mean blood flow in the common carotid artery |
| BFcap | mean capillary blood flow |
| BGA | blood gas analysis |
| BSR | blood sedimentation rate |
| c | concentration |
| CAO | central arterial occlusion |
| $CaO_2$ | oxygen content of the whole arterial blood |
| $CaO_{2chem}$ | oxygen content of chemically bound circulating oxygen |
| $CaO_{2phys}$ | oxygen content of physically dissolved circulating oxygen |
| CAT | computer-assisted tomogram |
| CBF | cerebral blood flow |
| CBV | cerebral blood volume |
| CCS | Canadian Cardiovascular Society |
| CHD | coronary heart disease |
| Cm | mean erythrocyte count per micrometer capillary |
| $CMRO_2$ | cerebral metabolic rate |
| CO | cardiac output |
| CPP | cerebral perfusion pressure |
| CT | computed tomography |
| CVC | central vein catheter |
| CVP | central venous pressure |
| d | erythrocyte column diameter |
| dia | diastolic |
| DBV | dye bolus velocity |
| DrH | duration of reactive hyperemia |
| E | erythrocyte |
| ECL | erythrocyte column length |
| EDTA | ethylenediaminetetraacetic acid |
| EF | ejection fraction |
| F | female |
| FIBc | free iron-binding capacity |
| FC | visual acuity to count fingers |
| GFR | glomerular filtration rate |

| | |
|---|---|
| Haes | hydroxyethyl starch |
| Hb | hemoglobin concentration |
| $Hb_{cap}$ | hemoglobin concentration in the microvascular system |
| Hct | systemic hematocrit |
| $Hct_{cap}$ | hematocrit in the microvascular system (capillary hematocrit) |
| HD | hemodilution |
| hyp | hypervolemic |
| HR | heart rate |
| ICB | intracranial bleeding |
| ICP | intracranial pressure |
| IM | intramuscular $pO_2$ (M. tibialis anterior) |
| Iø | scatter intensity |
| iso | isovolemic |
| Lactate | plasma lactate concentration |
| LDF | laser Doppler flux |
| LG | visual acuity to perceive gleam of light |
| M | male |
| MAVIS | mobile artery and vein imaging systems |
| MCHC | mean corpuscular hemoglobin concentration |
| MCV | mean corpuscular volume |
| Md | median |
| MICRO | microcirculatory disturbance |
| MW | molecular weight |
| MMn | mean molecule number |
| MMw | mean molecule weight |
| $n_{after}$ | erythrocyte count after hemodilution in the erythrocyte column |
| $n_{Pg}$ | missing number of erythrocytes in the plasma gap |
| $n_{before}$ | erythrocyte count before hemodilution in the erythrocyte column |
| NW | weight of the newborn |
| NYHA | New York Heart Association |
| OEF | oxygen extraction rate |
| p | significance level |
| $pCO_2$ | carbon dioxide partial pressure |
| pH | pH value in blood (arterial) |
| p.i. | post infusion (after the end of infusion) |
| $pO_2$ | oxygen partial pressure |
| $pO_2$-art | arterial oxygen partial pressure |
| $pO_2$-IM | intramuscular oxygen partial pressure in tibialis anterior m. |
| $pO_2$-cap | capillary oxygen partial pressure |
| $pO_2$-tc | transcutaneous oxygen partial pressure |
| $pO_2$-tca | anterior antebrachial oxygen partial pressure (transcutaneous) |
| $pO_2$-tcb | transconjunctival oxygen partial pressure |
| $pO_2$-tcf | dorsopedal oxygen partial pressure (transcutaneous) |
| $pO_2$-ven | venous oxygen partial pressure |
| PAI | plasminogen activator inhibitor |
| PAOD | peripheral arterial occlusive disease |
| PEG | pneumoencephalography |

| | |
|---|---|
| PET | positron emission tomogram/graphy |
| Pla | plasma gap length after hemodilution |
| Plb | plasma gap length before hemodilution |
| PM | perinatal mortality |
| Protein | total serum protein |
| PR | platelet reactivity index according to Grotemeyer |
| PRIND | prolonged reversible ischemic neurological deficit |
| PTT | partial thromboplastin time |
| PU | perfusion unit (unit of laser Doppler method) |
| PV | plasma viscosity |
| PW | weeks of pregnancy |
| Pyruvate | pyruvate concentration in plasma |
| r | erythrocyte columnar radius |
| RCF | ristocetin cofactor |
| RIND | reversible ischemic neurological deficit |
| RR | blood pressure (measured according to Riva Rocci) |
| SD | standard deviation |
| SEM | standord error of the mean |
| sTA | spontaneous thrombocyte aggregation |
| sys | systolic |
| SAE | subcortical ateriosclerotic encephalopathy |
| SAH | subarachnoid hemorrhage |
| SEA | standardized erythrocyte aggregation index |
| SER | standardized erythrocyte rigidity index |
| $SO_2$ | oxygen saturation |
| SPECT | single photon emission computed tomogram/graphy |
| SSSG | Scandinavian Stroke Study Group |
| OTc | oxygen transport capacity of arterial blood |
| t-PA | tissue plasminogen activator |
| T | thrombocyte |
| TC | thrombocyte count |
| TIBc | total iron binding capacity |
| TIA | transitory ischemic attack |
| UI | unbound iron binding capacity (serum iron) |
| v | mean capillary erythrocyte velocity |
| $v_{max}$ | mean maximum capillary erythrocyte velocity after 3 min of ischemia |
| $v_{rest}$ | mean capillary erythrocyte velocity at rest |
| vWF | von Willebrandt factor |
| $V_E$ | cell volume of an erythrocyte |
| X | mean value |

# Introduction

Hemodilution is a therapy for vascular diseases. In patients suffering from arterial occlusive diseases, hemodilution is often of clinical use if the systemic hematocrit value is 45% or higher.

In addition to its use in cerebral [10, 97, 131, 278, 348, 351], retinal [209, 210, 397, 398], otogenic [392], and peripheral circulatory disturbances [6, 55, 175, 176, 177, 228, 258, 266, 302, 388], hemodilution is often employed in gynecology in the case of placental restricted circulation [124], in cardiology in the case of coronary (ischemic) heart disease [178, 234] and recently in the case of cardiac insufficiency [226, 352] with hyperviscosity.

In 1989 cardiovascular diseases were involved in 50% of deaths in the Federal Republic of Germany (342 700), being the most frequent cause of death. Almost 40% of these patients died of coronary heart disease [349]. In recent years empirical studies have confirmed the connection between classical risk factors and blood fluidity [5, 188, 233]. The Aachen study [188] also found a significant frequency of pathologically increased rheologic parameters in vascular diseases with corresponding risk factors [191]. The incidence of arterial occlusion is doubled even in cases of slightly restricted blood fluidity [191, 197]. For blood flow in less perfused areas blood fluidity may even become a limiting factor [190, 195, 322].

Increased hematocrit and hemoglobin content of blood have also been identified as risk factors for vascular diseases in other epidemiologic studies [30, 38, 166, 345]. Treatment aimed at reducing hematocrit in circulatory disturbances has been practiced since antiquity [21]. A reduction in hematocrit is, in fact, identical with a reduction in oxygen carriers, that is, the oxygen capacity (oxygen content) of the blood. On the other hand, it causes an increase in blood fluidity and therefore decreases the apparent blood viscosity. The results of experimental animal and clinical studies suggest that the reduction in viscosity overcompensates the loss in oxygen capacity, leading to a hematocrit value between 38% and 42% in patients with circulatory disturbances and thereby even increasing the oxygen transport rate (oxygen transport capacity) [41, 105, 189, 278].

# 1 Iron Metabolism

J. Koscielny and H. Kiesewetter

## 1.1 Theoretical Principles

The mean iron concentration in men is 60 mg per kilogram body weight. This corresponds to a total of 4200 mg in a 70-kg man. In women the concentration is lower (about 50 mg per kilogram body weight), or 3000 mg in a 60-kg woman [201, 236, 335]. This iron is spread throughout the body of a 70-kg man (60-kg woman) as shown in Fig. 1.

The daily requirement depends on the daily loss; a man with a healthy metabolism needs 1 mg, a woman 2 mg, and a pregnant woman 3 mg iron per day [236, 335]. Of the iron lost daily, 66% is via the gastrointestinal tract, 30% through the skin with sweat, and probably 4% by microbleedings. [236, 335].

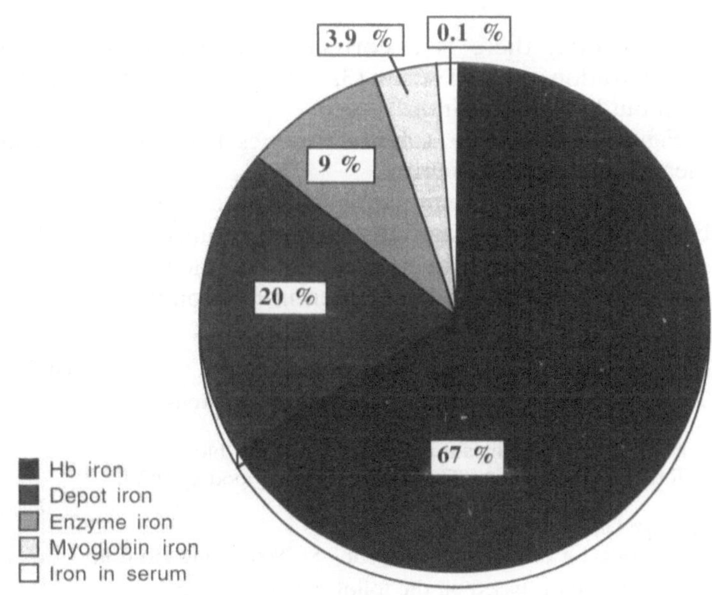


1. Hemoglobin-bound iron (Hb iron): 67% ≈ 2800 (2000) mg
2. Depot iron (ferritin/hemosiderin): 20% ≈ 840 (600) mg
3. Enzyme-bound iron (cytochromes, apoferritins, etc.): 9% ≈380 (270) mg
4. Myoglobin-bound iron (mainly in muscular tissue): 3.9% ≈ 170 (120) mg
5. Iron in serum (bound to s-transferrin and s-ferritin, unbound s-iron): 0.1% ≈ 5–7 mg

**Fig. 1.** Iron distribution in the human body (values for women in parentheses)

A 1000-kcal meal such as is typical in central Europe supplies about 6 mg absorbable iron. This corresponds to an average of 11–17 mg iron per day through food.

A maximum of 100 mg iron per day can be absorbed from appropriate ferriferous food (e.g., high meat portion) [236, 335]. Since at most 25 mg iron per day can be obtained through hemoglobin synthesis (highest iron requirement), the absorption of this quantity is sufficient; if more iron is absorbed, it can be stored [236, 329, 347].

The parameters of iron metabolism measured in blood serum are given below:

Serum transferrin: special depot iron protein of blood =
total iron-binding capacity (TIBc)
  Measured: bound quantity of iron
  Reference range: 250–400 μg/100 ml

Serum iron: unbound iron (UI) in blood = iron-binding capacity
  Measured: unbound quantity of iron in serum
  Reference range: 55–170 μg/100 ml
  (caution: circadian rhythm)
  Free iron-binding capacity (FIBc) = TIBc – UI

Serum ferritin: ubiquitous depot iron protein, measurable only in serum
  Measured: protein concentration
  Reference range: 1.2–30 μg/100 ml (12–300 ng/ml: WHO)

In general, there is a correlation between the ferritin and depot iron concentration in blood serum [329, 347]: 1 ng ferritin in 1 ml serum corresponds to about 8 mg depot iron.

Figure 2 shows the reference ranges for the iron metabolism parameters measurable in blood serum.

Estimation of the hemoglobin iron content of total blood volume (Hb iron) is based on the assumption that 1 g Hb contains 3.4 mg iron [201, 236, 329, 335, 347]. Furthermore, the estimated total blood volume and the hemoglobin concentration measured are taken into account:

Average values in men:
3.4 mg iron/1 g Hb × 15.5 g Hb/100 ml × 5250 ml ≈ 2800 mg Hb iron

The calculation is based on the following assumptions:
- Body weight: 70 kg
- Hemoglobin concentration: 15.5 g Hb/100 ml blood
- Total blood volume: 5250 ml (from 75 ml blood/kg BW)

Average values in women:
3.4 mg iron/1 g Hb × 15 g/Hb/100 ml × 3900 ml mg Hb iron

The calculation is based on the following assumptions:
- Body weight: 60 kg
- Hemoglobin concentration: 15.5 g Hb/100 ml blood
- Total blood volume: 3900 ml (from 65 ml blood/kg BW)

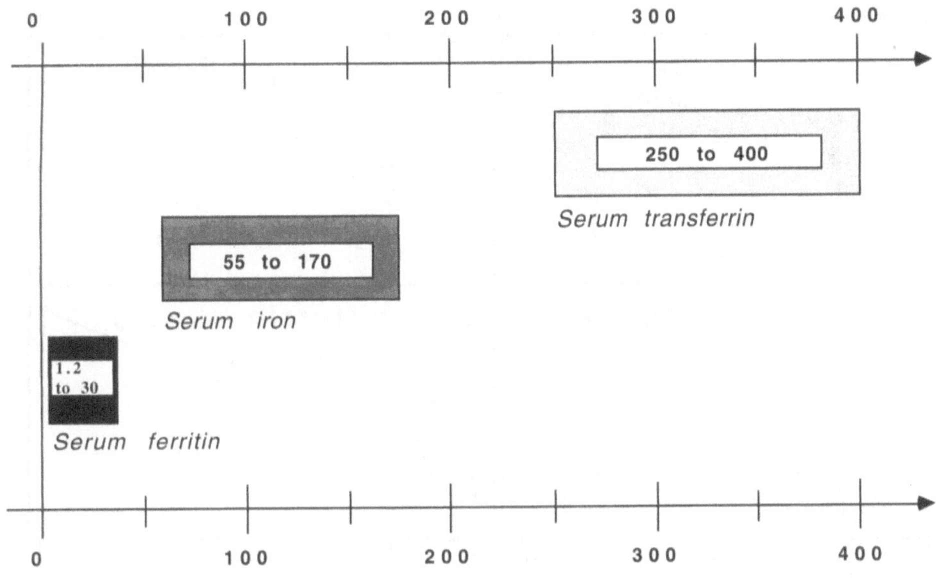


**Fig. 2.** Reference ranges in micrograms per 100 ml serum for iron metabolism parameters measurable in blood serum

## 1.2 Estimation of Hemodilution Intervals

A withdrawal of 500 ml blood (phlebotomy) is accompanied by the mean loss of 260 mg (230 mg) Hb iron. The blood values remain almost unchanged. The intravascular Hb iron loss is compensated out of the iron depot. [335, 347]. Consequently, there is a maximal withdrawal of 31% (38%) – from 840 mg (600 mg) to 580 mg (370 mg) iron – for the iron depot to be calculated, and for total iron a withdrawal of 6% (8%) – from 4200 mg (3000 mg) to 3940 mg (2770 mg) iron, and maximal a reduction in serum ferritin of 33 (29) ng/ml (in parentheses the values for women). A filling of the iron depot is to be expected by increased absorption over 2 weeks. An iron depot exhaustion is to be assumed in case of a blood loss of about 1500 (1300) ml. Further blood losses after an iron depot exhaustion lead to anemia [335, 347].

Estimation of hemodilution intervals takes an increased hemoglobin concentration of blood of 17 g/dl, depending on the listed average values for body weight, blood volume, total iron, hemoglobin-bound iron (Hb iron), serum iron (s-iron), serum transferrin (s-transferrin), and serum ferritin (s-ferritin).

The purpose of hemodilution is to achieve and maintain a hemoglobin concentration of 12–13 g/dl (hematocrit 40–42%).

The hemodilution steps should be carried out in combination with phlebotomies of 500 or 250 ml blood and complete volume substitution by hydroxyethyl starch (see Figs. 3, 4).

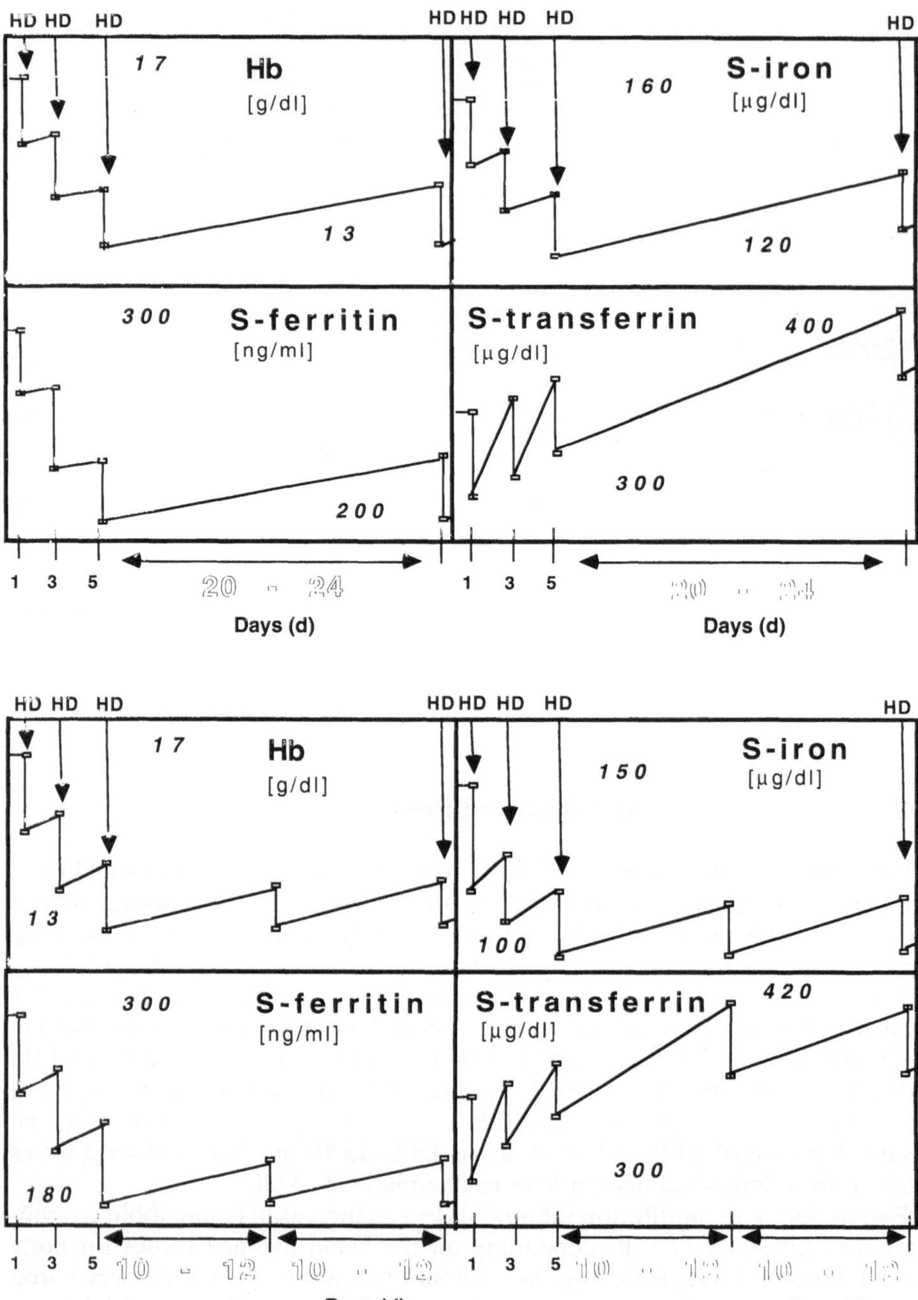


**Fig. 3.** Parameter changes and hemodilution intervals with 500 ml phlebotomy. Hb synthesis of 10 mg iron (*above*) and 25 mg iron (*below*) metabolism per day

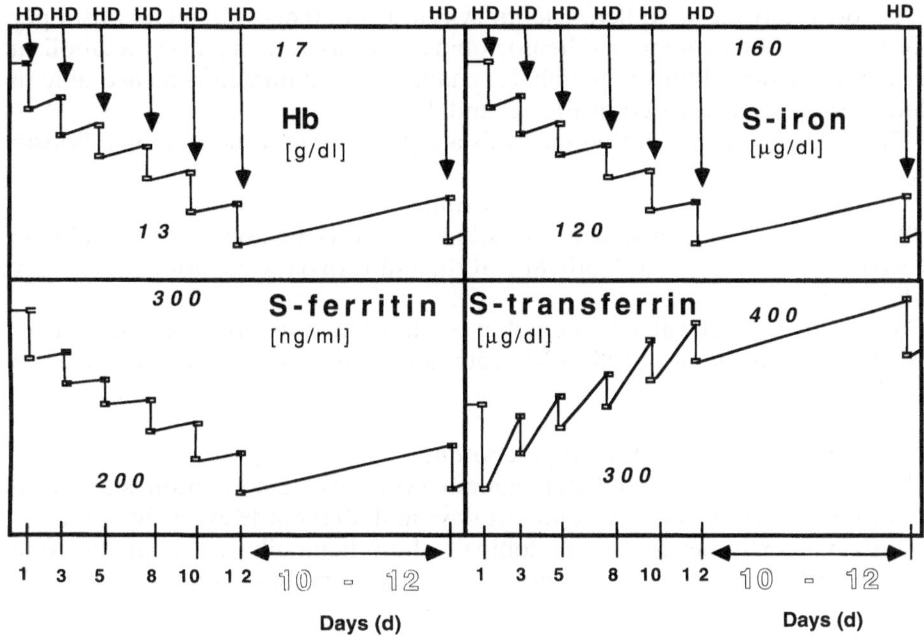


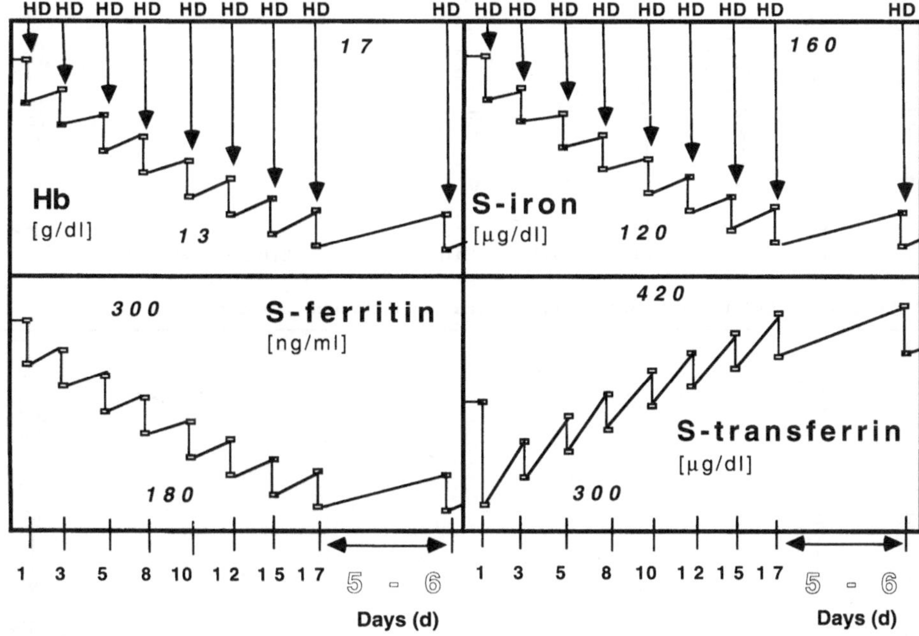


**Fig. 4.** Parameter changes and hemodilution intervals with 250 ml phlebotomy. Hb synthesis of 10 mg iron (*above*) and 25 mg iron (*below*) metabolism per day

A moderately elevated hemoglobin synthesis of 10 mg iron metabolism per day and a maximally increased hemoglobin synthesis of 25 mg iron metabolism per day are assumed for the parameter changes. The parameters measurable in blood serum are presented in Figs. 3 and 4.

The following hemodilution intervals are derived from the iron metabolism (see Fig. 5):

For a hemodilution with 250 ml phlebotomy:

- With moderately elevated hemoglobin synthesis hemodilution should be carried out on the 1st, 3rd, 5th, 8th, 10th, and 12th days and afterwards every 10–12 days.
- With maximally elevated hemoglobin synthesis hemodilution should be done on the 1st, 3rd, 5th, 8th, 10th, 12th, 15th, and 17th days and afterwards every 5 or 6 days.

For a hemodilution with 500 ml phlebotomy:

- With moderately elevated hemoglobin synthesis hemodilution should be carried out on the 1st, 3rd, and 5th days and afterwards every 20–24 days.
- With maximally elevated hemoglobin synthesis hemodilution should be done on the 1st, 3rd, and 5th days and afterwards every 10–12 days.

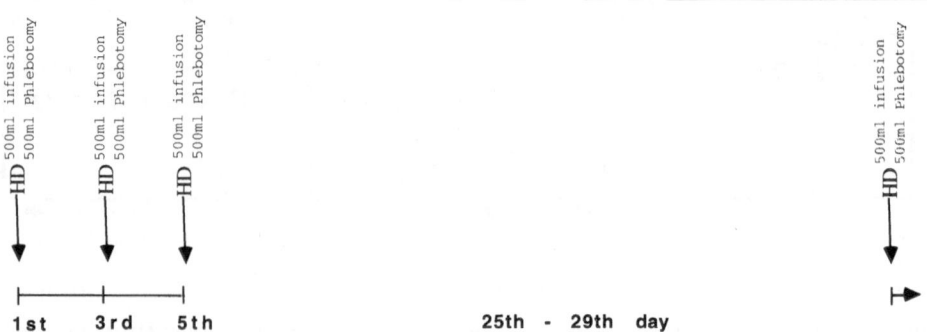


**Fig. 5.** Hemodilution intervals with moderately elevated hemoglobin synthesis with a phlebotomy of 250 ml and 500 ml (see Figs. 3 and 4)

# 2 Clinical Experience

In clinical use of hemodilution, the phlebotomy intervals correspond well with those determined theoretically [180, 182, 184, 187]. Therefore, a moderately elevated hemoglobin synthesis is taken as normal. Some clinical observations are described below. The desired hematocrit was 40%.

## *2.1 Hemodilution in Peripheral Arterial Occlusive Disease (PAOD)*

H. Kiesewetter, B. Angelkort, J. Blume, F. Jung, S. Spitzer, M. Gerhards, and E. Wenzel

### *2.1.1 Patients*

The five studies described below were carried out in patients with peripheral arterial occlusive disease stage II according to Fontaine (PAOD II) which had been evident for at least 6 months. The subjects were outpatients of both sexes, aged 40–75 years, and suffering from occlusions of the femoral and/or tibial type, with hemodynamically free external iliac artery and deep femoral artery. The mean walking distance without pain on admission was between 80 and 300 m (measured on the treadmill). The walking distances in the wash-out phase were not allowed to vary more than 30% in three measurements on different days. The Doppler pressure values over peripheral arteries at rest had to be greater than 50 mmHg.

Criteria for exclusion were: presence of hemodynamically effective stenoses in the external iliac artery or deep femoral artery, endangiitis obliterans, nonvascular walking impediment, operations in the previous 3 months, e.g., vascular operations or sympathectomy, condition after cerebral infarction with gait disturbances, severe cerebrovascular insufficiency, severe internal, not sufficiently compensated defects or dysfunctions of the heart, circulation, liver, kidney, or lung, nonadjustable hyper- or hypotension (RR systolic > 180 mmHg or < 110 mmHg), portal hypertension, renal insufficiency with a serum creatinine equal to or higher than 2.0 mg/dl, intake of anticoagulants, rheologically effective or vasoactive drugs, analgetics or antiphlogistics not discontinued at least 4 weeks previously, readjustment or correction of a therapy with cardiac glycosides, diuretics, antidiabetics, antiarrhythmics, or calcium antagonists [120].

### 2.1.2 Dilution in the Case of Decreased Hematocrit Values

H. Kiesewetter, J. Blume, F. Jung, S. Spitzer, M. Gerhards, and E. Wenzel

A double-blind, placebo-controlled, randomized study including two control groups [176] sought to clarify whether iso- and hypervolemic hemodilution with 10% Haes 200/0.5 (Haes-steril 10%; Fresenius) plus vascular exercise (with only moderately elevated hematocrit values of up to 46%) is more effective than iso- and hypervolemic hemodilution with Ringer lactate plus vascular exercise or vascular exercise alone. In all, 75 patients were selected from 108 outpatients.

The study period (Fig. 6) for each patient was 10 weeks (4 weeks of wash-out and 6 weeks of therapy. During this time the patients received physical therapy according to the program of Weidinger [387] three times per week (45 min each time). During the 6-week therapy phase the patients of the Haes and Ringer groups were additionally diluted. The dilutions were performed five times during the first 3 weeks and three times during the last 3 weeks. At hematocrit values of 43% and above, a phlebotomy of 250 ml was performed; at the same time the blood was substituted for 250 ml 10% Haes 200/0.5 or Ringer lactate via a second access. At hematocrit values less than 43% either 250 ml Haes or 250 ml Ringer lactate were given hypervolemically. Altogether, 6000 ml hydroxyethyl starch solution was infused per person. The mean withdrawal of blood was about 1200 ml. The third group served as second control group (see Fig. 6). Concerning

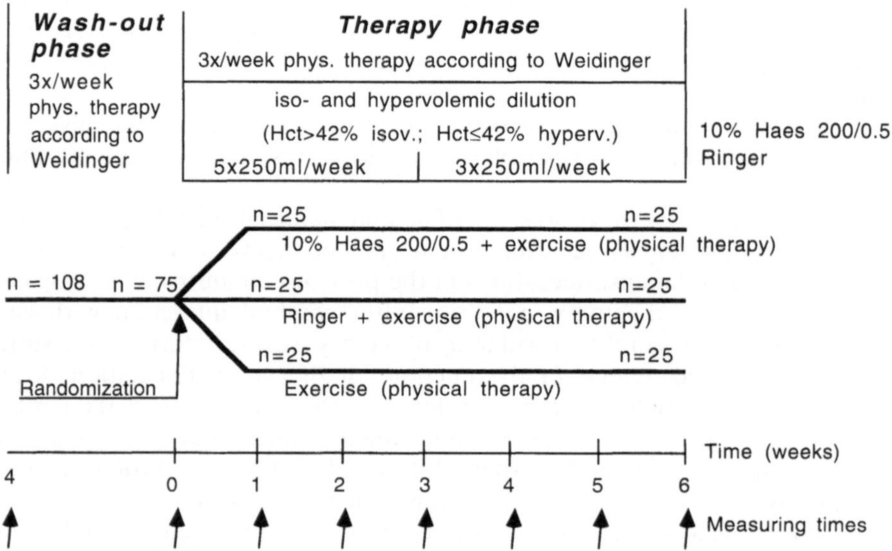


**Fig. 6.** Study design: combined iso- and hypervolemic hemodilution in PAOD II

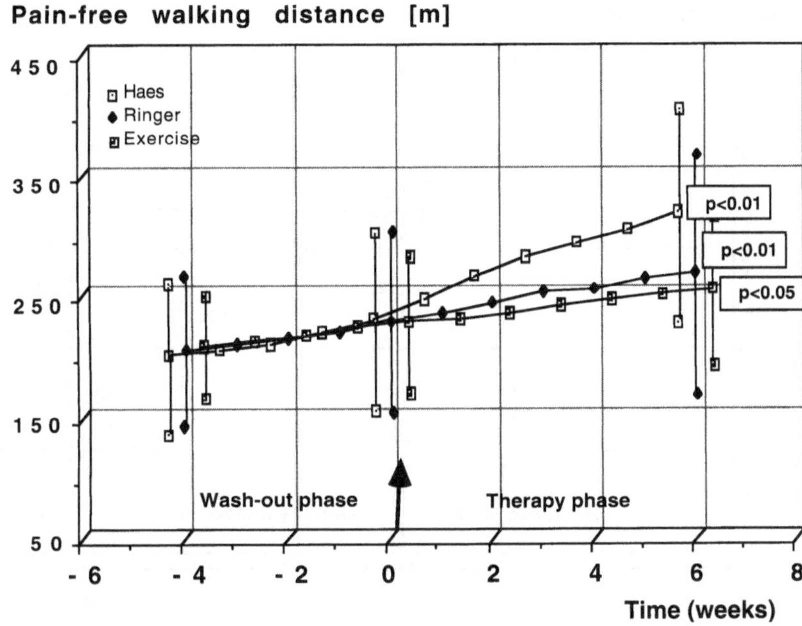


**Fig. 7.** Pain-free walking distances in the three groups for the time of treatment (*p*: significance level in time-series comparison – initial value to final value; limits of 1 SD, same symbols as the corresponding mean measuring points)

important demographic data, risk factors, concomitant diseases and medication the patients of the three groups were homogeneous.

The confirmatory parameter was the pain-free walking distance; essential exploratory parameters were plasma viscosity and erythrocyte aggregation.

The pain-free walking distance in the Haes group changed by 44% from 216 to 311 m, in the Ringer group by 20% from 214 to 258 m, and in the exercise group by 14% from 213 to 242 m (Fig. 7).

The increase in walking distance in the Haes group was significantly greater ($p<0.05$) than those in the other two groups.

The hematocrit values did not change after vascular exercise as monotherapy. Significant decreases in hematocrit were observed in the Ringer and Haes groups (Fig. 8).

The time course of plasma viscosity is shown in Fig. 9. The highest decrease (3%) was found in the Haes group. This was also the case concerning erythrocyte aggregation (decrease by 11%), 110 mm shown in Fig. 10.

This study demonstrated that a combined iso- and hypervolemic hemodilution with 10% Haes 200/0.5 is significantly superior to hemodilution with crystalloid solution.

> Even in the case of a decreased initial hematocrit value the clinical benefit by vascular exercise is also significantly increased by a combination with hemodilution.

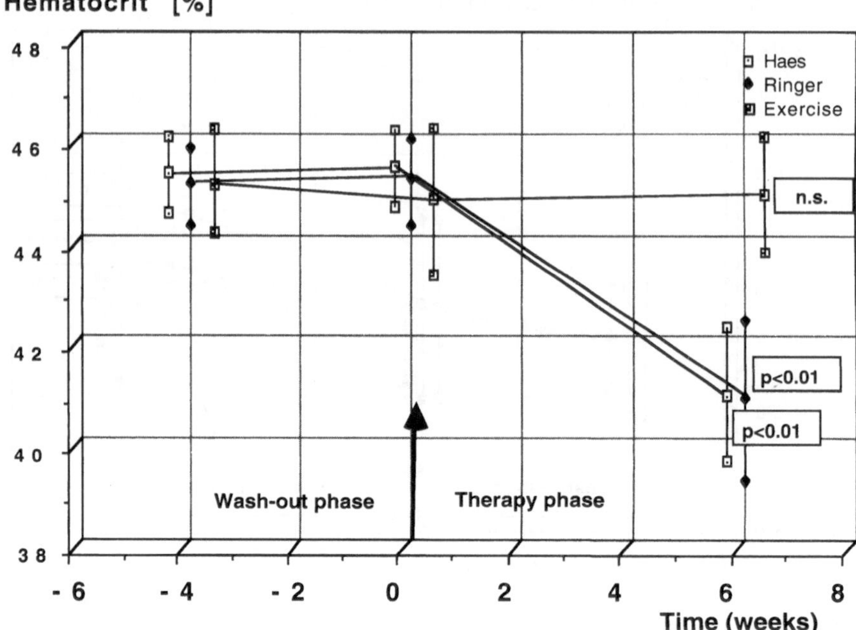


**Fig. 8.** Hematocrit values in the three groups ($p$: significance level in time-series comparison – initial value to final value; limits of 1 SD, same symbols as the corresponding mean measuring points)

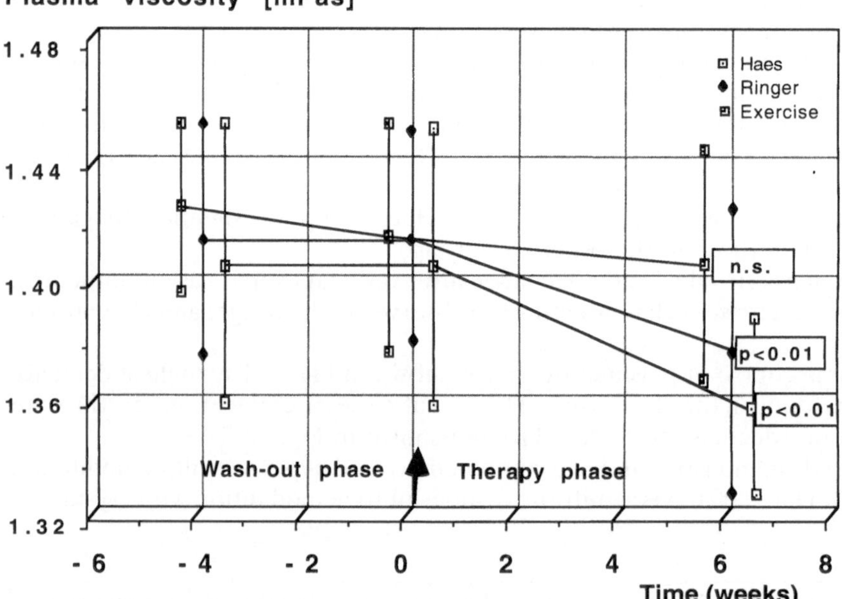


**Fig. 9.** Development of plasma viscosities in the three groups for the time of treatment. ($p$: significance level in time-series comparison – initial value to final value; limits of 1 SD, same symbols as the corresponding mean measuring points)

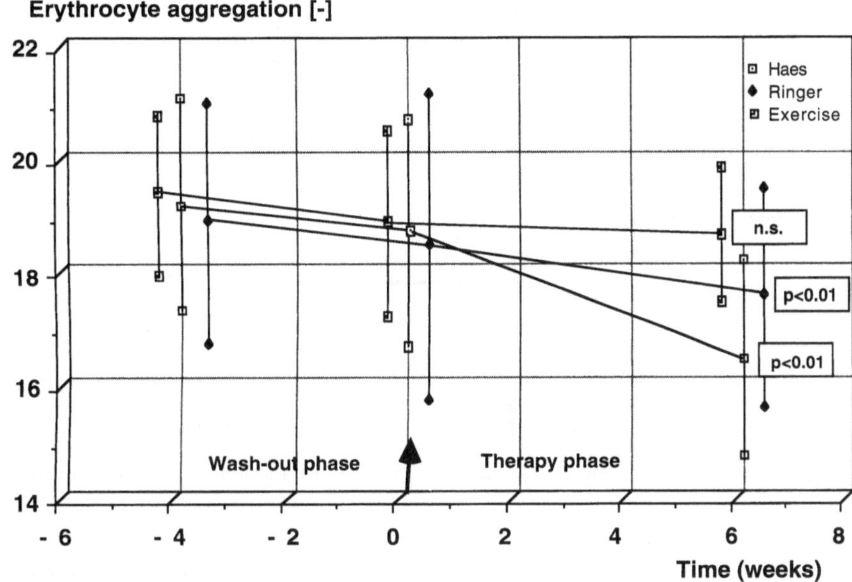


**Fig. 10.** Erythrocyte aggregations in the three groups for the time of treatment. ($p$: significance level in time-series comparison – initial value to final value; limits of 1 SD, same symbols as the corresponding mean measuring points)

## *2.1.3 Hydroxyethyl Starch or Dextran*

H. Kiesewetter, F. Jung, J. Blume, and M. Gerhards

The clinical efficacies of hydroxyethyl starch (Haes-steril 10%; Fresenius) and dextran 40 10% were compared in a double-blind study [187]. Increases in tibial circulation after the administration of dextran have been described repeatedly [32, 89, 313, 405].

Sixty outpatients suffering from PAOD II were selected at random in accordance with the criteria for inclusion described above. The patients received regular physical therapy for at least 6 months, three to five times per week according to the regimen of Weidinger [387]. At the beginning of the wash-out phase the patients were removed from the exercise groups. However, they were encouraged to maintain their customary pattern of movement.

Over the 6 weeks of therapy (Fig. 11) the hematocrit value was lowered isovolemically in four to eight sessions. In addition, 200–500 ml blood was removed each time and substituted isovolemically for 10% Haes 200/0.5 or dextran 40 10%. Phlebotomies were performed whenever the hematocrit was 43% or above; otherwise a hypervolemic hemodilution with 500 ml was

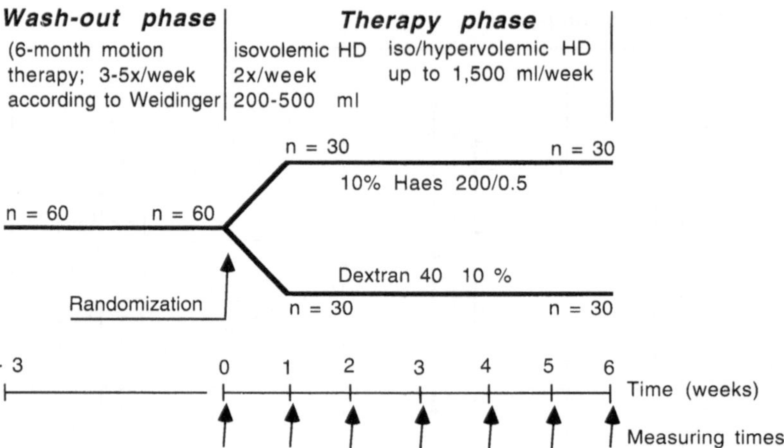


**Fig. 11.** Study design: comparative study of hydroxyethyl starch versus dextran in PAOD II

performed. In general, four to eight isovolemic and six to eight hypervolemic dilution sessions were necessary. The groups of patients were homogeneous with respect to demographic data, risk factors, concomitant diseases, and medication.

The pain-free walking distance in the Haes group changed by 44% from 189 to 281 m and in the dextran group by 28% from 193 to 246 m (Fig. 12). The difference is significant at the 5% level.

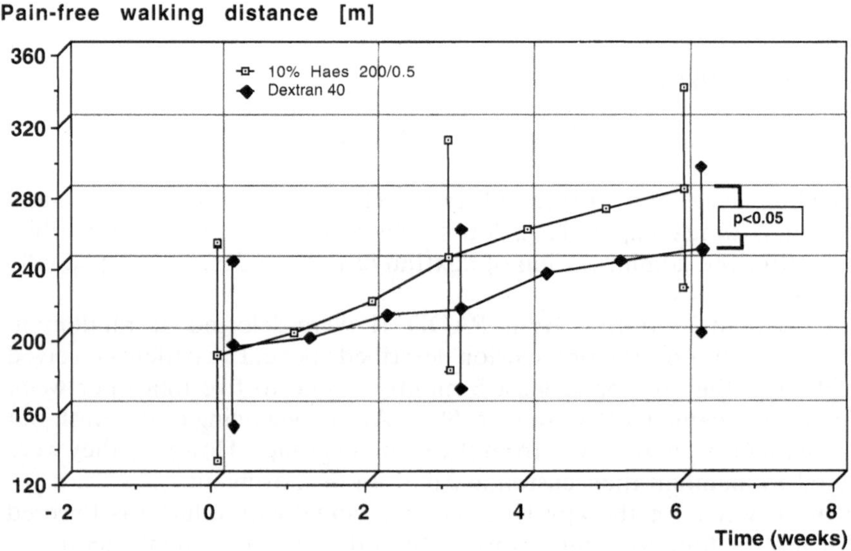


**Fig. 12.** Pain-free walking distance in the two groups for the time of treatment. ($p$: significance level in time-series comparison – initial value to final value; limits of 1 SD, same symbols as the corresponding mean measuring points)

Plasma viscosity in the Haes group decreased by 6% but remained almost constant in the dextran group. This was also observed for the erythrocyte aggregation, which fell by 13% in the Haes group.

| HAES-steril 10% (200/0.5) is clinically significantly superior to dextran 40 10% in the treatment of PAOD II. |
|---|

## *2.1.4 Rheologically Adjusted Therapy*

H. Kiesewetter and F. Jung

The studies presented here show that clinical improvement generally involved a clear increase in blood fluidity, especially in blood plasma. A series of 198 patients with PAOD II fulfilling the above criteria for inclusion underwent therapy in terms of rheologic factors [179]. On inclusion in the study all patients received intensive physical therapy, if possible, 1 h daily after a combination of programs designed by Krause [218], Schoop [328], and Weidinger [387] (Fig. 13).

***Wash-out phase***

***Therapy phase***

Physical therapy

intensively according to Schoop & Krause | according to Schoop,Krause & Weidinger

Naftidrofuryl

400 mg i.v. | 600 mg orally

10% Haes 200 0.5 iso/hypervolemically

200-400 ml 2-3x/week | 500 ml 2x/week | 500 ml 1x/week

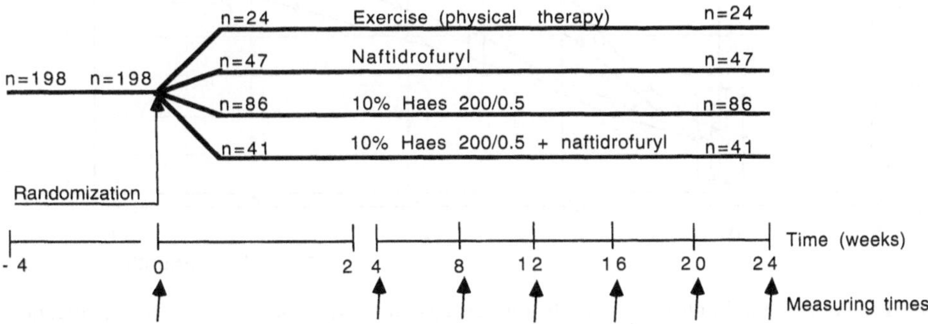


**Fig. 13.** Study design: combination therapy in PAOD II

In addition, a group of 47 patients with restricted erythrocyte deformability and plasma viscosity between 1.34 and 1.39 mPas were treated intravenously with 400 mg naftidrofuryl (Dusodril; Lipha) for the first 2 weeks and daily with 600 mg from the 3rd week on. A further group of 86 patients with hematocrit above 42% and plasma viscosity less than 1.39 mPas received a combined iso- and hypervolemic dilution. Moreover, 200–400 ml blood was removed twice per week during the first weeks and substituted isovolemically for 10% Haes 200/0.5 (Haes-steril 10%; Fresenius). After this adjustment phase 500 ml 10% Haes 200/0.5 was given hypervolemically twice per week for the first 3 months and once per week during the final 3 months. When hematocrit exceeded 42%, an isovolemic dilution was performed again. The fourth group consisted of 41 patients with severely restricted blood fluidity. These patients showed increased hematocrit and plasma viscosity, and several also had increased erythrocyte rigidity. This group were treated with the combination of the two therapeutic methods described above (hemodilution, naftidrofuryl). The groups were homogeneous except for the rheologic parameters.

The pain-free walking distance in the exercise group changed by 168% from 126 to 337 m, in the naftidrofuryl group by 233% from 188 to 393 m, in the Haes group by 227% from 132 to 431 m, and in the Haes + naftidrofuryl group by 315% from 134 to 514 m. Thus the highest increase in walking distance was in the group with vascular exercise, hemodilution, and naftidrofuryl, followed by that with hemodilution and vascular exercise or naftidrofuryl and vascular exercise. The smallest increase in walking distance was observed in the group which performed vascular exercise as monotherapy (Fig. 14).

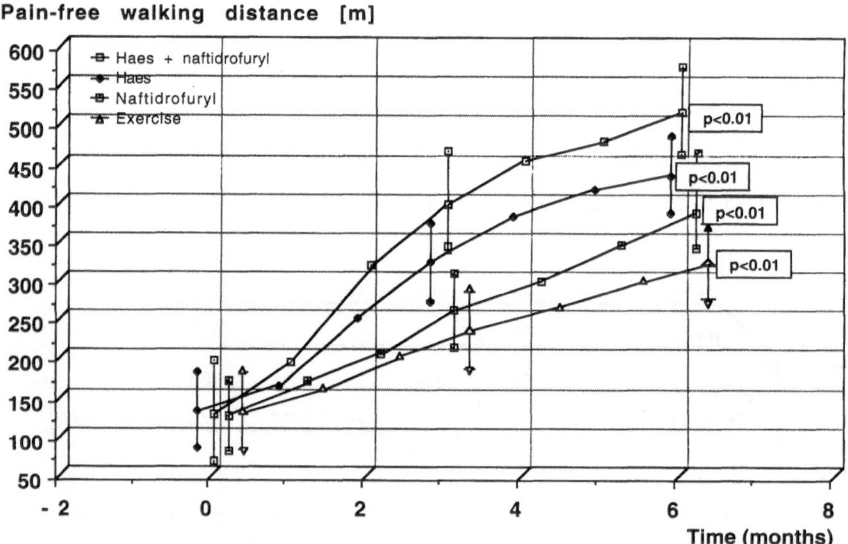


**Fig. 14.** Pain-free walking distance in the four groups for the time of treatment. ($p$: significance level in time-series comparison – initial value to final value; limits of 1 SD, same symbols as the corresponding mean measuring points)

In the hemodilution groups the hematocrit was adjusted to 40%. Plasma viscosity in the Haes group decreased significantly by 7% and by 10% in the Haes + naftidrofuryl group. In the naftidrofuryl groups the erythrocyte rigidity was also reduced by 12% in the naftidrofuryl group and by 14% in the Haes + naftidrofuryl group. Figures 15 and 16 show the rheologic parameters of the Haes and Haes + naftidrofuryl groups before and during therapy.

The considerable increases in walking distance are due to the fact that a very intensive walking exercise was performed in previously untrained patients, and a high percentage (more than 50%) were able to walk a distance of more than 1000 m without pain during the course of exercise. A tendency toward improved blood fluidity was achieved by this vascular exercise, but differences were not significant. Improved blood fluidity can be achieved only by additional rheologic therapy.

> A rheologic therapy in addition to vascular exercise adjusted to the specific defects in blood fluidity brings about a greater clinical benefit than vascular exercise alone.

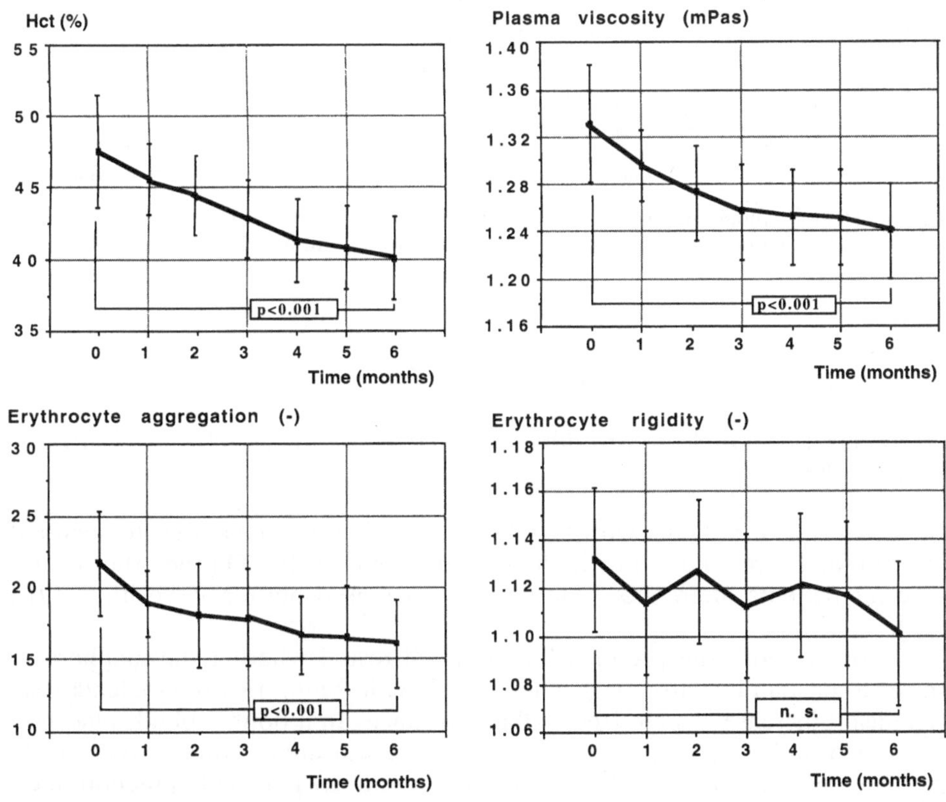


**Fig. 15.** Hemorheologic parameters in the Haes group for the time of treatment. ($p$: significance level in time-series comparison – initial value to final value)

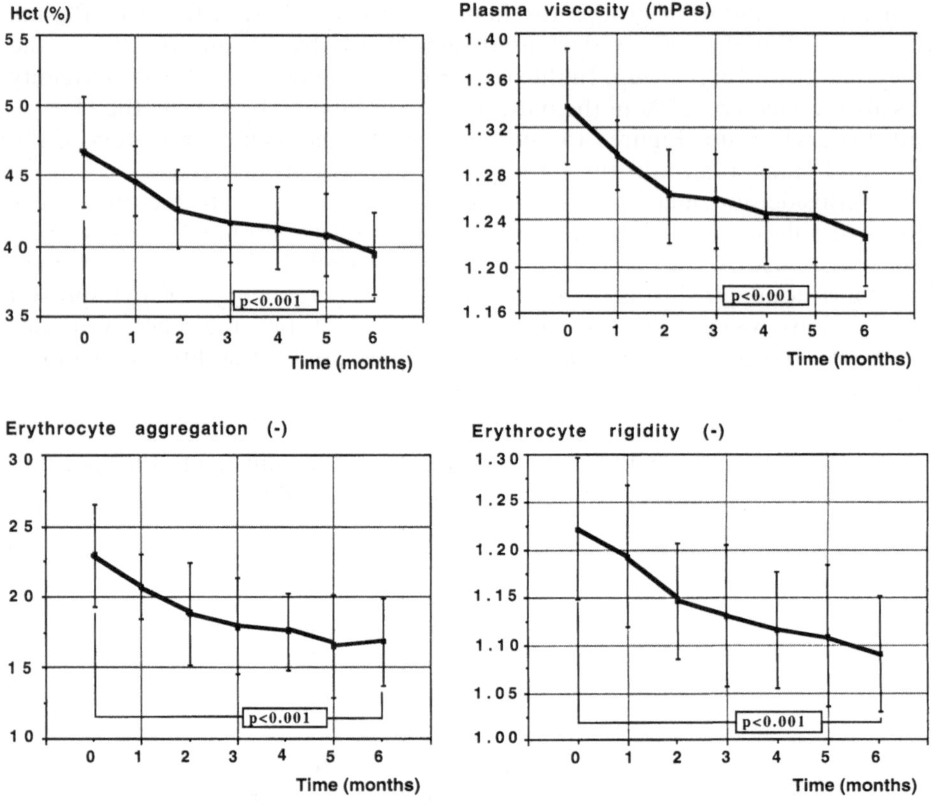


**Fig. 16.** Hemorheologic parameters in the Haes and naftidrofuryl group for the time of treatment. (*p*: significance level in time-series comparison – initial value to final value)

### 2.1.5 Bag Plasmapheresis as Useful Addition

H. Kiesewetter, J. Blume, F. Jung, M. Gerhards, G. Leipnitz, S. Spitzer, and E. Wenzel

In 40%–50% of patients with PAOD hematocrit is not increased to such an extent that a hemodilution with phlebotomy seems useful. On the other hand, vascular patients often show considerably increased plasma viscosities [191, 192].

For this reason, the presented study [173] tested whether plasmapheresis (given a constant hematocrit) in combination with gymnastic exercise leads to a significant increase in pain-free walking distance. In a double-blind, placebo-controlled study 60 patients with PAOD II were allocated to three groups of 20 patients each. Besides vascular gymnastics three times per week, phlebotomies of 300 ml blood were performed twice per week over 6 weeks. Plasma was rejected in the Haes and levulose groups and substituted for 10% Haes 200/0.5

(Haes-steril 10%; Fresenius) in the first group and substituted for levulose 5% in the second. In the third group, the autologous blood was autotransfused unchanged (Fig. 17).

The three groups were homogeneous with regard to essential demographic data, risk factors, concomitant diseases, and medication.

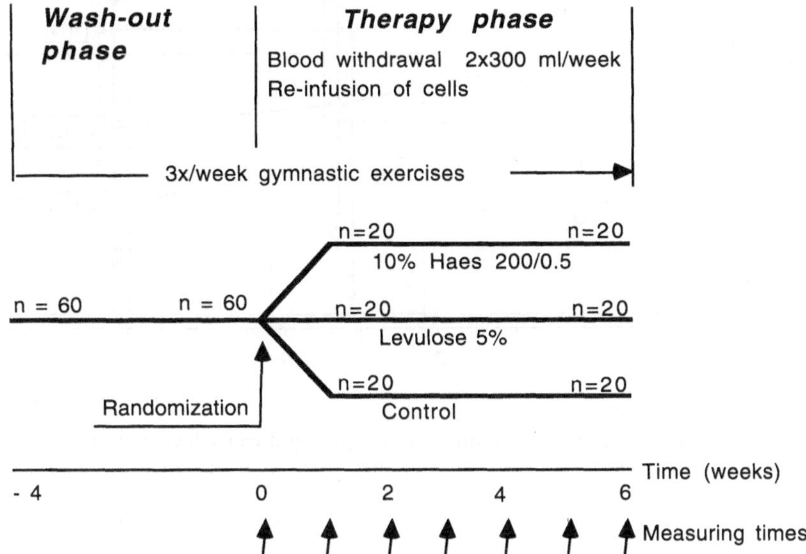


**Fig. 17.** Study design: bag plasmapheresis in patients with PAOD II

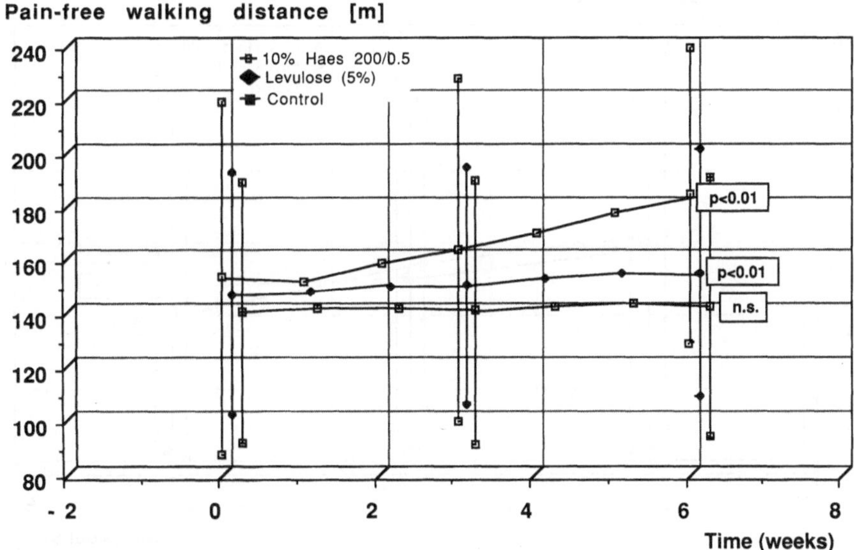


**Fig. 18.** Pain-free walking distances in the three groups for the time of treatment. ($p$: significance level in time-series comparison – initial value to final value; limits of 1 SD, same symbols as the corresponding mean measuring points)

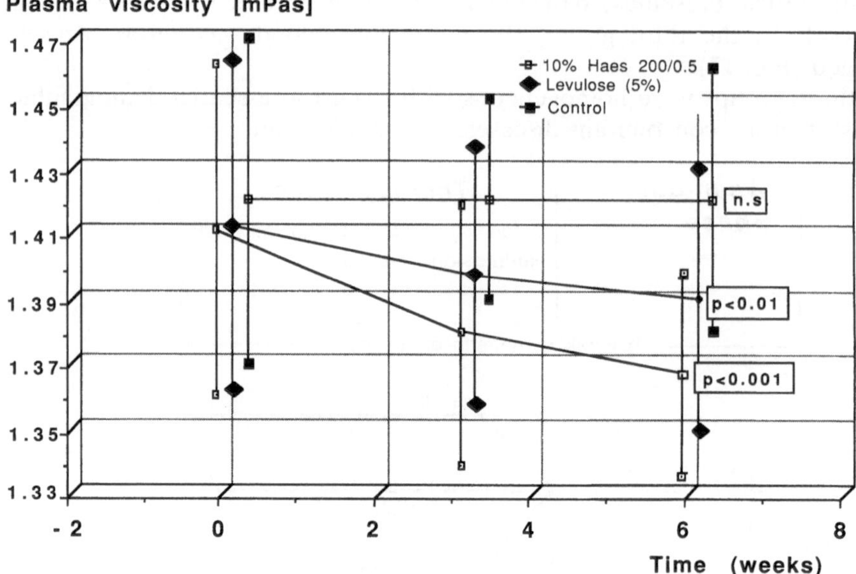


**Fig. 19.** Plasma viscosities in the three groups ($p$: significance level in time-series comparison – initial value to final value; limits of 1 SD, same symbols as the corresponding mean measuring points)

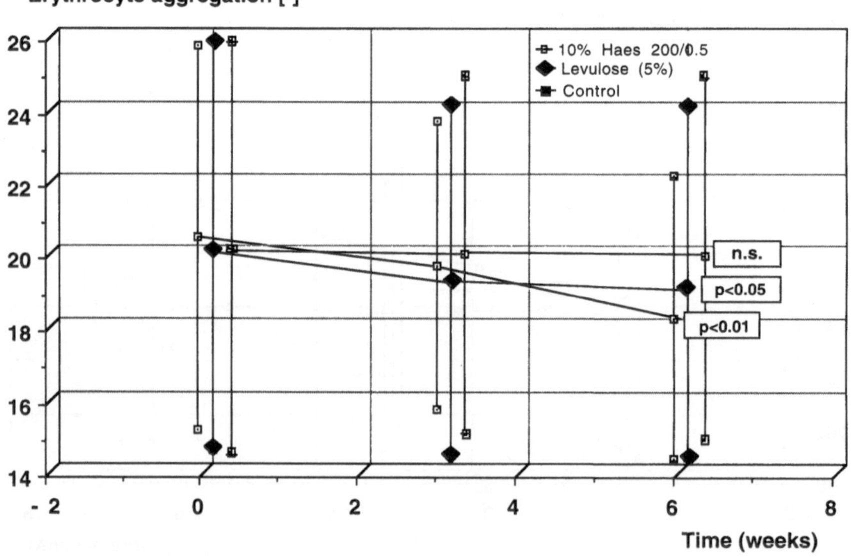


**Fig. 20.** Erythrocyte aggregations in the three groups for the time of treatment. ($p$: significance level in time-series comparison – initial value to final value; limits of 1 SD, same symbols as the corresponding mean measuring points)

The pain-free walking distance in the Haes group changed by 21% from 153 to 183 m, in the levulose group by 5% from 147 to 154 m, and in the plasma group by 1% from 140 to 142. Only the Haes group differed significantly from the other groups at the 5% level (Fig. 18).

Plasma viscosity in the Haes group decreased significantly by 3% and in the levulose group only by 1% (Fig. 19), the erythrocyte aggregation in the Haes group by 11% and in the levulose group by 5% (Fig. 20). The hematocrit value remained almost unchanged after 12 plasmapheresis sessions.

> The dilution of blood plasma alone leads to a significant decrease in pain-free walking distance.

### *2.1.6 Dilution in Multimorbid Patients*

H. KIESEWETTER, J. BLUME, F. JUNG, S. SPITZER, R. BACH, A. BIRK, H. SCHIEFFER, and E. WENZEL

The treatment of multimorbid patients with peripheral arterial occlusive disease (PAOD) may become problematic because of concomitant diseases such as coronary heart disease, chronic obstructive lung disease, arterial hypertension, or diabetes mellitus. Hemodilution can also be a clinically effective therapy for some of the concomitant diseases. But it is necessary to use a liquid colloidal solution which has, as an iso-oncotic substance, *no* additional intravascular volume effect. Hydroxyethyl starch 200/0.5 6% (Haes-steril 6%; Fresenius) meets these requirements.

The study was randomized, double-blind, placebo-controlled, and included 40 patients with PAOD stage II [175]. All patients performed gymnastic exercises for 10 weeks (twice per week). During the 6-week therapy phase the patients received hemodilution in addition to the physical therapy (Fig. 21).

The hematocrit value in all patients was adjusted to between 38% and 42%. For this, 250 ml blood was removed initially (on average over 2 weeks) two or three times per week and substituted hypervolemically. The hematocrit and plasma viscosity of all patients were then checked to be able to perform the appropriate hemodilution. At a hematocrit value above 42% a hypervolemic hemodilution (500 ml 6% Haes 200/0.5 or 500 ml sodium chloride) with a phlebotomy of 250 ml was performed; at hematocrit values equal to or less than 42% a single hypervolemic dilution (250 ml 6% Haes 200/0.5 or 250 ml sodium chloride).

Phlebotomies of about 1.7 l with volume substitution by sodium chloride lead to a significant increase in pain-free walking distance of 19% from 173 m to 206 m. The increase in pain-free walking distance in the Haes group was significantly higher and changed from by 36% 175 m to 238 m. The difference was significant at the 5% level (Fig. 22).

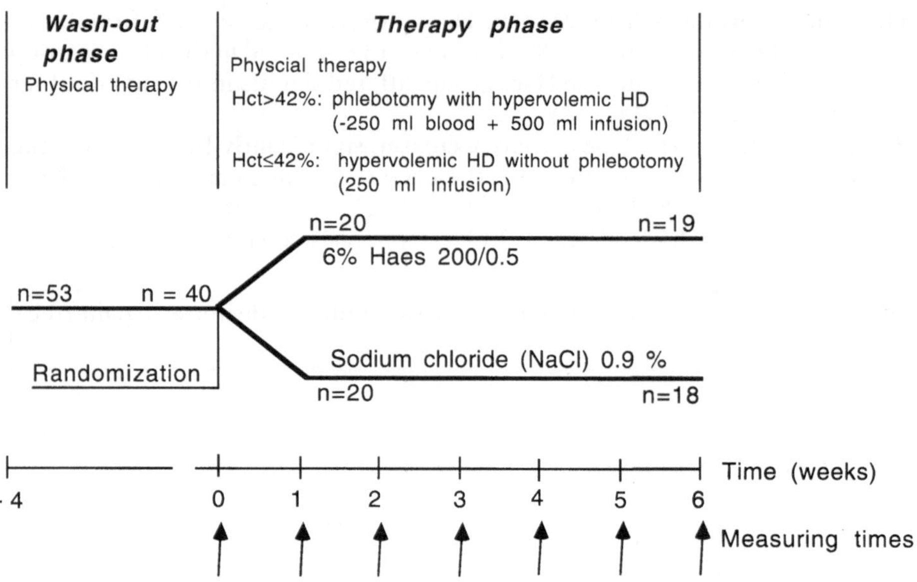


**Fig. 21.** Study design: hemodilution with 6% Haes 200/0.5 in multimorbid patients with PAOD II

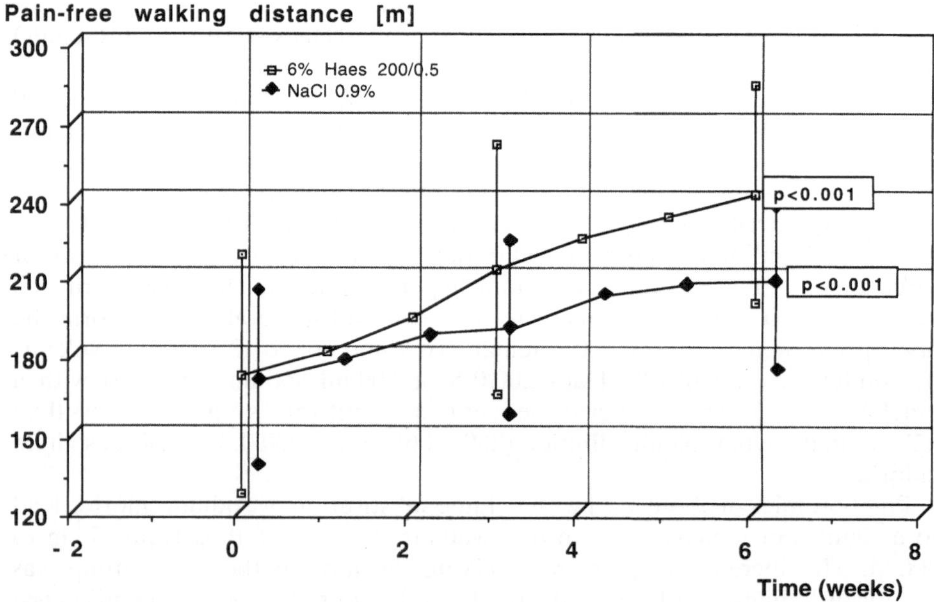


**Fig. 22.** Pain-free walking distances of the two groups for the time of treatment. (*p*: significance level in time-series comparison – initial value to final value; limits of 1 SD, same symbols as the corresponding mean measuring points)

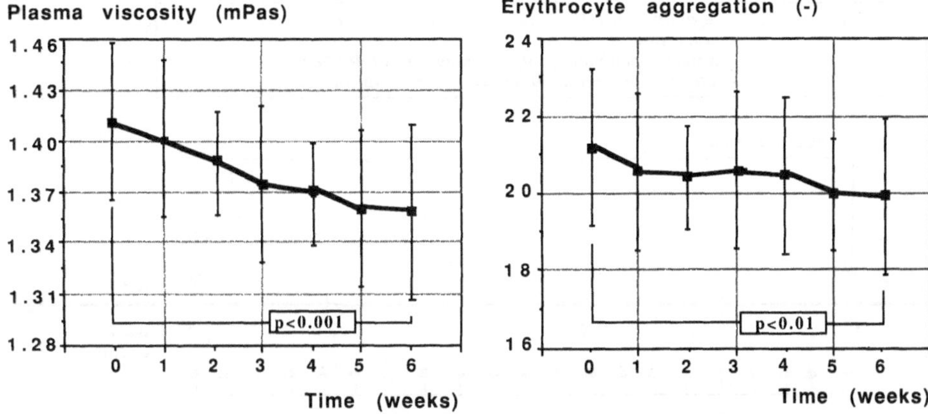


**Fig. 23.** Hemorheologic parameters (plasma viscosity, erythrocyte aggregation) in the group treated with Haes for the time of treatment (*p*: significance level in time series comparison – initial value to final value)

The decreases in plasma viscosity by 3.5% in the active substance group and by 1.4% in the placebo group differed significantly; the decreases in erythrocyte aggregation of 6.1% in the active substance group and of 4.4% in the placebo group were only tendencies (Fig. 23).

Ten patients in the active substance group presented a reduction in systemic arterial hypertension. The frequency of angina attacks decreased in the active substance group.

> Hemodilution with an iso-oncotic Haes-steril 6% (200/0.5) solution in multimorbid patients with PAOD brings about a significant increase in walking distance and a benefit concerning concomitant diseases.

### 2.1.7 *Dilution in Patients with PAOD (Stages II–IV) and Coronary Heart Disease*

H. Böhme and I. Bulik

Because of the high coincidence of peripheral arterial occlusive disease (PAOD) and coronary heart disease (CHD) almost all patients with PAOD stage III or IV (more than 90%) also suffer from CHD [265]. CHD can also be observed in 50% of the patients with PAOD stage II [44]. The study presented here [29] tested whether patients with CHD or PAOD benefit from hemodilution.

The patients in stages II and III received hemodilution with 250 ml 10% Haes 200/0.5 over a period 25 days. In stage IV, dilution was performed until the ulcers were healed, but not longer than 25 days (Fig. 24). The parameters measured were: ejection fraction (echocardiographically), body weight, walking distance

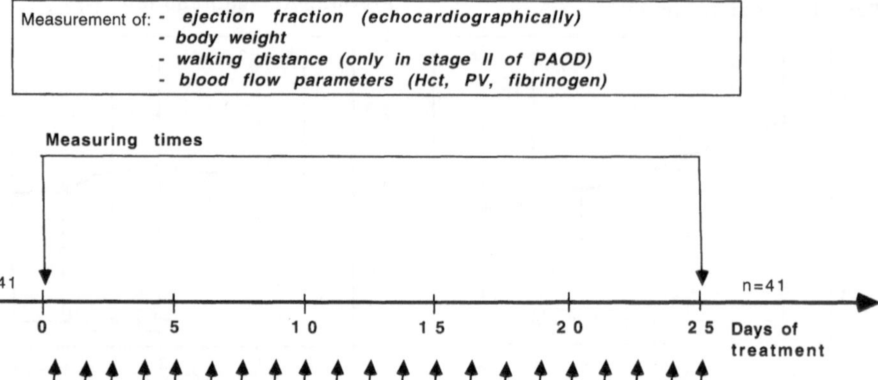


**Fig. 24.** Hemodilution design with 10% Haes 200/0.5 in patients with PAOD (stages II–IV) and coronary heart disease

(only in stage II of PAOD), and blood flow parameters (Hct, PV, fibrinogen).

All patients with PAOD stages III or IV ($n$ = 16) were examined by angiography. A conservative therapy was indicated since vascular surgical recanalization, percutaneous transluminal angioplasty, or a fibrinolysis (local or systemic) could not be performed due to the criteria for inclusion. Most of the patients in stages III or IV had a condition after posterior infarction ($n$ = 12) and four after extended anterior infarction with restricted ejection fraction. All other patients ($n$ = 25) suffered from PAOD stage II; 24 had a case history of posterior infarction and only one an extended anterior infarction.

After 3–14 days of the above hemodilution scheme the five patients with extended anterior infarction and restricted ejection fraction suffered from an insufficiency of the left ventricle although diuretics had been administered. The patients with PAOD stage II and condition after posterior infarction ($n$ = 24) showed a 108% improved walking distance (without increase in frequency of angina pectoris attacks) from about 198 m before the initiation of the therapy to 412 m after the end of the therapy.

The two patients in stage III were transformed stage II. The rest pain could be removed in 10 out of 14 patients with PAOD stage IV. In six cases the necrosis healed completely, in five only partially, and in three cases it remained unchanged.

In all, systemic hematocrit was significantly reduced. Plasma viscosity was lowered in almost all patients, especially when it had been considerably high before. In patients with anterior infarction, plasma viscosity and fibrinogen concentration increased under the hemodilution treatment due to decompensation.

Even in stage IV of PAOD with coronary heart disease a daily hypervolemic hemodilution can be performed over 25 days and leads to a clinical success. However, patients with condition after extended anterior infarction and restricted ejection fraction should not receive hemodilution hypervolemically.

### 2.1.8 General Conclusions

H. Kiesewetter, B. Angelkort, and H. Böhme

Iso- and hypervolemic hemodilution and bag plasmapheresis are useful substitutes or additional measures to physical exercise in the case of PAOD stage II [55, 173, 175, 177, 183, 187, 266, 389]. Dilution is also possible as additional treatment for ulcers of stage IV, according to Fontaine [28, 302, 303]. Analysis of these studies allows a fundamental therapy recommendation adjusted to hemorheologic aspects (Table 1). Hematocrit and plasma viscosity must be measured as rheologic parameters (special therapy recommendations in Sect. 4.6).

**Table 1.** General therapy scheme

| | Hemodilution (creatinine <2 mg/dl) | | |
|---|---|---|---|
| Hct (%) | 40–42 | 43–45 | >45 |
| Infusion (ml) | 250–500 | 500 | 500 |
| Phlebotomy (ml) | – | 250 | 250–500 |
| PV (mPas) | ≤ 1.39 | | >1.39 |
| Colloid | 10% Haes 200/0.5 | | 6% Haes 200/0.5 |
| | Bag plasmapheresis (creatinine< 2 mg/dl) | | |
| PV (mPas) | ≤ 1.39 | | >1.39 |
| Colloid | 10% Haes 200/0.5 | | 6% Haes 200/0.5 |

The most important contraindications for hemodilution with hydroxyethyl starch are summarized in Table 2.

If the vasomotor reserve is still preserved, an overloading of the vascular system causes a peripheral vasodilation and thus a reduction in peripheral resistance [55]. At hematocrit values above 45% and with distinct clinical symptoms hypervolemic hemodilution with phlebotomies is effective. In multimorbid patients and in those with plasma viscosity above 1.39 mPas the 6% Haes 200/0.5 is to be given preference [175]. For patients with possible cardiac decompensation by hypervolemia isovolemic hemodilution presents an alternative if hematocrit values are above 42%. This also applies to patients with distinct arteriolosclerosis (exhausted vasomotor reserve).

**Table 2.** Contraindications

- Severe hemorrhagic diathesis
- Cardiac infarction within the last 6 weeks
- Ejection fraction below 30%, truncus stenosis or equivalents > 60%
- Unstable angina pectoris, crescendo angina, angina CCS stage IV
- cardiac insufficiency stage III and IV (NYHA)
- Hemodynamically relevant cardiac abnormality
- Condition after cardiac decompensation, syncope cardiac genesis
- Arrhythmia Lown IVb and V, high-grade SA and AV blockage
- Heart rate below 50/min or above 10/min at rest
- Significantly reduced state of health
- Other severe diseases, e.g., hematologic system disease, cirrhosis of the liver, renal insufficiency (creatinine > 2 mg/dl), cerebral convulsions
- known "Haes allergy"

At hematocrit values below 40% and plasma viscosities of up to 1.39 mPas the administration of vascoactive substances with rheologically effective components is useful as monotherapy if, in addition, attention is paid to a **sufficient fluid supply**.
Naftidrofuryl (Dusodril) or pentoxifylline (Trental) are recommended [172, 174]. On exceeding a critical plasma viscosity (values above 1.39 mPas) bag plasmapheresis should be performed since the risk of occlusion increases significantly with such increased plasma viscosity. In the case of markedly restricted blood fluidity (Hct > 45%, PV ≥ 1.39 mPas) a combination of hemodilution or plasmapheresis and rheologic drugs is promising. Attention must be paid to an additional sufficient fluid supply.

## 2.2 Hemodilution in Patients with Ischemic Heart Disease

R. Bach, S. Erlenwein, W. Vogel, J. Dyckmans, G. Berg, H. Schieffer, and L. Bette

In 1969, after studies with dextran, Ditzel and collaborators [46] detected in patients with recent cardiac infarction a higher lethality in the active substance group than in the control group. Since then coronary heart disease (CHD) has been regarded as a contraindication for hemodilution treatment. In a recent study Leschke and collaborators [234] also warn against performing hemodilution with a hematocrit reduction to 30% in patients with CHD [321].
Due to the availability of hydroxyethyl starch, which is tolerated much better than dextran, and the positive experiences with mild isovolemic hemodilution (target hematocrit 38%–40% in patients with peripheral arterial occlusive disease (PAOD) [55, 176, 182, 388] the clinical efficacy was examined in patients with ischemic heart disease.

### 2.2.1 Patients

A total of 100 patients with coronary one–, two–, three-vascular disease or cardiac microangiopathy and stable angina pectoris were included (mean age 56 years; blood pressure 140/80 mmHg; pulse rate of 72 bpm). All patients had been hospitalized due to suspected or confirmed CHD to perform diagnostic coronary angiography. A detailed patient description is presented in the original work [178]. The contraindications listed in Table 2 (Sect. 2.1.8) served as criteria for exclusion.

### 2.2.2 Isovolemic Single Dilution

On hemodilution, 500 ml (Haes-steril 10%; Fresenius) was injected into a brachial vein over 30 min. A phlebotomy of 500 ml was performed simultaneously in a contralateral brachial vein. The total duration of the hemodilution including the preparations was 45 min. Before and after hemodilution nail-fold capillaroscopy [163], phlebotomy with determination of rheologic parameters, and ergometer exercise were performed. The time courses of the individual measures are given in Fig. 25. It was attempted during ergometer exercise to keep the circulatory parameters constant; as a rule this was achieved after 3 min, first at the first level (1 Wkg body weight), then at the second (1.5 Wkg BW), and finally at the third level (2 Wkg BW). The exercise breaking was performed with regard to the general criteria for this [243], exercise-limiting symptoms, or muscular exhaustion. The recovery phase lasted until circulation values approached the initial resting values, and the possible cardiac symptoms had passed.

The resting and exercise pressures decreased significantly after hemodilution; the maximum frequency under exercise increased significantly.

Clinical benefit was determined when one or more of five criteria were improved by hemodilution (Table 3). The symptom of dyspnea was decreased

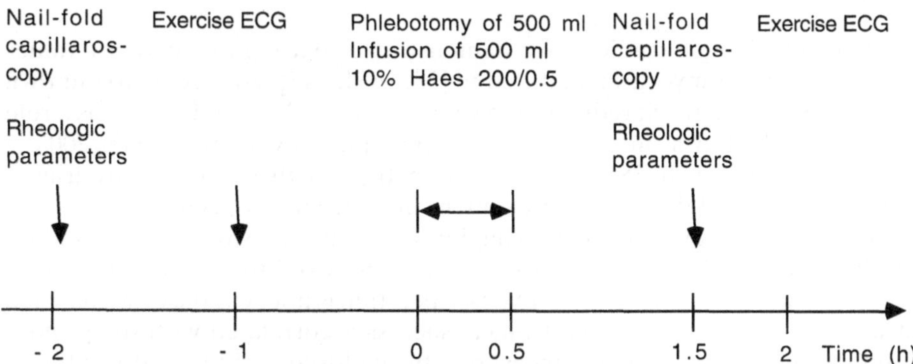


**Fig. 25.** Study design: hemodilution in ischemic heart disease

**Table 3.** Clinical criteria before and after hemodilution

| | Before | After | Significance |
|---|---|---|---|
| Angina pectoris | 28 | 16 | NS |
| Dyspnea | 31 | 15 | <0.01 |
| Arrhythmia | 17 | 13 | NS |
| Negative ST segment displacement | 18 | 17 | NS |
| Pressure × frequency (mmHg/min) | 22 983 | 21 803 | <0.05 |

significantly by hemodilution (at the 1% level), as did that of pressure × frequency product (at the 5% level). Prior to hemodilution 71 patients terminated due to muscular exhaustion and the remaining 29 due to cardiac symptoms or other criteria. After hemodilution 80 patients terminated due to muscular exhaustion and the 20 due to cardiac symptoms or other criteria. The clinical evaluation of isovolemic hemodilution was good if one of the five parameters (Table 3) was improved, very good if more than one parameter was improved, no improvement in the case of constant parameters, slight worsening if one parameter deteriorated and severe worsening in the case of more than one deteriorated parameter. According to this classification 10 patients showed a very good improvement, 42 a good improvement, 30 no improvement, 15 a slight worsening, and 3 a severe worsening.

The resting velocity in the nutritive main capillaries increased significantly by 26.5% from 0.34 to 0.43 mm/s on average ($p<0.01$) and the mean maximum velocity after 3 min of ischemia by 58% (from 0.67 to 1.06 mm/s; $p<0.01$). The duration of reactive hyperemia was increased only as a tendency from 125 to 138 s. Systemic hematocrit was reduced significantly from 45% to 38% ($p<0.01$), plasma viscosity from 1.36 to 1.34 mPas ($p<0.05$), and erythrocyte aggregation from 15.2 to 12.4 ($p<0.05$). Erythrocyte rigidity and spontaneous thrombocyte aggregation did not change.

### 2.2.3 Conclusions

Several epidemiologic studies have demonstrated that high hematocrit values are a risk factor for myocardial infarction [38, 1654, 345]. According to our own experiences, a hematocrit reduction to values between 38% and 40% is as a rule well tolerated. After a single isovolemic hemodilution with 10% Haes 200/0.5 (hematocrit reduction to 38%) over 50% of patients with ischemic heart disease showed a very good or good improvement in their angina pectoris.

In patients with severe CHD and angina symptoms an isovolemic hemodilution should be tried if a conservative therapy improved the exercise tolerance only insufficiently, or if a PTCA or bypass operation is not possible or was carried out without satisfactory results. Clinical success is correlated with the prolongation of reactive hyperemia measured by nail-fold capillaroscopy after a congestion of 3 min at the upper arm (at 300 mmHg).

The reservations toward hemodilution in ischemic heart disease should not be maintained. However, the clinical benefit of the first hemodilution must be checked by means of an exercise ECG before and after hemodilution.

## *2.3 Hemodilution in Ischemic Cerebral Infarction from a Neurologic Point of View*

A. Haass

The aim of hemodilution is to improve the regional cerebral circulation in acute and chronic circulatory disturbances. In acute ischemic infarction it increases the circulation in the penumbra. Furthermore, it supports the recanalization, increases oxygen transport, and reduces reperfusion damages. Since the autoregulation in the penumbra of the cerebral infarction (Sect. 3.3) is disturbed, not only hemorrheologic parameters such as Hct, PV, SEA, thrombocyte aggregation and leukocyte adhesivity must be optimized by hemodilution but also the hemodynamics by an increase in CO. Hemodilution does not consist simply of increased circulation by filling the cardiovascular system at hemoconcentration and improvement of blood flow.

Hydroxyethyl starch 200/05 is a suitable plasma substitute since it decreases PV and SEA significantly. It does not cause an increase in PV or SEA, as do dextran and high-substituted starch solutions (Sect. 3.4.4).

The hypervolemic infusion method increases CO whereas an improper isovolemic hemodilution can cause a negative hemodynamic effect (details see Sect. 3.3.5). For this reason, the method of choice is hypervolemic hemodilution adjusted to the cardiac load capacity. Isovolemic hemodilution is appropriate only at an extremely high Hct level and not in acute cerebrovascular accidents.

Early initiation of therapy is important for a successful outcome, including in myocardial infarction. The use of hydroxyethyl starch 200/05 hardly changes the coagulation parameters (Sect. 3.4.5.4), which also allows a direct action by the family or emergency physician without previous exclusion of intracerebral bleeding. The initiation of therapy with a rapid infusion, such as the so-called "*loading dose*," is useful even if the clinical findings reveal an increased intracranial pressure, which is not a contraindication (details see Sect. 3.4.6).

The "loading dose" can consist, for example, of 500 ml 6% Haes 200/0.5 or in the case of stronger cardiac load capacity of 1000 ml 6% or 500 ml 10% solution, but in the latter case 500 ml low-sodium electrolyte solution must be added (details see Sect. 3.4.7).

A *long-term infusion treatment* follows the loading dose and depends on the cardiac load capacity. A standardized dose cannot be established, and an infusion scheme can provide only the basis. The dose must be adjusted to the individual conditions (compare other therapies). A volume that is too small diminishes the success of therapy while too much volume can endanger the patient. Therefore, hemodilution requires a certain amount of expertise or experience in the procedure.

Hemodilution does not compete with other therapies but is an essential step for supplementary forms of treatment such as inhibition of thrombocyte aggregation with acetylsalicylic acid (ASA). However, intracerebral bleeding should be excluded before the use of ASA. Drugs for the reduction of reperfusion damages are also optimally transported by hemodilution for reaching the damaged tissue. Furthermore, after admission to hospital it can be decided whether fibrinolysis or total heparinization is possible, especially in a clinical situation involving increased embolism relapse rates or other special cases (Sect. 3.6). The recently newed critical discussion about hemodilution has the advantage that the fundamental pathophysiologic principles of this therapy have been stated more precisely (Chap. 3). The points of criticism adduced by Back and von Kummer [16] are unjustified since they exclude serious objective methods (Haaß and Jung [106]) and are based on experiments with healthy cats which do not apply directly to the conditions in patients. Their allegations about hemodynamic oxygen transport capacity (OTC), Hct, SEA, and PV are basically not valid. A comparison of the different studies on hemodilution (Sect. 3.4.2) shows that the failure demonstrated by several studies was due to a late initiation of therapy and an increasingly isovolemic method of infusion. This became evident in the unfavorable results of Mast and Marx [250], who performed a hypovolemic hemodilution which lasted several hours. Other studies report positive results with hypervolemic hemodilution (the studies of Strand et al. [351]; the Hemodilution in Stroke Study Group [94]; Goslinga [85, 86]; Koller et al. [213]; Haaß et al. [103, 104]. Moreover, the positive results of hypervolemic hemodilution in subarachnoid hemorrhage and noncerebral indications such as retinal infarction, PAOD, and CHD support the efficacy of this therapy. To meet the complexity of this topic the details of pathophysiology, hemodynamics, hemorheology, and additional therapy in ischemic cerebral infarction are described in detail in Chap. 3.

### 2.3.1 Hemodilution in Ischemic Cerebral Infarction from a Geriatric Point of View

J. Schwab

Cerebrovascular accidents occur predominantly in advanced age. Approximately 75% of all ischemic attacks occur in patients over 65 years of age. Subarachnoid hemorrhages and hemorrhagic forms of bleedings are seldom found in advanced age (fewer than 5%) whereas ischemic infarctions are predominant (e.g., arterial thromboses of cerebral vessels, arterio-arterial embolism, cardio-arterial embolism) [384]. More recent studies on the treatment of cerebrovascular accidents do not necessarily reflect the conditions in elderly people. Grotta [94] treated patients with an average age of 65 years, in the Scandinavian Stroke Study Group [316]; the mean age of patients was 72 years. In the study of the Italian Study Group [147] 75% of patients were younger than 75 years and 49% younger than 65 years.

The recommendation given here stems from a study involving 84 patients with an average age of 80 years (66–90 years). The confirmatory parameter of this study is the Barthel index as a measure for the proper daily routine and is closely correlated with the paresis scores of the Scandinavian Stroke Study Group [316] and a score for the recording of mental performance (functional psychosis scale B [330]. This study included only patients in whom ischemic cerebral infarction was determined exclusively from the vascular distribution of the middle cerebral artery by computer-assisted tomography.

The treatment of cerebrovascular accidents in advanced age includes an attempt at causal therapy. However, it is also necessary to consider a large number of possible complications and to treat them in time. Such complications are:

- Phlogistic diseases: such as bronchopneumonia (oral hygiene!), aspiration pneumonia, catheter infections (urinary passages and veins), often secondary septicemia
- Exsiccation tendency: in case of senile drinking weakness
- Fluid overload cardiac decompensation: under infusion therapy
- Upper gastrointestinal bleeding (rarely): stress ulcers or erosions, e.g., by anti-inflammatory agents
- Decubital ulcers (rarely): at improper positioning
- Thrombosis and pulmonary embolism (rarely): at immobilization

The diagnosis of cerebrovascular accidents in elderly persons includes several studies of origin:

- Computer-assisted tomogram (CAT) of the cranium: hemorrhagic bleeding or ischemic attacks
- Doppler examination of the brain supplying arteries [76]: extracranial: arterio-arterial embolism, carotid obliteration, stenoses; transcranial: stenoses or obliterations in the area of circle of Willis or basilar artery
- Long-term ECG: tachy- and/or bradycardic arthythmia
- Blood pressure control: hypotonic dysfunction in arterial hypertension or hypertensive crisis with "breakthrough phenomenon"

The clinical course pretreatment parameters of the threatening diseases are:

- Rheologic parameters: plasma viscosity (PV) – increase in dehydration, often synergistic with plasma osmolality; increase in inflammatory processes, often synergistic with erythrocyte aggregation (SEA)
- Red and white blood cell counts: inflammatory processes, bleeding
- Blood sedimentation rate (BSR): increase in inflammatory processes
- Creatinine clearance: renal function
- Central venous pressure (CVP): cardiac function, dehydration
- Examination of the feces for occult blood: gastric hemorrhages
- Control of parts vulnerable to decubital: in all patients!
- Blood gas analysis (BGA): impaired ventilation and/or perfusion

The basic therapy of cerebrovascular accidents is to avoid complications:

- Positioning according to Bobath [255] or changing 30°C storage for decubitus prophylaxis
- Controlled administration of fluid: determination of central venous pressure (CVP)
- Prophylaxis of stress ulcer: antacids in patients without dysphagia, pirenzepine in patients with dysphagia

- Supply of at least 1000 kcal daily: orally or by central vein catheter (CVC), possibly gastric tube/PEG
- Intensive oral hygiene and prophylactic antibiotics: recommendation for the use of a second-generation cephalosporin (especially in patients with dysphagia)
- Individual blood pressure control: essential hypertension in arterial occlusions (corrective measurement in the case of media sclerosis or calcinosis)

It is difficult to standardize causal therapy of cerebrovascular accidents in the elderly. In the following all possible therapeutic measures are on the basis of results among 84 patients with an average age of 80 years:

1. The administration of rheologic drugs would be ideal in the treatment of apoplexy in elderly patients since these pharmaceutics normally do not strain the circulation and are effective without the risk of hemorrhage. In contrast to the encouraging results in younger patients [2, 135] rheologic drugs showed no efficacy exceeding the placebo effect in this study on elderly people.
2. Hemodilution treatment with hydroxyethyl starch was also not very successful in elderly persons, who generally do not have cardiac reserves. Out of 85 patients assigned to stage 2 (NYHA cardiac disease classification) 57 received daily 250 ml 10% Haes 200/0.5; the cardiac- risk healthy patients received 500 ml 10% Haes 200/0.5 for 2 weeks. While the cardially vulnerable patients showed a clearly better Barthel index after the administration of 250 ml 10% Haes 200/0.5 after 2 weeks (from 27.6 to 43.6; $p<0.0003$), this index did not increase significantly in the patients with healthier hearts after the infusion of 500 ml 10% Haes 200/0.5. Simultaneous phlebotomy for further reducing hematocrit was even damaging for the elderly patients in both groups. The improvement rates without phlebotomy were significantly higher; with phlebotomy the lethality was even increased by 30%. The administration of hydroxyethyl starch is clinically and pathophysiologically useful, predominantly in very recent attacks, if the hematoencephalic barrier has not collapsed [401]. Therefore, mild hypervolemic hemodilution with 250 ml is to be prefered. With clinical improvement it can be continued if the contraindications are observed.
3. Acetylsalicylic acid (ASA) can be administered successfully for the prophylaxis of recurrent cerebrovascular accidents, as confirmed by the *Europäische Studie zur Prävention des Schlaganfalls* [56]. (Note: dipyridamole is not a successful treatment for the prophylaxis of recurrent cerebrovascular accidents [33, 284].) In 1977 Fields and collaborators [63] presented relevant data. These were modified by the results of the Canadian Cooperative Study (1978) [36] since women did not seem to benefit from the administration of ASA. In this study ASA was used for the prophylaxis of recurrent cerebrovascular accidents [330] and proven to be an effective therapeutic agent. Under treatment with ASA the Barthel index improved from 35 to 74 ($p<0.0001$); without ASA it improved from 39 to only 65 ($p<0.0001$). Women did, without doubt, benefit from the administration of ASA since the Barthel index increased from 37 to 76 and without ASA from 36 to only 58. The percentage of patients who died during the administration of ASA (average Barthel index on admission, 6.1), was lower by 20% than the corresponding

percentage of patients not receiving ASA (average Barthel index on admission, 39.3).

A dose of 500 mg twice weekly or 100 mg daily was given. The discussion about dosage of ASA is still pending or incomplete [90]. However, the gastrointestinal tolerance of the low dose is better, with angiologic equivalent efficacy.

The administration of ASA is contraindicated in intracerebral hemorrhages. Therefore, a cranial computer-assisted tomogram is required in every cerebrovascular accident which is to be treated with ASA. ASA has no fibrinolytic effect. Thus there is no recurrent bleeding in an area in which the lesions have already been closed with fibrin. This also explains why there are no deteriorations in patients who had experienced early intracerebral bleedings under ASA. Overall, the intracerebral bleeding [384] in advanced age is very seldom (3.2%). ASA has no influence on rheologic parameters [54], especially in the elderly [330].

The danger of secondary bleeding with primary ischemic attack is significantly higher in patients with arterial hypertension especially with recurrent hypertensive relapses.

4. Oral anticoagulants are not considered in the treatment of cerebrovascular accidents in elderly persons.
5. Heparin should be used in low doses (twice daily 5000 IU subcutaneously) for the prophylaxis of thromboses. Total heparinization in the case of thromboembolic processes has been tested in several centers.
6. Fibrinolytic agents, now being tested in occlusions of the area of the middle cerebral artery and thromboses in the basilar artery of younger patients, should not be used in elderly patients at present.
7. Nimodipine seems especially useful in hypertensive patients and those with ischemic attack [80]. The relevance of this to elderly persons cannot be assessed at present.

A further peculiarity in the process of cerebrovascular accidents in elderly persons is an alteration of the sympathic hormonal system. In such an event high noradrenaline levels in plasma are measured, whereas the dopamine levels increase in plasma during the course of disease [391]. This often leads to dysregulations of the circulation while standing. Because of this it is advisable to perform a Schellong test in every patient before the remobilization. If a decrease in blood pressure of more than 20 mmHg with insufficient increase in heart rate and without increase in diastolic blood pressure is found, the administration of a peripheral effective dopamine antagonist is indicated [84].

> Cerebrovascular accidents in advanced age entail a high mortality and frequently immobilize the patient. Only proper initiation of therapy (considering the reduced functional reserves) can sometimes help to prevent hopeless fates and may benefit the elderly. Mild hypervolemic hemodilution in combination with acetylsalicyclic acid – besides being a concomitant basic therapy – has proven an effective therapy in advanced age.

### 2.3.2 *Hemodilution in Ischemic Cerebral Infarction from an Internalist and Point of View*

H. Kiesewetter and B. Angelkort

The aim of hemodilution is the quick restoration of sufficient perfusion of brain areas affected by hypoxia. Hypervolemic hemodilution with hydroxyethyl starch 200/0.5 supports hemodynamic and hemorheologic effects [131]. This is confirmed in our own studies on patients with peripheral arterial occlusive disease [183]. The results show that hemodynamic and hemorheologic effects are rather equally pronounced. The administration of dextran exerts only the hemodynamic effect since blood fluidity in the microvascular system is even worsened [108].

The choice of the proper plasma substitute is equally as decisive as the time of treatment. According to the program of Haaß, who also treats subarachnoid and intracerebral hemorrhages with hemodilution (if no contraindication is given), a hypervolemic hemodilution should be started immediately after the evidence of a cerebrovascular accident or a transitory ischemic attack [105]. At least 500 ml 6% Haes 200/0.5 must be infused within about 30 min as a so-called "loading dose" regardless of whether the accident is hemorrhagic or ischemic.

In the hitherto published studies hemodilution was unfortunately not started until 6 or 24 h after the attack.

> The initiation of hemodilution is required as soon as possible after the occurrence. The "loading dose" should be administered immediately after it is determined that the patient is neither comatose nor dyspneic.

This is supported by findings from the treatment of retinal infarctions [398]. After a loading dose of 500–1000 ml 6% Haes 200/0.5 it must be determined at the hospital which differential treatment should be continued, dependent upon clinical and, if necessary, computed tomographic findings. After the exclusion of intracerebral or subarachnoid hemorrhages a local lysis as ultima ratio may be considered in occlusions in the basilar vascular area [410]. Systemic lysis in the treatment of cerebrovascular accidents of the middle cerebral artery area is now being tested [131, 294]. Intravenous continuous total heparinization must be performed if no contraindication exists in the case of progressive symptoms, confirmed embolisms, confirmed atrial thromboses or serverely reduced ejection fraction [97, 105].

If these therapeutic measures are not considered, hemodilution must often be combined with the administration of acetylsalicyclic acid or "rheologic drugs" since a distinct thrombocyte aggregation can be observed during the acute-phase reaction [91, 92]. According to the latest literature [105], 250 mg acetylsalicylic acid should be given every 12 h. In another study 600 mg naftidrofuryl (Dusodril) per day proved effective [350].

Table 4 presents all studies which meet the clinical and statistical requirements.

**Table 4.** Study survey: clinical efficacy of hemodilution in patients with ischemic attack

| | Year | Colloidal solution | Clinical efficacy |
|---|---|---|---|
| *Hypervolemic dilution* | | | |
| Gilroy [81] | 1969 | Dextran 40 | – |
| Spudis [346] | 1973 | Dextran 40 | – |
| Matthews [251] | 1976 | Dextran 40 | + |
| Italian Study [147] | 1988 | Dextran 40 | – |
| Grotta [94] | 1989 | Hydroxyethyl starch 250 | +/– |
| *Iso- and hypervolemic dilution* | | | |
| Strand [351] | 1984 | Dextran 40 | + |
| Asplund [10] | 1986 | Dextran 40 | – |

Important points of criticism in all these studies are that hemodilution was started too late, that the reduction in systemic hematocrit was too pronounced, and that the groups of patients had been too inhomogeneous with respect to the small number of cases. Six of the seven studies used dextran as colloidal solution. It has been proven that blood fluidity in the terminal vascular bed decreases with the administration of dextran, and therefore the circulation is reduced if the vasomotor reserve is exhausted [108]. This applies to almost all patients with arterial hypertension or arteriolosclerosis in the area of the cerebrovascular accident and penumbra.

The only valid study with mean molecular weight hydroxyethyl starch was performed by Grotta [94]. Here, 1500 ml hydroxyethyl starch was given per day. The hematocrit target was 33%. The active substance group presented the best clinical efficacy but also the highest mortality. A lethal result was quite often accompanied by the appearance of cerebral edema. This shows that the benefit of hemodilution in cerebrovascular accidents depends upon the patient's general state of health (concomitant diseases) and on the initiation of hemodilution. If the latency period is too long (several hours after beginning of the cerebrovascular accident) the vascular walls could be damaged so that parenteral fluid administration is accompanied by the development of or increase in cerebral edema with clear signs of an increased intracranial pressure.

The points of criticism adduced by Back and Kummer [16, 224, 318] concerning hemodilution in cerebrovascular accident are not justified since they are based on hardly useful animal experiments, and their pathophysiologic examinations on hemodynamics, oxygen transport capacity and blood fluidity are furthermore incorrect. Nevertheless, better studies are required to demonstrate the clinical efficacy with regard to the described procedure.

After the first hemodilution in the form of a "loading dose" of at least 500 ml Haes-steril 6% in the case of apoplexy, further treatment should be carried out on an individualized basis according to the pathophysiology. The possible treatment schemes are hypervolemic hemodilution, local or systemic fibrinolysis, heparinization, administration of vasoactive substances, and bag plasmapheresis.

## 2.4 Hypervolemic Hemodilution in High-Risk Pregnancies

L. HEILMANN

The hemodynamic and hemorheologic changes during pregnancy include an increase in plasma volume and cardiac output and a decrease in viscosity and hematocrit value. There is a close correlation between the increase in plasma volume and the weight of the newborn [12]. Liley [235] discovered an inverse relationship between plasma volume and hemoglobin content during pregnancy. Low hemoglobin values in the second and third trimesters reflect maximal hemodilution and are accompanied by a sufficient uteroplacental perfusion and big children [73, 74, 77, 269].

With the existing epidemiologic data there are sufficient results to verify the relationship between hemoglobin content or hematocrit during gravidity and the weight of the child (Table 5).

In order to test the clinical efficacy of hemodilution with colloidal solutions during pregnancy the following studies were performed.

**Table 5.** Pregnancy-related complications due to lack of physiologic hemodilution in the second trimester (from [77, 254, 269, 270, 277])

| | Without hemodilution | Normal pregnancy population |
|---|---|---|
| Intrauterine growth retardation | 10%–15% | 4%–7% |
| Pregnancy-related hypertension | ca. 30% | 10% |
| Perinatal mortality | 3%–4% | <1% |

### 2.4.1 Open Study Comparing Colloidal Solutions: Low Molecular Weight Dextran, 10% Haes 200/05, and Human Albumin 20%

A total of 144 female patients with sonographically verified intrauterine growth retardation were treated as described below. After clinical diagnosis, sonography, and determination of rheologic parameters (hematocrit, plasma viscosity, erythrocyte aggregation) 90 patients received 10% Haes 200/0.5 for 8 days, 40 patients low molecular weight dextran for 8 days, and 14 patients 100 ml 20% human albumin for 8 days [125]. The clinical data are presented in Table 6.

Patients with intrauterine growth retardation (IUGR) are characterized by hemoconcentration, reduced cardiac output, and increased plasma viscosity. The erythrocyte aggregation was normal compared to apparently healthy women in the same week of pregnancy. The use of colloidal solutions resulted in reduction in perinatal mortality of 2.5%–3.3%. The administration of 20% human albumin proved advantageous with respect to the placental perfusion, such experience was also recorded by Jouppila [152] and Zondervan [411].

**Table 6.** Hemodilution therapy with different colloidal substances (1979–1984)

| Colloidal solution | Number | NW< 2500 g PM | | NW > 2500 g PM | |
|---|---|---|---|---|---|
| 10% Haes 200/0.5 | 90 | 24.4% | 3.3% | 75.6 | 0% |
| Low molecular weight dextran | 40 | 40.0% | 2.5% | 60.0 | 0% |
| Human albumin 20% | 14 | 57.1% | 21.4% | 42.9% | 0% |

NW, weight of the newborn; PM, perinatal mortality.

### *2.4.2 Randomized Prospective Study Comparing Low Molecular Weight Dextran and 10% Haes 200/0.5 in Women with Suspected Placental Insufficiency*

In each of two groups we examined 30 pregnant women with sonographically verified growth retardation [69, 126]. These women received a hemodilution of 10% Haes 200/0.5 or low molecular weight dextran for 8 days during the second trimester. The daily dosage was 500 ml, but the pregnant women were

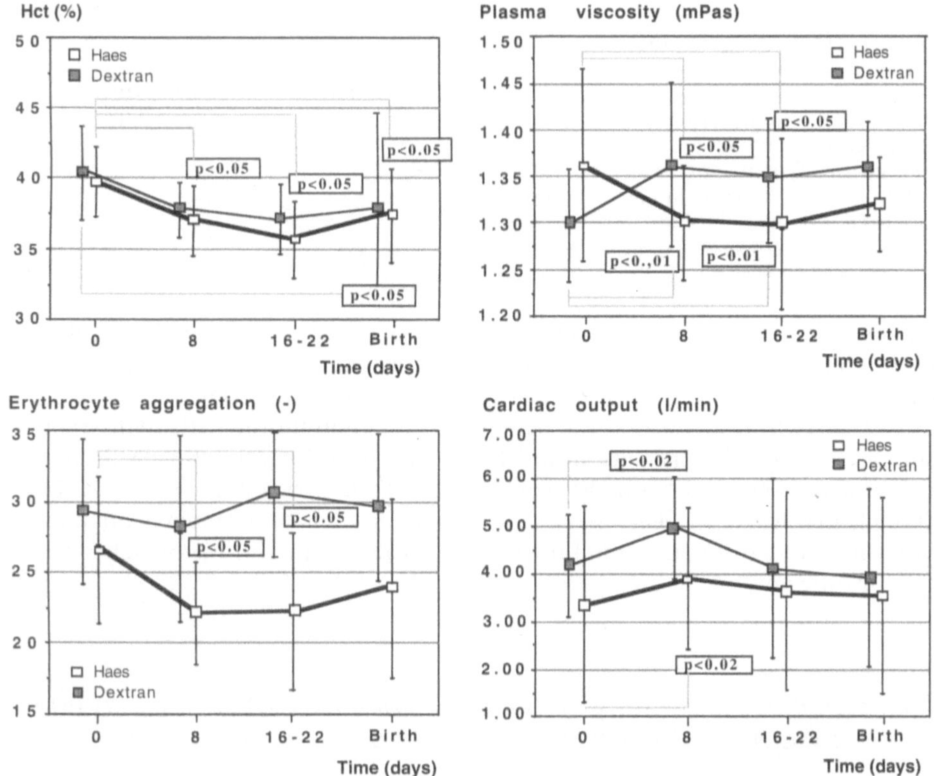


**Fig. 26.** Time courses of hemorheologic and hemodynamic parameters in the Haes and dextran groups in until day of birth ($p$: significance level in time-series comparison with reference to the initial value)

**Table 7.** Course of the hemorheologic and one hemodynamic arameter before, during, and after the infusion therapy

| Parameter | Colloidal solution | 0 days | 8 days | 8–14 days after end of infusion | Day of birth |
|---|---|---|---|---|---|
| Hematocrit (%) | Haes | 39.3±2.1 | 37.2±2.2* | 36.1±2.2* | 37.3±3.4* |
| | Dextran | 40.1±2.8 | 38.1±1.2 | 38.1±2.1 | 37.9±6.1* |
| Plasma viscosity | Haes | 1.36±0.1 | 1.30±0.07* | 1.30±0.09* | 1.33±0.03 |
| (mPas) | Dextran | 1.30±0.06 | 1.36±0.08*** | 1.35±0.07*** | 1.36±0.03 |
| Erythrocyte | Haes | 26.8±6.3 | 22.1±3.5* | 22.2±5.3* | 23.9±6.5 |
| aggegation (–) | Dextran | 29.4±5.4 | 28.4±7.4 | 30.1±5.2 | 29.5±7.2 |
| Cardiac output | Haes | 3.21±1.95 | 3.91±1.54** | 3.54±1.85 | 3.40±1.9 |
| (l/min) | Dextran | 4.15±0.91 | 4.95±1.67** | 4.04±1.89 | 3.85±2.1 |

* $p<0.05$; ** $p<0.02$; *** $p<0.001$

**Table 8.** Clinical success

| Parameter | Dextran 40 | 10% Haes 200/0.5 |
|---|---|---|
| Birth weight< 10th percentile | 20 | 15 |
| Perinatal mortality | 4 (13%) | 1 (3%) |
| Weight of the newborn | 2184±804 | 2480±910 |
| pH value in umbilical artery | 7.21±0.07 | 7.24±0.08 |
| Repeated hemodilutions | 15 | 12 |
| Incompatibility reactions 1st degree | 4 | 1 |
| Additional human albumin administration | 5 | 1 |
| Occurrence of hypertension | 5 | 1 |

encouraged to drink 2 l fluid each time. The risk factors were equally distributed between the two groups. Besides plasma viscosity and erythrocyte aggregation, cardiac output was also measured by impedance cardiography.

The best clinical success was achieved by hemodilution with hydroxyethyl starch (Fig. 26). The maternal and fetal complication rates during 8 days of infusion of 500 ml dextran 40 were untenably higher than with 10% Haes 200/0.5 (Tables 7, 8). The causes lie in an inadequate influence on plasma viscosity and cardiac output. Furthermore, the compensation of dehydration was insufficient.

### *2.4.3 Double-Blind Study with Naftidrofuryl and 10% Haes 200/0.5 in Women with Fetal Growth Retardation*

In each of two groups 15 female patients with fetal growth retardation (IUGR) were examined. These women received either 400 mg naftidrofuryl (active substance) or placebo per day. Both groups were given 500 ml 10% Haes 200/0.5

for 10 days. We tested whether the combination therapy with naftidrofuryl has an effect on erythrocyte deformability. Further parameters of blood fluidity as well as the cardiac output as hemodynamic parameter were determined prior to therapy and on the 5th and 10th days of infusion (hematocrit, erythrocyte aggregation, plasma viscosity) [121].

The erythrocyte filtration rates did not differ between active substance and placebo groups. There was a relative increase in the naftidrofuryl group in comparison to the placebo group, indicating a tendency to improvement in the erythrocyte filtration rate; however, this was not statistically significant. Examination specifically among preeclampsia patients showed a considerably clearer result in pregnant women with worse initial situation ($p<0.08$).

The combined medication of naftidrofuryl and hypervolemic hemodilution with 10% Haes 200/0.5 during pregnancy showed an improvement in the erythrocyte deformability only in the group of patients with pregnancy-related hypertension. The group with idiopathic fetal growth retardation (IUGR) did not benefit from this combination therapy. The other clinical and rheologic data did not differ between the two groups (Table 9).

**Table 9.** Results of hemorheologic and one hemodynamic parameter

| Parameter | Group | 0 days | 5 days | 10 days | *p* |
|---|---|---|---|---|---|
| Hematocrit | Active substance | 39.0±0.4 | 37.5±0.8 | 35.4±0.3 | <0.001 |
| (%) | Placebo | 39.1±0.3 | 35.0±0.6 | 35.5±0.7 | <0.003 |
| Plasma viscosity | Active substance | 1.37±0.02 | 1.38±0.02 | 1.33±0.08 | <0.08 |
| (mPas) | Placebo | 1.33±0.03 | 1.31±0.01 | 1.32±0.01 | NS |
| Erythrocyte aggregation | Active substance | 27.9±1.0 | 24.4±2.3 | 23.9±2.0 | NS |
| (–) | Placebo | 28.0±1.8 | 25.3±1.6 | 25.9±1.7 | <0.06 |
| Erythrocyte filtration | Active substance | 8.8±0.09 | 9.7±0.5 | 9.3±0.3 | NS |
| (ml/s) | Placebo | 10.9±0.8 | 12.0±1.1 | 10.1±0.6 | NS |
| Cardiac output | Active substance | 3.32±0.4 | 4.37±0.4 | 3.94±0.4 | <0.05 |
| (l/min) | Placebo | 3.75±0.1 | 3.86±0.3 | 3.81±0.3 | NS |

### *2.4.4 Prospective Study with 10% Haes 200/0.5 in Women with Fetal Growth Retardation and Isolated Plasma Volume Concentration*

In this study 30 patients without hemodilution and 38 with sonographically verified fetal growth retardation were treated. The pregnant women received 500 ml 10% Haes 200/0.5 and 500 ml Ringer solution for 10 days. Prior to therapy, on the 5th and 10th days of infusion, and at the time of birth hematocrit, plasma viscosity, erythrocyte aggregation, and cardiac output were determined. [122, 123, 127, 129]. Tables 10 and 11 present the rates of success from these and other data.

**Table 10.** Rates of success of hemodilution with 10% Haes 200/0.5 in combination with Ringer solution

| Criteria | Number (percentage) | Incidence in cases without hemodilution |
|---|---|---|
| Birth weight > 2500 g | 37 (57.4%) | ND |
| Gestation period > 37th WP | 54 (79.4%) | ND |
| Prolongation of therapy > 14 days | 49 (72.1%) | ND |
| Repetition of hemodilution | 10 (14.7%) | ND |
| IUGR at birth | 23 (33.8%) | 53% |
| Hypertension at birth | 5 (7.4%) | 30% |
| Hct > 38% at birth | 9 (13.2%) | ND |
| Perinatal mortality | 2 (2.9%) | 4% |

WP, weeks of pregnancy; IUGR, idiopathic growth retardation; ND, not determined.

**Table 11.** Rates of success of hemodilution with 10% Haes 200/0.5 in combination with Ringer solution in the rheologically abnormal subgroups

| Grouping | Number | Hypertension at diagnosis | IUGR at birth | Hypertension at birth |
|---|---|---|---|---|
| Plasma volume contraction in the second trimester | 30 | 0 | 0 | 0 |
| Fetral growth retardation (IUGR) in the second trimester | 38 | 2 | 23 | 5 |

With adequate hemodilution therapy and compensation of multiple iatrogenic dehydration there were fewer immature babies and pregnancy-related complications than expected. Therapy failures occured if the plasma viscosity was not reduced, and the cardiac output did not increase in spite of hematocrit reduction.

### *2.4.5 Comparison of Two 10% Hydroxyethyl Starches 200/05 with Regard to Starch Accumulation in the Placenta*

In this study we compared a hydroxyethyl starch I (classic production method) with a hydroxyethyl starch II (levosin production method) with regard to their side effects and histologically confirmed accumulation phenomena in the placenta. The preparations did not differ in concentration, mean molecular weight, or substitution degree [123, 129].

A total of 36 women (Table 12) received hydroxyethyl starch I (Haes I), 21 because of pregnancy-related hypertension and 15 because of fetal growth retardation (IUGR). A second group of 24 women received hydroxyethyl starch II (Haes II); here hemodilution was indicated due to pregnancy-related

**Table 12.** Characteristics of patients in the comparative study: Haes I versus Haes II

| Characteristics | Haes I | Haes II |
|---|---|---|
| Age (years) | 27.6 (17–41) | 28.0 (20–40) |
| Weight (kg) | 74.7 (50–115) | 79.2 (53–106) |
| Initiation of hemodilution (WP) | 35.6 (25–40) | 37.4 (33–40) |
| Infused quantity of Haes (g starch) | 464 (50–1400) | 408 (50–1220) |
| Time: end of therapy – birth (days) | 7.1 (0–77) | 0.3 (0–1) |

WP, Weeks of pregnancy.

hypertension in 14 patients and fetal growth retardation (IUGR) in the other 10 women.

Due to the varying production methods of hydroxyethyl starch there are differences in clinical use with regard to coagulation and tissue accumulation despite equal concentration, mean molecular weight, and substitution degree. The hydroxyethyl starch (Haes-steril 10%; Fresenius) produced by the classic method has lower accumulation and complication rates (Tables 13, 14).

**Table 13.** Starch accumulation in the trophoblast or stroma of the chorionic villi and hemostatic complications in terms of the infused Haes volume

| Preparation quantity | | Accumulation trophoblast | | Stroma | | Hemostatic complications |
|---|---|---|---|---|---|---|
| | | No | Yes | No | Yes | |
| Haes I | ≤ 150 g | 8 | 1 | 9 | 0 | 0 |
| Haes I | > 150 g | 6 | 11 | 9 | 8 | 0 |
| Haes II | ≤ 150 g | 3 | 2 | 5 | 0 | 1 |
| Haes II | > 150 g | 1 | 19 | 2 | 18 | 3 |

**Table 14.** Complications during hemodilution therapy with different hydroxyethyl starch solutions

| Complications | Haes I Number (percentage) | Haes II Number (percentage) |
|---|---|---|
| No complications | 30 (83.4%) | 13 (54.1%) |
| Vomiting | 0 (0%) | 1 (4.2%) |
| Increase in uric acid > 5 mg/dl | 4 (11.1%) | 1 (4.2%) |
| Increase in blood pressure and uric acid | 2 (5.6%) | 3 (4.2%) |
| Thrombocyte count< 150 000/mm$^3$ | 0 (0%) | 0 (0%) |
| Afterbleeding | 0 (0%) | 4 (16.6%) |
| Premature removal of the placenta | 0 (0%) | 1 (4.2%) |

Regarding complications, extensive blood loss in the puerperal uterus and damage to the perineum during birth were observed. A relationship to the infused Haes quantity was obvious, while the time interval between the final administration of starch and birth was of secondary importance.

### 2.4.6 Use of 10% Haes 200/0.5 for Perioperative Thrombosis Prophylaxis in Cesarian Section

The incidence of thrombosis after cesarian sections is between 0.7% and 3.0%. Most studies have reported the postoperative thromboses according to clinical aspects. In this study of 106 pregnant women it was attempted to record the thrombosis rate prospectively by means of impedance plethysmography. A general thrombosis prophylaxis with 3 × 500 ml 10% Haes 200/0.5 was carried out. The clinical results are summarized in Tables 15 and 16.

**Table 15.** Course of hemorheologic and several coagulation parameters until the 10th postoperative day under perioperative thrombosis phrophylaxis with 10% Haes 200/0.5

| Parameter | 0 days | 5 days | 10 days |
|---|---|---|---|
| Hematocrit (%) | 32.8±4.2 | 31.0±4.0 | 35.4±4.0 |
| Plasma viscosity (mPas) | 1.33±0.1 | 1.35±0.1 | 1.37±0.1 |
| Erythrocyte aggregation (–) | 24.9±6.5 | 23.0±6.8 | 20.2±6.9 |
| Antithrombin III (AT III; IU/ml) | 11.8±2.1 | 13.1±1.6 | 13.2±1.8 |
| Factor VIII R: Ag (%) | 163 ±70 | 159 ±55 | 138 ±96 |

**Table 16.** Preoperative risk factors of three patients with postoperative deep leg phlebothrombosis

| Preoperative risk factors | Number (percentage) |
|---|---|
| Anamnestic risk factors | 1/3 ( 33.3%) |
| Maternal diseases | 2/3 ( 66.6%) |
| AT III < 8 (IU/ml) | 2/3 ( 66.6%) |
| Plasma viscosity > 1.30 (mPas) | 3/3 (100 %) |
| Erythrocyte aggregation > 28 (–) | 2/3 ( 66.6%) |

A proximal deep leg phlebothrombosis was diagnosed in three patients (2.8%). The following preoperative risk factors were found in these three patients, with an average age of 27.8 years and a body weight between 83 and 103 kg.

Changes in blood fluidity are important as additional risk factors in gravidity-related postoperative thrombosis morbidity. Due to the frequency rates the patients with cesarian section must be included in a low-risk group. For this operation hydroxyethyl starch serves as an alternative means for thrombosis prophylaxis since – besides improving the venous circulation – it can also reduce erythrocyte aggregation. The reduction in the activity of the coagulation factor VIII R:AG after the period of hemodilution indicates that hydroxyethyl starch apparently also has a small influence on thrombocyte aggregation. Thus, two features of Virchow's triad are positively influenced by hemodilution.

### *2.4.7 Summary of Therapy Recommendations*

#### 2.4.7.1 Hemodilution in Suspected Placental Insufficiency

A systemic hematocrit value above 38% is a criterion for exclusion. Over a period of 2 weeks 500 ml 10% Haes 200/0.5 and 500 ml electrolyte solution should be infused per day within at least 4 h. If systemic hematocrit exceeds 38% after 2 weeks, a repeated dilution should be carried out.

> The hemodilution must always be hypervolemic since maternal hypovolemia occurs in the case of placental insufficiency.

#### 2.4.7.2 Hemodilution in Pregnancy-Related Hypertension

Besides the basic therapy with hydralazine (3 ml/h) and magnesium sulfate (1 g/h) 500 ml 10% Haes 200/0.5 should always be infused together with 500 ml Ringer solution.

> The vasodilation by hydralazine causes an increase in hypovolemia. Therefore, Ringer solution should be given in addition to the administration of 10% Haes 200/05.

#### 2.4.7.3 Hemodilution as Thrombosis Prophylaxis in Cesarian Section

During the preparation of the anesthesia 500 ml 10% Haes 200/0.5 is infused. The infusion should be finished at the end of the operation. On the evening of the operation day 500 ml 10% Haes 200/0.5 must be given again. The third and final infusion of 500 ml 10% Haes 200/0.5 is carried out on the evening of the first postoperative day (end of thrombosis prophylaxis). If the patients are insufficiently mobilized after the 7th postoperative day this scheme must be repeated.

> The administration of 10% Haes 200/0.5 allows an effective perioperative thrombosis prophylaxis in cesarian sections.

## *2.5 Hemodilution in Venous Circulatory Disturbances of the Retina*

S. WOLF, B. BERTRAM, and M. REIM

The continuing lack of understanding in regard to the pathophysiologic processes during central vein thrombosis of the retina may explain why there is no established therapy. Although after diabetic retinopathy retinal phlebemphraxis is the most frequent cause of circulatory disturbances of the retina, little has changed concerning the prognosis of this disease with regard to the central visual acuity since its discovery.in Venous Circulatory Disturbances

Therapie with anticoagulants, thrombocyte aggregation inhibitors, and vasodilators was discontinued due to unsatisfying results. The efficacy of fibrinolytic therapy by an increase in central visual acuity was demonstrated by Metzler and collaborators [260]. In this case it has not been accepted to this day because of the multitude of contraindications and the danger of severe side effects. The therapeutic attempt to improve the microcirculation is by hyper- or isovolemic hemodilution in combination with the administration of rheologic drugs [396, 399].

To assess this therapy a randomized controlled study was performed in 40 patients with central vein thromboses of the retina (Fig. 27). The frequency of ischemic ($n$=7, hemodilution group; $n$=7, control group) or nonischemic ($n$=12, hemodilution group; $n$=14, control group) central vein thromboses was

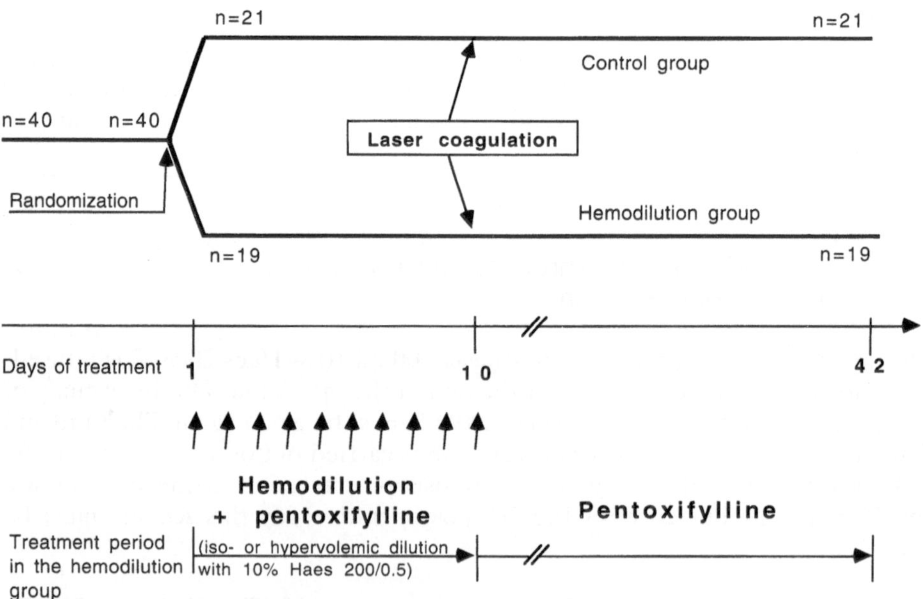


**Fig. 27.** Study design: hemodilution with 10% Haes 200/0.5 in patients with retinal vein thromboses

comparable in the two groups; with respect to cardiovascular risk factors, angiographic values, and measured laboratory parameters the groups were also homogeneous.

Figure 28 shows the correlation of the visual values before and after 6 weeks of therapy. Points above the diagonal indicate an improvement in vision during the observation period, points below the diagonal a deterioration of central visual acuity.

After 10 days there was a significant decrease in arteriovenous passage time (active substance group, $p<0.05$) in comparison to the initial values (Fig. 29).

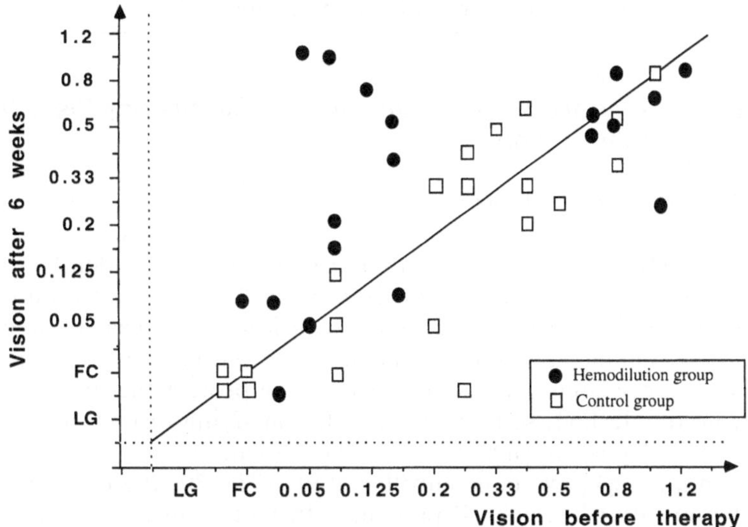


**Fig. 28.** Development of vision within 6 weeks. *Points* above the *diagonal line* represent improved vision; *points* below, deteriorated vision. *FC*, Visual acuity to count fingers; *LG*, visual acuity to perceive gleam of light

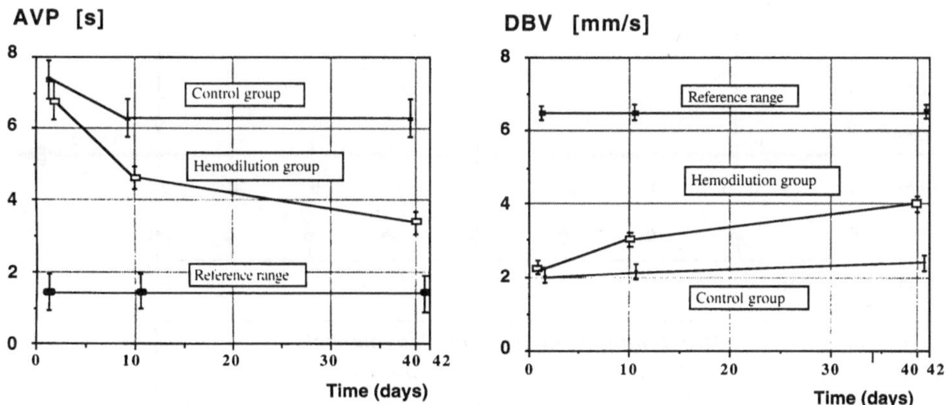


**Fig. 29.** Mean arteriovenous passage time (*AVP*) and mean arterial dye bolus velocity (*DBV*) of the hemodilution and control groups over 6 weeks (X±SEM) with reference ranges

Further, during the time course AVP continued to decrease significantly in the active substance group but not in the control group. The arteriovenous passage times in the active substance group were smaller than in the control group during and after the therapy ($p<0.01$ each).

After 10 days and after 6 weeks the arterial dye bolus velocity of the groups differed significantly ($p<0.01$). In the active substance groups this was higher than in the control group during and after the therapy (Fig. 29).

> In addition to the effectiveness of laser coagulation, hemodilution in combination with pentoxifylline is of clinical benefit in patients suffering from central vein thrombosis of the retina.

### *2.5.1 Hemodilution in Acute Arterial Circulatory Disturbances of the Retina*

S. Wolf and M. Reim

Obstruction of the central retinal artery causes a sudden loss in visual ability. Concerning prognosis it is decisive whether there is a total obstruction or a high-grade stenosis with residual perfusion. In the case of an obstruction with total ischemia irreparable damage to the retina occurs as early as 15–30 min. However, a small residual perfusion may protect the nerve cells of the retina from the decline, so that functionally satisfying results can be achieved in the case of a quick recanalization of the obstruction.

In a prospective noncontrolled study (Fig. 30) the efficacy of hemodilution therapy was assessed in 40 patients with acute central arterial occlusions ($n=20$) or arterial branch occlusions ($n=20$) in the retina [397]. The parameters

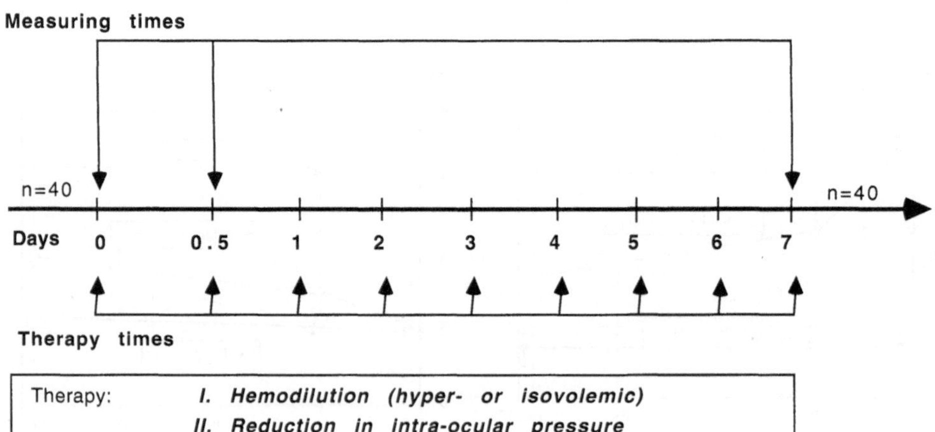


**Fig. 30.** Study design: hemodilution with 10% Haes 200/0.5 in patients with acute central artery or arterial branch occlusions of the retina

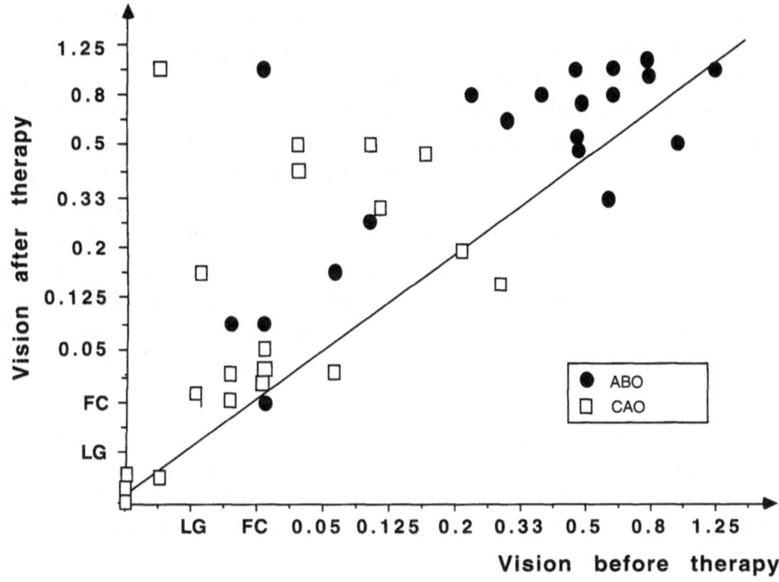


**Fig. 31.** Difference in visual acuity before therapy and after 42 days depending on the latency period until therapy initiation in patients with central arterial occlusions (*CAO*) or arterial branch occlusions (*ABO*) *FC*, Visual acuity to count fingers; *LG*, visual acuity to perceive gleam of light

measured were: vision, visual field; video-fluorescein angiographic values; blood flow parameters HcT, PV, SEA, and SER.

Figure 31 presents the visual acuity of patients with central arterial occlusions and arterial branch occlusions before and after 6 weeks of therapy. The points above the diagonal line indicate an improvement in vision during the course of therapy. The patients ($n$=4) in whom therapy was started a few hours after occurrence achieved an increase in vision of more than three levels. This improvement was achieved during the first 24 h after the initiation of therapy; afterwards it changed only insignificantly. At a later initiation of therapy the increases in vision were smaller and were achieved only if a residual perfusion was confirmed by video-angiography. Deteriorations of more than one visual level with regard to the initial findings were not observed.

In patients with arterial branch occlusions the increase in vision was higher. Under the conditions of a residual perfusion or at least a retrograde supply situation, the patients with a longer latency period did not show a worse course than patients with an early initiation of therapy. This was confirmed by video-angiography in five cases.

The initial values for arm-retina time (ART), arteriovenous passage time (AVP), and dye bolus velocity (DBV) were significantly worse with respect to normal values. In the course of the disease ART, AVP, and DBV improved significantly. The improvements were significant ($p<0.01$) compared to initial values. Even after 6 weeks a significant increase ($p<0.05$) was observed compared to the values after 10 days.

Initially, significantly prolonged circulation times in the supply area of the arterial branches concerned were found in patients with arterial branch occlusion compared to the areas which were not affected. In comparison to the normal values the blood flow parameters of both areas were disturbed ($p<0.01$). During the course of the disease the circulation times improved. Six weeks after the occurrence of the occlusion the AVP value did not differ significantly from normal; the DBV value continued to be significantly decreased.

In none of the patients examined was a reocclusion of the retinal arteries observed clinically or angiographically. Since hemodilution should begin as soon and as hypervolemically as possible after the occurrence of the occlusion, the therapy schedule (Fig. 30) was changed in such a way that the infusion quantities were increased in the beginning and reduced later (see Sect. 4.6).

> Concerning the prognosis of retinal artery occlusions it is decisive to improve hemodynamics as soon as possible after occurrence of the occlusion in order to prevent the retina from suffering irreversible damage. This is achieved by hypervolemic hemodilution through an increase in microcirculation.

## 2.6 Hemodilution in Idiopathic Sudden Hearing Loss

H.-J. Wilhelm and R. Hubertus

To evaluate the possible prognostic significance of several possible factors an epidemiologic study in 312 patients with idiopathic sudden hearing loss was begun in 1983 [392].

All patients received hemodilution treatment with hydroxyethyl starch (Haes-steril 10%; Fresenius) or dextran 40 10% 1000 ml for at least 10 days in combination with naftidrofuryl (per infusion 400 mg Dusodril PI plus 600 mg/day orally; Lipha). The treatment was performed hypervolemically up to a hematocrit of 47%; in cases of higher hematocrit a simultaneous phlebotomy of 500 ml whole blood was carried out.

Included in the study were 155 men and 157 women, with an average age of 48 years. Of these, 88 had a recurrent sudden hearing loss and 40 a vestibular involvement. Mean blood pressure was 140/80 mmHG. On average the therapy was begun after 16 days. In 38% there were increased serum lipid concentrations, 23% hypertension, and 11% abnormal fasting blood-sugar concentration; 29% were obese, and 28% were smokers.

### 2.6.1 Results

Of the 312 patients, 119 showed no improvement, and 193 had a mean increase in hearing of at least 6 dB (improvement rate about 62%) after 10 days of treatment. Age, sex, adiposity, smoking, and alcohol did not have a significant influence on the success of therapy.

In the group with an increase in hearing, 20% showed a recurrent sudden hearing loss, but in the group without increase 35%. Therefore, the evidence of a recurrent sudden hearing loss reduces therapy success significantly ($p<0.05$) and is an important predictor.

Forty patients showed a vestibular involvement; 19 of these had an increase in hearing while the remaining 21 patients showed no increase.

Early treatment of sudden loss of hearing is an important factor for increasing hearing; this has been demonstrated in numerous studies. This was also the case in the study presented here. The group of patients with increased hearing was treated after 7.7±12.4 days and the group without increase only after 30.1±73.3 days. This difference is highly significant ($p<0.002$; Fig. 32).

Blood fluidity was worsened in about 60% of patients with sudden hearing loss. Especially plasma viscosity was frequently increased (51%). Mean plasma viscosity in the patients with an increase in hearing after the infusion therapy was significantly higher (1.31 mPas; $p<0.05$) than that of the patients without increase in hearing (1.28 mPas). The infusion therapy with Haes 200/0.5 10% and naftidrofuryl (Dusodril) led to significantly higher increases in hearing in the group with arterial hypertension ($p<0.01$).

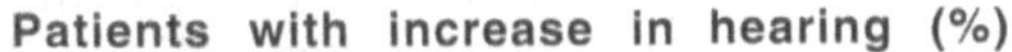

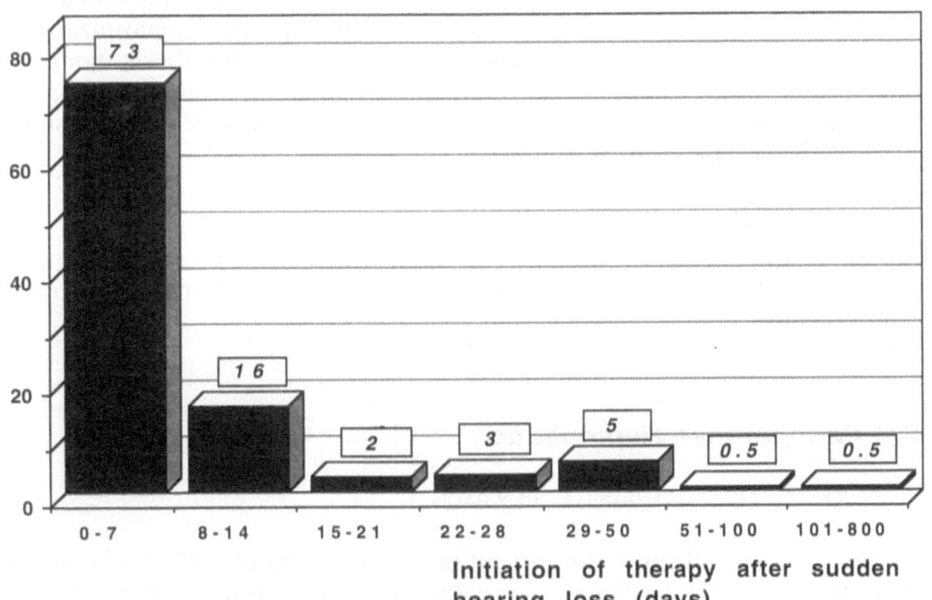


**Fig. 32.** Relative percentage of patients with increase in hearing in terms of the time of initiating therapy

### 2.6.2 Conclusions

Vasospasms in the area of the anterior arteries and arterioles or changes in the capillary system of the internal ear can reduce the perfusion pressure to such an extent that blood fluidity becomes a limiting factor. The clinically relevant parameters are plasma viscosity and erythrocyte aggregation. A rise in both parameters above 1 (>1.29 mPas) increases the risk of arterial occlusion by a factor of 2 [191]. Furthermore, plasma viscosity seems to be of prognostic importance; if it is above 1.29 mPas, the success of rheologic therapy is more probable. In these cases the etiology of sudden hearing loss also seems to have a hemorheologic component since these patients generally show a restricted plasma volume. These findings are confirmed by examinations in patients with retinal occlusions [397, 398]. Moreover, treatment with hydroxyethyl starch and naftidrofuryl to increase the microcirculation leads to a significantly better results than the use of dextran, especially in hypertensive patients with microangiopathies. Dextran increases the perfusion pressure but causes disturbances in the blood volume by increasing plasma viscosity and erythrocyte aggregation [392]. On the administration of 1 kg hydroxyethyl starch without an additional infusion of fluid (e.g., crystalloid solution) more than 50% of patients presented pruritus; this was often only transitory and hardly disturbing. Because of the frequent pruritus a different hemodilution scheme with less hydroxyethyl starch is now being evaluated (see Sect. 4.6). A previously damaged vascular circulation in the case of a recurrent sudden hearing loss diminishes and a quick initiation of therapy increases the success rate of therapy. Total heparinization in patients with the strong suspicion of otogenic venous thrombosis (condition after passed venous thromboses – retina, extremities, portal vein, etc. – or recurrent phlebothromboses) must be taken into account. Even systemic fibrinolysis therapy could be discussed.

In the case of an early initiation of hemodilution, high plasma viscosity, and arterial hypertension the prognosis of therapy with hydroxyethyl starch and naftidrofuryl is promising. The prognosis of a recurrent sudden hearing loss is always worse.

## 2.7 Perioperative Hemodilution

J. Simon, T. Tormann, and T. Holbach

In the case of small surgical interventions without considerable blood loss an infusion of crystalloid solutions is usually carried out. However, the volume as well as the rheologic effect of the electrolyte solutions is restricted [341].

From the studies of Rudofsky it is known that even small surgical interventions can cause considerable changes in the fluidity of blood [311]. For this reason, the choice of a rheologically effective colloidal plasma substitute improves the probability of a better perioperative supply of the tissue.

### 2.7.1 Patients

Patients who were to undergo micro-intervertebral disk operation were examined. After randomization 13 men and 7 women with an average age of 52 years were in the Haes group, 12 men und 8 women with an average age of 48 years in the dextran group, and 10 men and 10 women with an average age of 47 years in the electrolyte group.

### 2.7.2 Hypervolemic Single Dilution

In a controlled, randomized, single-blind, clinical comparative study the effect was examined of the infusion solution on the intraoperative oxygen supply (by measuring the conjunctival oxygen partial pressure) and blood fluidity (by measuring the rheologic parameters such as hematocrit, plasma viscosity, erythrocyte aggregation, erythrocyte rigidity, and thrombocyte aggregation). One group received an electrolyte solution (Elomel), the second group dextran 40 10% (Rheomacrodex), and the last group 10% Haes 200/0.5 (Haes-steril 10%).

Measurement of the conjunctival oxygen partial pressure was started after initiation of the anesthesia but before the infusion. Before and 1, 2, 4, 6, and 24 h after the operation the rheologic parameters were quantified (Fig. 33). A detailed record of the study can be taken from the original work [341].

At the beginning of the operation the mean oxygen partial pressure was equal in all three groups (about 64 mmHg). Immediately after the initiation of the

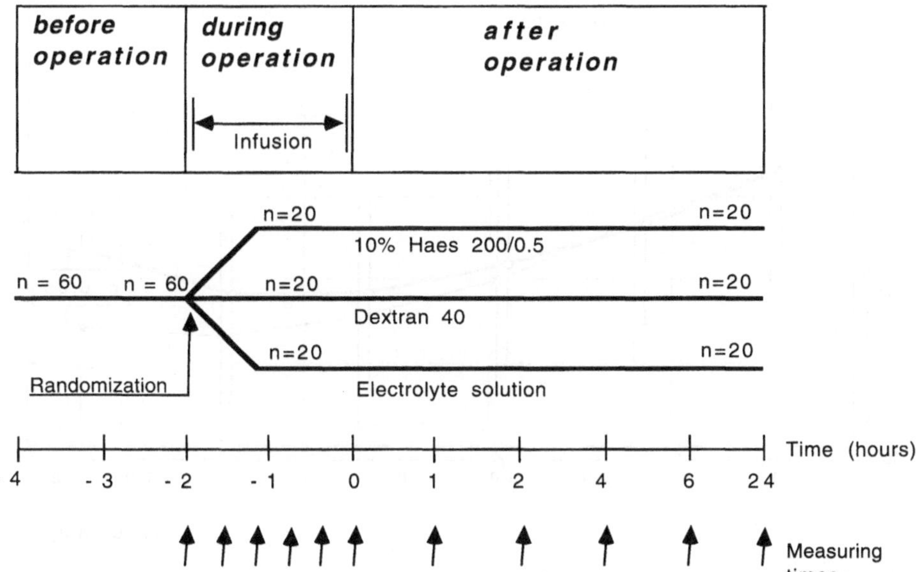


**Fig. 33.** Study design: perioperative hemodilution

infusion the oxygen partial pressure started to drop in all three groups although the blood flow parameters (blood pressure and heart rate) remained constant. In the three groups the minimum was achieved at different times, but first in the Haes group. The oxygen partial pressure then increased significantly ($p<0.05$) in this group. The drop in oxygen pressure was more distinct in the dextran and electrolyte groups. The time courses of oxygen pressure are almost identical for the electrolyte and dextran solutions (Fig. 34).

Figure 34 compares the course of the two colloidal infusion solutions. A slight reincrease in the oxygen partial pressure is also recognizable in the dextran

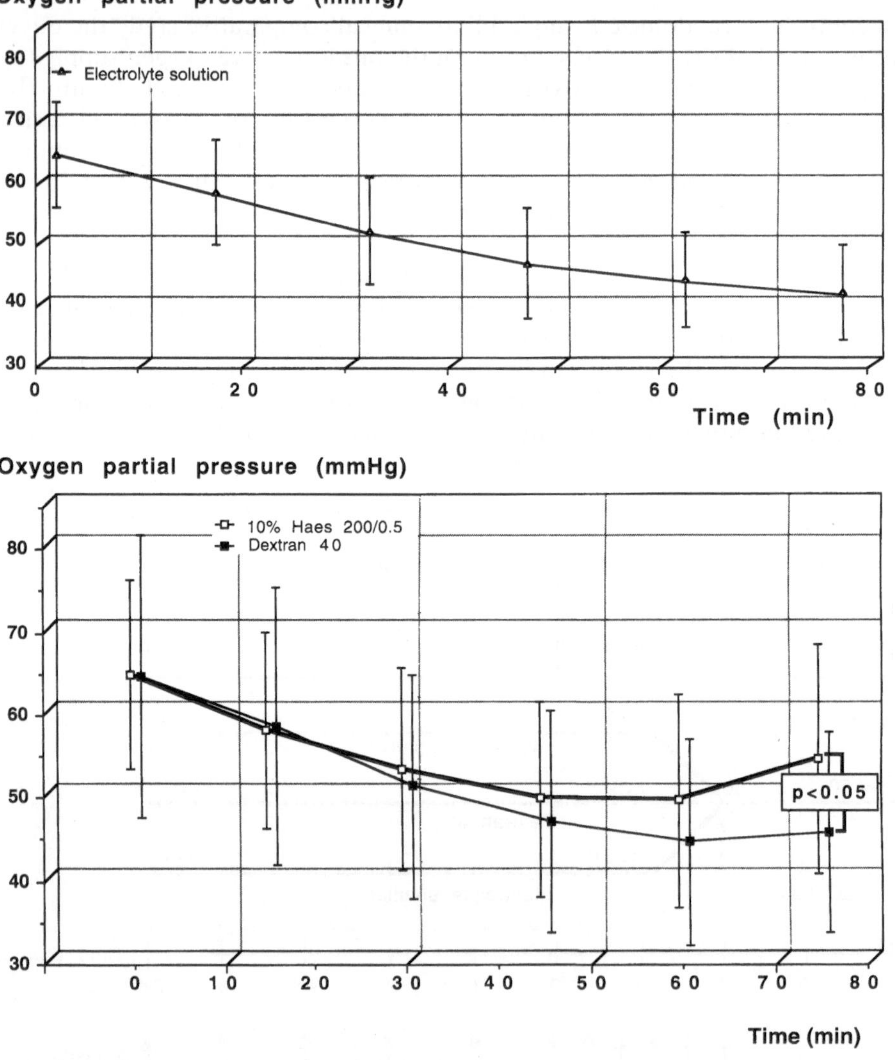


**Fig. 34.** Intraoperative course of conjunctival oxygen partial pressure in the electrolyte, Haes, and dextran groups ($p$: significance level for the group comparison)

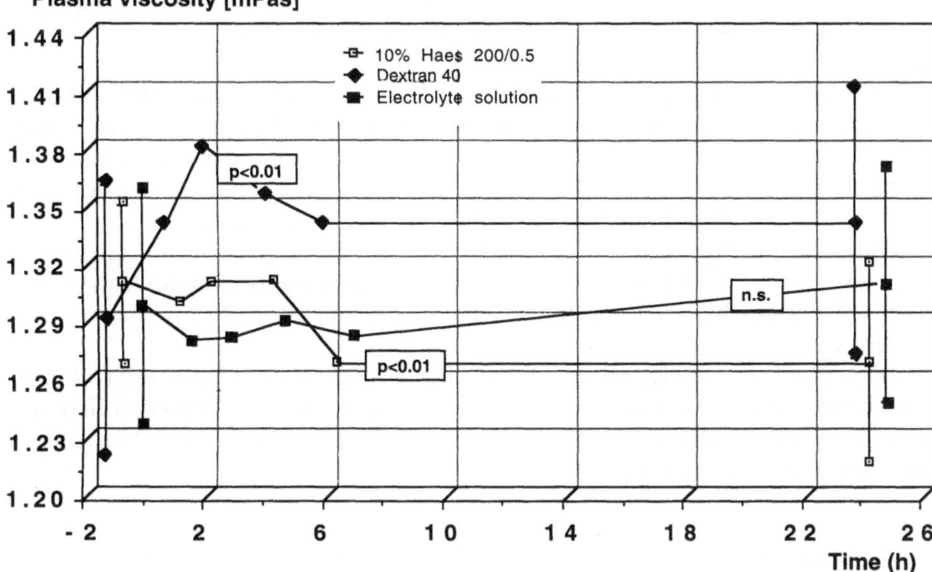


**Fig. 35.** Course of plasma viscosity for 24 h in the three groups (*p*: significance level in time-series comparison – initial value to later value; limits of 1 SD, same symbols as the corresponding mean measuring points)

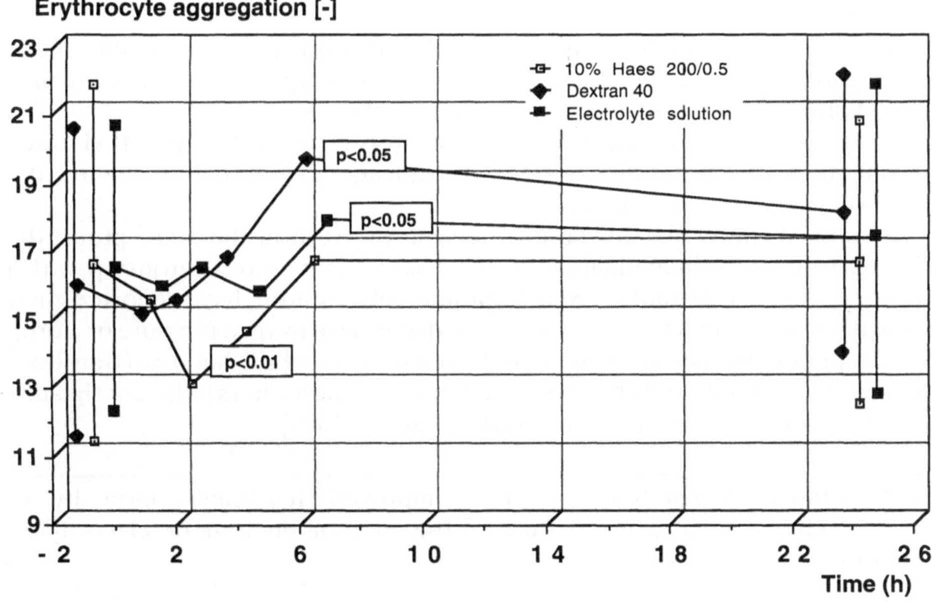


**Fig. 36.** Course of erythrocyte aggregation in the three groups for 24 h (*p*: significance level in time-series comparison – initial value to later value; limits of 1 SD, same symbols as the corresponding mean measuring points)

group. But this was considerably less pronounced than in the Haes group. The Haes and dextran groups differed significantly until the final measuring time.

The highest volume effect was found in the dextran group. The minimal hematocrit was achieved 2 h after the operation; the difference to the initial hematocrit was 13.6%. A significant reduction in hematocrit was also found in the Haes group, but it was less pronounced (11%) than in the dextran group. The electrolyte solution did not influence the systemic hematocrit.

While plasma viscosity remained constant in the electrolyte group, it decreased in the Haes group later up to 24 h, and increased in the dextran group. Figure 35 shows the postoperative course of plasma viscosity for the infusion solutions.

The erythrocyte aggregation increased postoperatively in the dextran and electrolyte groups (here significantly); in the Haes group it decreased at first and then increased slightly. The initial values in the dextran and electrolyte groups were not achieved again (Fig. 36).

### 2.7.3 Conclusions

Although blood pressure and heart rate remained constant during the operation, conjunctival oxygen partial pressure reacted differently depending on the plasma substitute used. With both colloidal solutions an increase in the oxygen pressure occurred after 1 h of the operation. After the administration of the electrolyte solution the conjunctival oxygen partial pressure decreased until the end of the operation.

The increase after administration of the plasma substitute was probably due to the hemodynamic effect. Increases in cardiac output after hypervolemic hemodilution have been observed in several other studies [67, 158, 258]. The greater reincrease in conjunctival oxygen partial pressure by hydroxyethyl starch – compared to the administration of dextran – is probably due to the improvement in blood volume.

Because of the earlier increase in oxygen pressure in the Haes group the minimal value in the individual case was not as low as in the dextran group, with a decrease of up to 30 mmHg. Weisskopf and collaborators have reported their casuistic experience; if there is an extreme decrease in oxygen pressure or a drop in certain conjunctival oxygen partial pressures, cerebral failures (transitory unilateral symptoms) must be expected. However, the authors point out that this observation must be confirmed in further studies [390].

> Perioperative oxygen tissue supply is improved significantly more by a hydroxyethyl starch infusion than by the use of dextran or electrolyte solutions.

# 3. Hemodilution in Cerebral Circulatory Disturbances: Indications, Implementation, Additional Drug Treatment, and Alternatives

A. Haass, M. Stoll, and J. Treib

Disturbances of the cerebral circulation are the third most frequent cause of death [349]. The largest group of these are ischemic strokes followed by intracerebral hemorrhage, subarachnoid hemorrhage, sinus venous thrombosis, and other cerebrovascular lesions (Table 17). Ischemic strokes have a high incidence of 150/100 000 and an estimated prevalence of 600/100 000. They present a challenge to prevention, acute treatment, and rehabilitation; however, compared with the management of myocardial infarction they have received relatively limited attention.

## 3.1 Classification of Ischemic Strokes

### 3.1.1 Aetiological Classification of Ischemic Strokes

From a pathological point of view strokes can be classified into macro- and microcirculatory disturbances.

The causes of *macrocirculatory disturbances* are embolism, thrombosis, and hemodynamically significant stenosis (Table 18). According to a survey of five cerebral stroke registers, about 21% of all ischemic strokes are due to embolism [252, 253]. The lowest frequency was 8%, and the highest frequency was 31%. Embolisms may arise from the heart, large vessels or be due to particular causes such as cholesterol crystal embolism. According to the findings of six studies, about 14% of all ischemic strokes result from cardiac embolism, with a range of 6% and 23% [39, 101].

There are various causes, such as an atrial embolus in the case of absolute arrhythmia and atrial fibrillation, cerebral infarction in the case of myocardial infarction, and rare paradoxic emboli in the case of leg or pelvic phlebothrombosis with patent foramen ovale. Thrombosis of the cerebral arteries are

**Table 17.** Frequency of the most important cerebral circulatory disturbances

| | |
|---|---|
| Ischemic stroke | 62% |
| Intracerebral hemorrhage | 16% |
| Subarachnoid hemorrhage | 12% |
| Sinus venous thrombosis | 5% |
| Miscellaneous lesions of the cerebral vessels | 5% |

**Table 18.** Causes of ischemic strokes

---

*Cardiac embolism*

Atrial fibrillation
Other cardiac dysrhythmias
Valvular disease, prosthetic heart valves
Myocardial infarction
Myocardial aneurysm
Cardiomyopathy
Endocarditis
Patent foramen ovale with paradoxic emboli
Atrial myxoma

*Arterio-arterial embolism*

Atherosclerosis of the large vessels with plaques and stenoses
Dissection or trauma of the large vessels
Fibromuscular dysplasia
Aneurysms of the large cerebral arteries
Fat, air, cholesterol crystal embolism

*Thrombosis of cerebral arteries*

Atherosclerosis of the large intracranial cerebral arteries
Dissection or trauma of the large vessels
Compression or aneurysm of the large vessels
Arteritis
- Syphilitic (Lues)
- Lyme disease
- Drug abuse
- Arteritis of different aetiology including systemic diseases

*Hemodynamic cerebral infarctions*

High-grade stenosis of the large vessels with drop in blood pressure or cardiac output
Cardiac arrest, asphyxiation

*Microcirculatory disturbances*

Arteriolosclerosis with lacunar strokes
Subcortical arteriosclerotic encephalopathy (SAE)

*Hemorheological and hemostasological causes*

Polycythemia, haemoconcentration
Sickle cell anemia
Smoking and contraceptives
Migraine
Hyperviscosity (dysproteinemia, SAE)
Thrombocytosis
Coagulopathies in cases of neoplasms, leukemia, X-ray therapy, and other causes

---

the most frequent cause of acute ischemic strokes, and atherosclerosis is the most important aetiology. Hemodynamic infarctions due to a high-grade stenosis of the large cerebral arteries are uncommon; these are called watershed infarcts or terminal zone infarction. A different infarction pattern arises after circulatory interruptions during cardiac arrest or asphyxia.

*Microcirculatory disturbances* are the second most frequent cause. These consist mainly of lacunar strokes and often result from hypertension-induced arteriolosclerosis. Subcortical arteriosclerotic encephalopathy (SAE) is rarer, with interesting disturbances of autoregulation and hemorheology (Sect. 3.2.2). Various hemorheological causes, such as haemoconcentration or dysproteinaemia, and hemostasological ones, such as coagulopathies in the case of neoplasm, leukemia, X-ray therapy, or other causes, can lead to infarctions. The increased risk of cerebral infarction due to the use of oral contraceptives and simultaneous smoking or migraine with intracerebral vasospasm is based on the same mechanisms.

### *3.1.2 Classification of Stroke by Clinical Stage and Duration of Neurologic Deficit*

This common classification must be regarded as inadequate especially due to the lack of understanding regarding the pathophysiological basis (Table 19) because it considers only the duration of the neurologic deficit. As Caplan [37] has pointed out, this classification says nothing about prognosis, treatment, or prevention, and therefore cannot constitute the only classification in studies investigating cerebral infarction.

### *3.1.3 Pathophysiological Classification of Acute Ischemic Strokes*

The clinical classification of strokes according to pathophysiological criteria can be difficult. Naturally, the occurrence of infarctions in different brain areas indicates an embolism, but this could also be the expression of repeated lacunar strokes. The frequent occurrence of atrial fibrillation also does not confirm cerebral embolism. Only the nature and extent of the clinical picture

**Table 19.** Classification of ischemic cerebral strokes by clinical stage and duration of neurologic deficit

| | |
|---|---|
| Ia | Transient ischemic attack (TIA): reversal of the neurologic deficit within 24 h |
| Ib | Reversible ischemic neurologic deficit (RIND): reversal within 3 days |
| | Prolonged reversible ischemic neurologic deficit (PRIND): reversal within 7 days |
| II | Progressing stroke: fluctuating, slowly worsening clinical picture |
| III | Completed stroke: "minor stroke" (patient unfit for work, slight symptoms), "major stroke" (patient unfit for work and handicapped) |

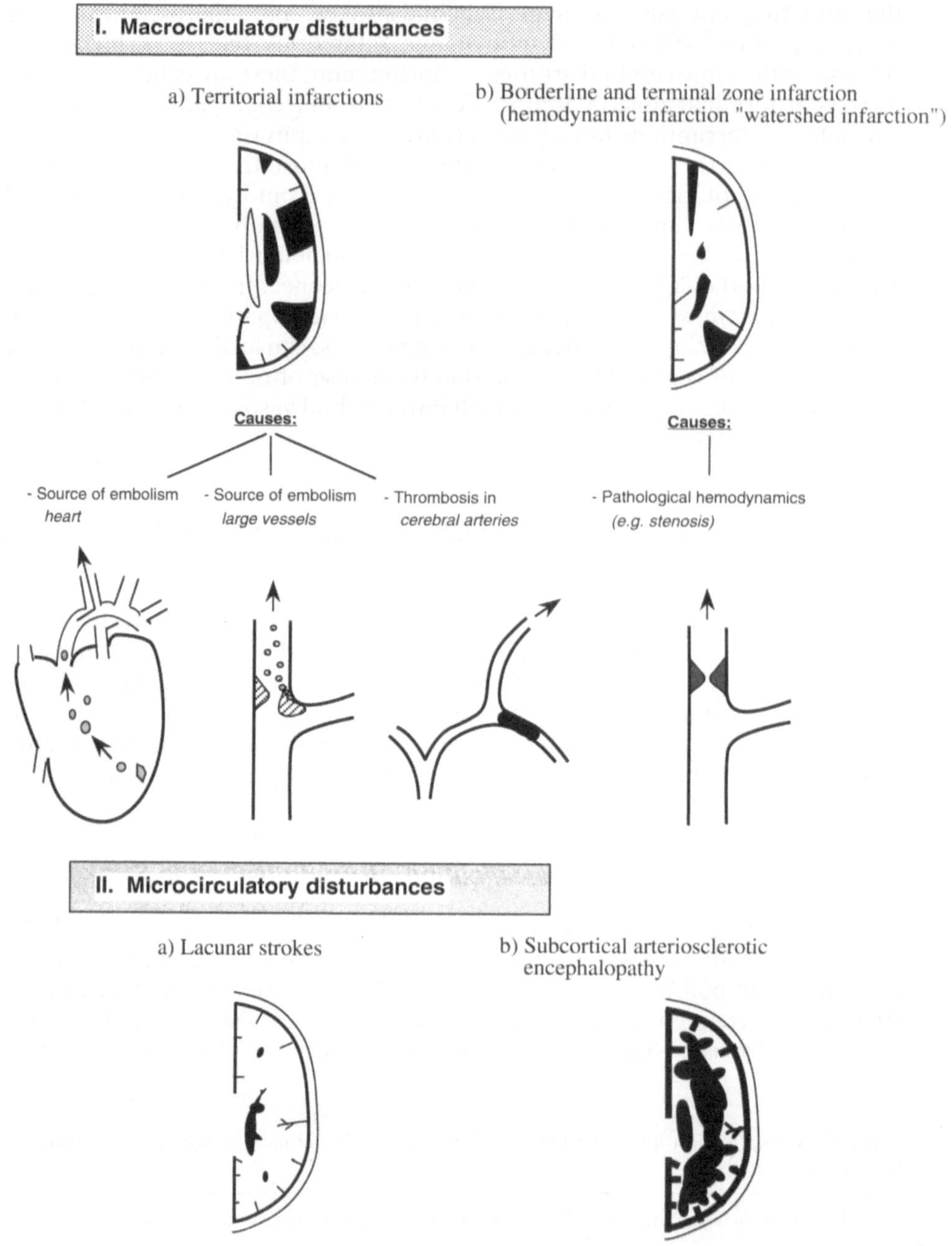

**I. Macrocirculatory disturbances**

a) Territorial infarctions

b) Borderline and terminal zone infarction (hemodynamic infarction "watershed infarction")

Causes:

- Source of embolism *heart*
- Source of embolism *large vessels*
- Thrombosis in *cerebral arteries*

Causes:

- Pathological hemodynamics *(e.g. stenosis)*

**II. Microcirculatory disturbances**

a) Lacunar strokes

b) Subcortical arteriosclerotic encephalopathy

**Fig. 37.** Pathophysiological classification of acute ischemic strokes. (Modified from [307, 309])

allows a partial differentiation between macro- and microangiopathic pathology and symptomatology, and there is an unmistakable overlap due to the fact that two-thirds of all patients with lacunes also suffer from arteriosclerosis of the large vessels [65, 106]. A decisive help are examinations by computed tomography and magnetic resonance tomography (Fig. 37) [307, 309].

*Macrocirculatory disturbances* consist of territorial infarcts which can be provoked by embolism or thrombosis or by hemodynamically produced watershed or terminal infarcts. Territorial infarcts affect a more or less large area supplied by leptomeningeal vessels, an embolus lodged peripherally in one of these vessels often results in rhomboid or cuneiform areas of infarction which include the cortical area in a characteristic way.

Lacunar infarcts in the basal ganglia and thalamic area may on CT scan resemble subcortical territorial infarcts in the lentiform nucleus and thalamus and thus be difficult to distinguish one from the other.

Hemodynamic infarcts occur in only 15% of cases. This includes watershed infarcts between the areas of supply of two or more cerebral arteries and terminal infarcts in the distribution of long, penetrating arteries of the central white matter. The latter, which are infarctions of functional end-arteries, are difficult to differentiate from lacunar infarcts in the individual case.

*Microcirculatory disturbances* are the cause of cerebral infarctions in 11%–23% of cases according to cerebral stroke registers and in 34% according to findings by CT scan [252, 253, 309]. These lacunes are about 1–20 mm in size and result from occlusion of long penetrating arteries. The

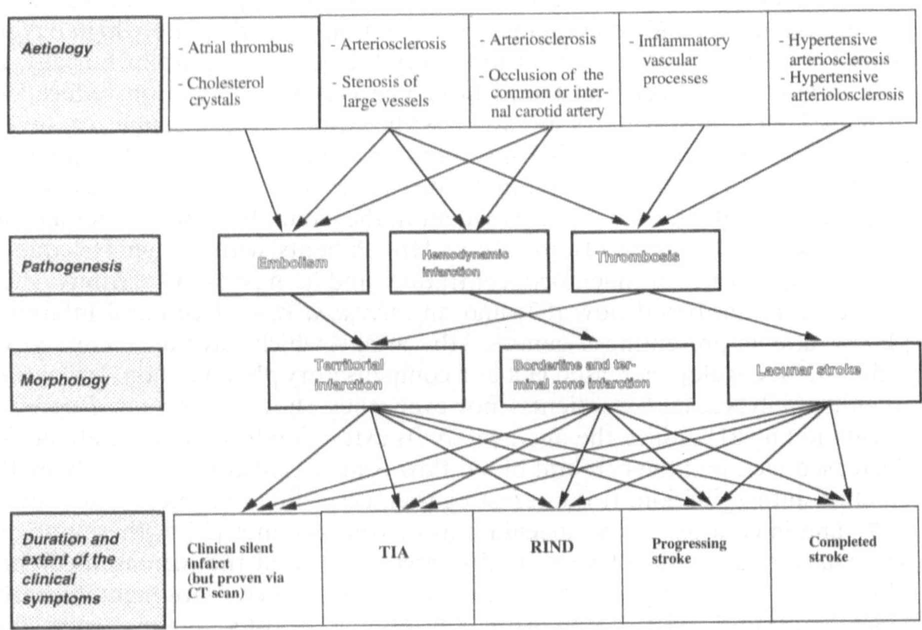


**Fig. 38.** Relationship between aetiology, pathogenesis, morphology, and clinical course of ischemic strokes

vessels concerned are the lenticulostriata, thalamoperstriate, long penetrating arteriols of the central grey and white matter, and the brain stem arteries. These are especially long, small vessels, often taking disadvantageous right-angle courses with regard to circulatory dynamics. The causes especially lipohyalinosis and fibrinoid necrosis of the small arteries and arterioles are often the result of hypertension. Small, circumscribed motor or sensory functional disturbances are typical of these infarctions. A special case is SAE, which is accompanied by an arterio- and arteriolosclerosis.

Mixed forms are seen in 10% and diffuse hypoxic lesions in 1% of cases.

Figure 38 presents the relationship between aetiology, pathogenesis, morphology, and time course.

## 3.2 Hemorheological Risk Factors as a Basis for Hemodilution

### 3.2.1 Haematocrit

#### 3.2.1.1 Clinical Studies

Time after time in daily practice it is clear how increased hematocrit (Hct) and decreased volume of the intravascular and extracellular space (e.g., in elderly patients with dehydration) can lead to acute cerebral circulatory disturbances and cause focal-neurologic deficit or general symptoms such as disturbances of consciousness and behaviour. As a rule the symptoms recede quickly after having restoration of the blood volume. Marschall [249] pointed out that in the prevention of TIA and cerebral infarctions not only an adequately high oxygen transport capacity in the form of many erythrocytes is important but also an appropriately rapid cerebral blood flow. The cerebral circulation reduced by increased Hct causes in combination with a poor hemodynamic or severe atherosclerosis an increased risk of cerebral infarction (Table 20). The relationship between Hct value and cerebral blood flow as well as its importance for the risk of a cerebral infarction is also evident in the example of polycythemia with and without a disturbed $O_2$ affinity of Hb. Patients with a high Hct due to polycythemia vera or haemoconcentration and a normal $O_2$-affinity show *reduced* cerebral blood flow [87] and an *increased risk* of cerebral infarction [288]. Patients presenting a genetic Hb variant, which have an increased $O_2$ affinity, also develop increased Hct as a compensatory phenomenon. In contrast to other polycythaemic patients, however, they show an *increased* cerebral circulation by 81% since the aggravated $O_2$ extraction has the same effect as a decreased Hct, and the cerebral blood flow is increased compensatorily by the cerebral autoregulation. It is interesting that, according to clinical observations [380] and in contrast to the speculations of von Kummer [223], these patients show *no increased risk* of a cerebral infarction, so that the increased cerebral blood flow apparently compensates the danger which is thought to result from increased Hct. Similarly, an increased blood flow can also be expected from treatment by hemodilution. It should be used in the prevention of ischemic strokes not only in patients with polycythemia but also in

**Table 20.** Haematocrit as a risk factor for ischemic stroke

| | |
|---|---|
| *Clinical studies* | |
| Pearson and Wetherly-Mein (1978) [288] | Polycythemia, haemoconcentration |
| Pearce et al. (1983) [287] | Lacunes in cases of polycythemia |
| Harrison et al. (1981) [116] | The higher the Hct the sooner the carotid occlusion |
| Nardini et al. (1983) [271] | Hct $\uparrow$ in cases of arteriosclerosis of the carotid |
| Lowe et al. (1983) [244] | Hct $\uparrow$ in cases of atrial fibrillation and cerebral infarction |
| Bogousslavsky and Regli (1986) [31] | Hct $\uparrow$ in cases of arteriosclerosis of the carotid and terminal zone infarctions |
| La Rue et al. (1987) [230] | Hct $\uparrow$ in cases of lacunes and hypertension |
| *Epidemiologic studies* | |
| Kannel et al. (1972) [166] | Hb $\geq$ 14% F; 15% M |
| Walker et al. (1981) [384] | Hct $\uparrow$ = 47.1%; Hct normal 27.6%; Hct $\downarrow$ = 28.3% |
| Böttiger and Carlson (1982) [30] | Hb $\uparrow$ M |
| Kiyohara et al. (1986) [199] | Hct $>$ 45% F; Hct $<$ 30% F<br>Hct $>$ 35%–45% M |
| Toghi et al. (1978) [367] | Stroke rate: Hct $<$ 30 = 6.6%<br>Hct 36%–40% = 18.3%; Hct 45%–50% = 43.6% |
| Harrison et al. (1982) [117] | Hct, hypertension, smoking-dependent and independent risk factors in case of TIA |
| *Stroke prognosis and Hct* | |
| Harrison et al. (1981) [116] | The higher the Hct, the greater the infarction (CT) |
| Sundt et al. (1967) [360] | The higher the Hct, the greater the infarction (CAT) |
| Pollock et al. (1982) [295] | The higher the Hct, the greater the infarction (monkeys) |
| Lowe et al. (1983) [244] | The higher the Hct on admission to hospital, the higher the infarction mortality |
| Kiyohara et al. (1985) [198] | Hct $<$ 35%; Hct $>$ 45% = lactate $\uparrow$ + ATP $\downarrow$; optimal Hct 40%; Hypertensive rats: autoregulation disturbed, more ischemic-sensitive |
| Sakai et al. (1989) [315] | According to SPECT, the higher the Hct in cases of TIA and RIND, the worse the clinical prognosis |

those with haemoconcentration of other aetiology. The Hct reduction depends on the primary disease, and drastic decreases must be avoided. Approximate values are to be derived from the treatment of polycythemia in which a Hct value of 45% or lower and a thrombocyte count below 400 $\times$ $10^9$/l is recommended [256, 288].

Wade et al. [379] demonstrated that the reduction in Hct from 54% to 44% by isovolemic hemodilution in these patients increases the cerebral $O_2$ supply by 8%. This is due to the increase in the cerebral blood flow, which compensates more than adequately the decrease in the $O_2$-transporting erythrocytes. The acute positive effect of such hemodilution treatment on brain function was confirmed by Willison et al. [393] by psychological examinations. After a Hct reduction (previously above 46%) in these patients the alertness and speed and accuracy of performance increased significantly.

Harrison et al. [116] and Nardini et al. [271] discovered an increased Hct in patients with TIA or RIND and carotid occlusion or carotid stenosis. In neither case was the Hct increase correlated with the degree of arteriosclerosis of the common or internal carotid artery. Therefore, the Hct increase was a risk factor independent of arteriosclerosis, which was perhaps alone responsible for the clinical manifestation of the vascular disease. This view is supported by the observation that a Hct of 50% or higher occurs more frequently in carotid occlusions. Lowe et al. [244] also discovered an increased Hct in patients with atrial fibrillation and cerebral infarction. Bogousslavski and Regli [31] found an increased Hct very frequently in patients who had suffered a watershed cerebral infarction due to a high-grade arteriosclerotic carotid stenosis. This was due mainly to abuse of smoking and chronic respiratory tract disease. On the one hand, these four studies show that increased Hct, as dependent but also as independent risk factor, can lead together with secondary diseases such as atrial fibrillation or arteriosclerosis of the major vessels to cerebral infarctions belonging to the group of microcirculatory disturbances. On the other hand, the pathologico-anatomical findings of Toghi et al. [176] and studies using computed tomography by Harrison et al. [117] and LaRue et al. [230] demonstrate that an increased Hct, as dependent and independent risk factor, together with hypertension or polycythemia also causes microcirculatory disturbances with lacunar infarcts.

### 3.2.1.2 Epidemiologic Studies

The prospective Framingham study showed that Hct is a weak risk factor. Highly pathologic Hct values together with hypertension and smoking represented an increased risk of cerebral infarction; in women with Hb values of 14% or higher and in men with Hb values of 15% the probability of suffering cerebral infarction was doubled [166]. Böttiger and Carlson [30] also found a generally increased risk of cerebral infarction in men with increased hemoglobin concentration. Similar findings have also been reported by Walker et al. [384], who found an infarction probability of 27.6% at a normal Hct, 47.1% at an increased Hct, and 28.3% at low Hct. Kiyohara et al. [199] also confirmed the danger of a Hct above 35%–45% in men and above 45% and below 30% in women. Although the two latter studies revealed a decreased Hct as risk factor, these are not "controversial" findings which disprove the risk of increased Hct, as was pointed out by Back and von Kummer [16]. These are rather two different kinds of risk, not mutually exclusive. No one would reject hypertension as a risk factor since low blood pressure values can also cause problems. The Hct level depends on various factors, and low Hct is not necessarily accompanied by a good prognosis [285] as regards cerebral infarction.

An increased Hct, especially in TIA patients, depends on hypertension and smoking and is an independent risk factor [117]. Furthermore, after pathologico-anatomical examinations the infarction rate increases by three or six times if Hct (in contrast to values below 30%) is increased to 36%–40% or 45%–50% [367]. It is interesting that high Hct values are often accompanied by small subcortical infarctions.

#### 3.2.1.3 Findings from Clinical and Animal Experiments Concerning Cerebral Infarction: Prognosis and Hematocrit

The negative influence of high Hct on the extent of an infarction have been demonstrated using CT scan [116]: the higher the Hct was on admission of the patient the greater the area of infarction. The correlation between these parameters meant that a patient with Hct of 46%–48% develops an area of infarction which is ten times greater than a patient with a value of 40%–42%. After two additional examinations the prognosis of patients with infarctions was worse, the higher the Hct value was. On the one hand, mortality increased with the Hct value [244]. On the other hand, after examinations of the ischemic area by single photon emission computed tomography (SPECT) the clinical prognosis of TIA and PRIND patients was more unfavourable the higher their Hct [315]. In standardized animal experiments the extent of infarction increased with the level of erythrocyte concentration [295, 359]. Important conclusions for hemodilution treatment can also be drawn from examination of the cerebral metabolism at different Hct values [198]. There is an optimal Hct (about 40%) which is dependent on factors such as cardiac output and the degree of arteriosclerosis. Any rise above or fall below the optimal Hct leads to a disturbance in the cerebral metabolism, which results in a decrease in ATP content and an increase in the lactate concentration (Sect. 3.1.4.1).

> Numerous clinical, epidemiological, and experimental studies reveal a Hct above a value within the upper normal range as a risk factor for ischemic strokes. In addition, the level of Hct is also decisive for the extent and prognosis of cerebral infarction.

This is not disproven by the EC-IC Bypass study [381] since it must be considered that all the patients in this study received acetylsalicylic acid (ASA) for prophylaxis of cerebral infarction. Thomas showed with the ASA and placebo groups of the United Kingdom TIA study that thrombocyte aggregation inhibition with ASA normalizes the increased risk of a cerebral infarction due to increased Hct [114].

The example of polycythemia patients reveals that hemodilution can improve the acute clinical condition of patients and decrease the risk of cerebral infarction. In agreement with Harrison [115], ASA can be administered alternatively for prophylaxis in the case of increased Hct.

> According to clinical, computer-tomographic and pathologico-anatomical examinations, the negative effect of increased Hct as a dependent and an independent risk factor superimposes itself on the primary disease. Thus, in the case of atrial fibrillation or arteriosclerosis of the large vessels (regardless of degree of severity) cerebral infarctions occur as typical for macrocirculatory disturbances, whereas in the case of polycythemia or simultaneously existing hypertension lacunar strokes result as an expression of microcirculatory disturbances.

### 3.2.2 Plasma Viscosity and Erythrocyte Aggregation

Plasma viscosity (PV) is influenced mainly by large molecules such as fibrinogen or alpha-2-macroglobulin. The importance of very large molecules is further increased by the fact that the increase in PV is not linear but exponential with the molecular weight of the substances. These large molecules also lead to erythrocyte aggregation (SEA) if they are able to overcome the physiological distance of 30 nm between the erythrocytes. The MW and the length of fibrinogen are, for example, 340 kDA and 47.5 nm, and of dextran 80 kDA and 53 nm. The PV, fibrinogen concentration, and SEA are closely related concerning their effects, and therefore they are discussed together in this study. An effect is observed especially in the microcirculation if shear stress is reduced [99, 100–101]. Moreover, the degree of PV is a limiting factor for the Fahraeus-Lindqvist effect when the blood viscosity falls to plasma viscosity values in order to facilitate the microcirculatory perfusion. Epidemiological studies such as the Framingham study [167] reveal fibrinogen as an important independent factor and as a risk factor for stroke dependent on Hct, hypertension, a pathological glucose tolerance test, smoking, and obesity. However, the risk of cerebral infarction in men is tripled if their fibrinogen concentration is 2.65–3.10 g/l instead of 1.26–2.64 g/l.

An impressive clinical proof of the importance of PV and fibrinogen concentration in strokes was ascertained in patients with SAE [308]. Due to arteriosclerosis and increased PV these patients suffered from such a severe cerebral circulatory disturbance that the cerebral vasomotor reserve was reduced by 25%, and the authors spoke about a "preischaemic state". The reduction in PV from 1.38 to 1.31 mPas by a reduced fibrinogen concentration from 3.26 to 1.52 g/l alone normalized the cerebral perfusion reserve and improved the microcirculation by 30%, as determined by the arteriovenous passage time of the retina. They were understandably called "striking improvements" by the authors. But this treatment did not lead to an acute improvement in cerebral capacity so that we cannot generally assume a chronic penumbra in the SAE patients. Furthermore, the number of fresh lacunar infarcts had not decreased after 6 months, but this could not be expected since the therapy lasted only one month and the effect receded immediately afterwards.

> The hemorheological factors PV, SEA, and their most important basis, the fibrinogen concentration, are clinically important for the prophylaxis and acute treatment of strokes according to epidemiological and functional examinations. The constant decrease in PV and fibrinogen concentration should reduce the risk of cerebral infarction and improve the circulation in the area of the microcirculation disturbance in the penumbra by the acute treatment.

## 3.3 Pathophysiological Basis of Circulatory Disturbances in Acute Ischemic Cerebral Infarctions

### 3.3.1 Cerebral Autoregulation

Hemodilution treatment in ischemic cerebral infarctions is based on the observation that haemoconcentration or polycythemia patients with increased Hct show reduced cerebral blood flow (CBF), and that patients with anaemia and decreased Hct show increased CBF (Fig. 39). This resolves the resulting question of whether the increase in cerebral blood flow is based primarily on vasodilation or a reduction in whole blood viscosity. Under normal circulatory conditions and a normal vasomotor reserve, that is to say, in the case of an intact cerebral autoregulation, vasodilation dominates at first. The data in Figure 39 show that cerebral autoregulation increases the CBF compensatorily by vasodilation if the Hct, the oxygen transport capacity and the cerebral oxygen supply are decreased. Since the increase in the CBF is proportionally more pronounced than the decrease in the oxygen transporting erythrocytes, a slightly increased $O_2$ supply results. When this so-called cerebral vasomotor reserve is exhausted, or the cerebral autoregulation, for example, in the penumbra of the cerebral infarction or in patients with SAE (Sect. 3.2.2) is disturbed, hemorheological factors are of increased importance.

The different conditions in cases of intact and disturbed cerebral autoregulation must be differentiated for a better understanding of the hemodilution

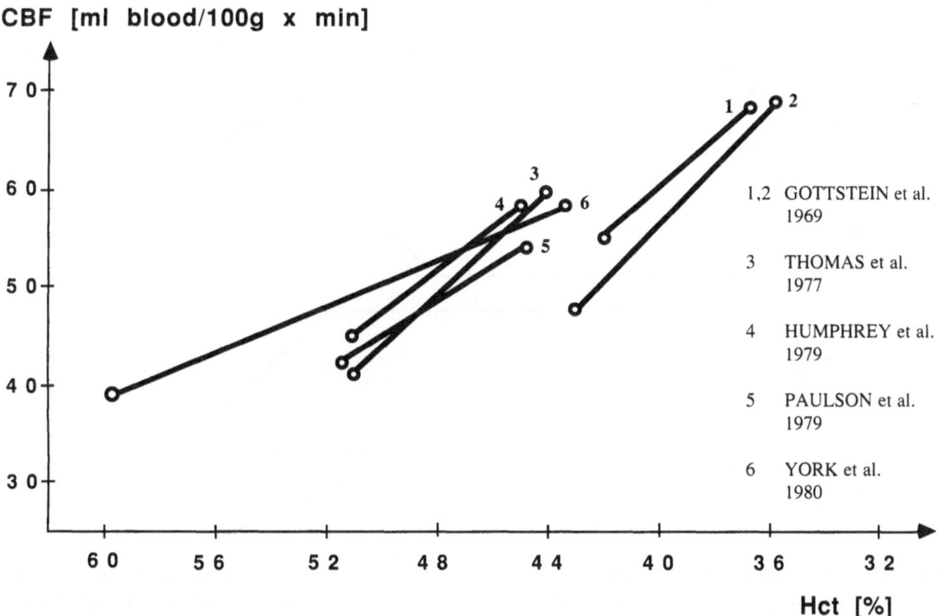


**Fig. 39.** Relationship between Hct and cerebral blood flow according to measurements of the different study groups (From [87])

treatment. In case of *intact autoregulation* hemodilution by vasodilation leads to an improved cerebral circulation. In addition, the whole blood viscosity is decreased by the reduction in Hct, and the cardiac output is therefore improved since the peripheral resistance decreases, and the cardiac filling volume increases by a facilitated venous return. The prophylactic effect of the *isovolemic* hemodilution in polycythemia vera and haemoconcentration results from these mechanisms, but an additional volume deficiency is not allowed. In cases of *disturbed autoregulation* the cerebral circulation, apart from an increase in blood pressure, is increased mainly by an elevated cardiac output (CO) and secondly by an improvement in the hemorheological factors. Thus, *hypervolemic* hemodilution is more useful in these cases (Sect. 3.3.5).

The different steps in the intact cerebral regulation were illustrated by Powers and Raichle [297] with the help of positron emission tomography (PET) (Fig. 40). If the cerebral perfusion pressure (CPP) decreases during stroke,

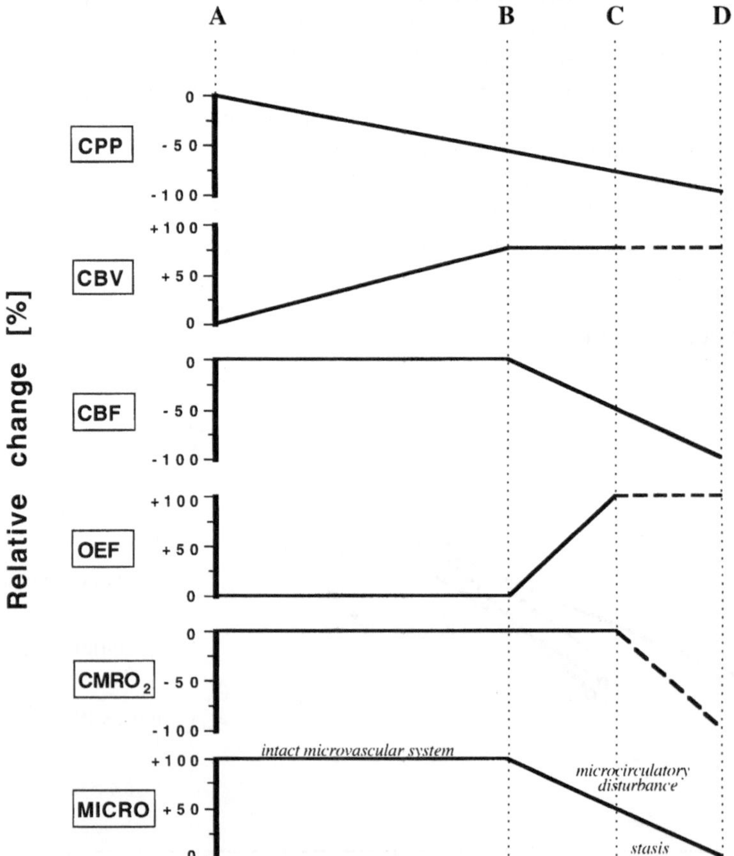


**Fig. 40.** Schematic illustration of the autoregulation mechanisms in disturbed local cerebral perfusion after PET examinations plus indication of the concomitant microcirculatory disturbances (*MICRO*), cerebral perfusion pressure (*CPP*), cerebral blood volume (*CBV*), cerebral blood flow (*CBF*), oxygen extraction fraktion (*OEF*), and cerebral metabolic rate of oxygen (*CMRO*$_2$). (From [297])

autoregulation will bring about vasodilation, thus reducing the peripheral resistance. Therefore, more blood flows through the brain, influencing the PET by an increase in the cerebral blood volume (CBV) and keeping CBF constant for the moment despite a decreased CPP (Fig. 40 A-B). If this cerebral vasomotor reserve is exhausted and CPP continues to fall, CBF is also reduced (B-C). Now the oxygen extraction fraction (OEF) can be increased as a second compensatory mechanism so that in this phase the cerebral metabolic rate ($CMRO_2$) still guarantees a normal cell function (B-C). If CPP and CBF continue to decrease, an oxygen deficiency occurs, leading for the moment to a reversible loss of function and in the case of further decrease to irreversible cell damage. Studies with PET in humans refer only to nonacute cerebral perfusion. In patients with carotid occlusion and TIA the decrease in CBF from a normal value of 48 ml/min × 100 g to 22 ml/min × 100 g despite compensatory vasodilation leads to a cerebral $O_2$ metabolism that is reduced by half (1.43 ml/min × 100 g). According to animal experiments, a reversible loss of function occurs at a CBF of 16–18 ml/min × 100 g; irreversible damages are to be expected at 6–8 ml/min × 100 g, and, in addition, the degree of damage depends on the duration of the circulatory disturbance [272]. PET examinations in cerebral infarctions have shown very different perfusion conditions and still allow no final evaluation since they have generally not been carried out early enough after the acute stroke [169, 395]. On the basis of the PET experiences of Heiss [132] hemodilution treatment is to be preferred. Further mechanisms concerning the regulation of the cerebral blood flow involve osmo-, volume-, pressure-, $O_2$-blood-, $O_2$-tissue-, and $CO_2$- receptors [142].

### *3.3.2 Acute Disturbed Microcirculation as a Further Attempt at Hemodilution*

For the understanding of hemodilution treatment it is also decisive that microcirculatory disturbances result from the CBF decrease during the phases B-D (Fig. 40), which are also known in circulatory disturbances of other organs (coronary heart disease, arterial occlusive disease, dermal muscle transplantation, or multiple failure of organs in a disturbed cardiovascular system). These microcirculatory disturbances lead to an inhomogeneous circulation by opening arteriovenous shunts, hyperperfusing short capillaries, and hypoperfusing long capillaries [324]. Thereby, a sufficient circulation of the tissue can be simulated, but the important parts of the tissue are not adequately supplied with oxygen. This uneven, defective blood flow is also reflected in the already mentioned SPECT examinations in TIA and infarction patients; the higher the Hct in the ischemic area, the worse circulation in this part of the tissue. The high Hct was negative for the area since the clinical course of the infarcted patients was increasingly unfavourable corresponding to the elevated Hct in the area of infarction [315]. Also, in the case of multiple organ failure due to circulatory disturbances local tissue hypoxia could occur due to a disturbed microcirculation despite a systemic oversupply of oxygen [242]. Here, too, the reperfusion is achieved first by volume substitution and subsequent improvement in hemodynamics by substances of positive inotropic effect so that a further important attempt at *hypervolemic hemodilution* results from these pathomechanisms. Inhomogeneous circulation where extremely extended, hyperperfused, short capillaries are present in an area with hypoperfused capillaries, was shown anatomico-pathologically in microscopic brain sections after repeated hypoxia [375]. That the microcirculatory disturbances could not be assessed by the previous noninvasive methods, including PET, due to a too small resolving power explains some of the apparently contradictory results on the cerebral circulation. Microcirculatory disturbances are especially intensified by increased PV, SEA, thrombocyte aggregation (s-TA), and leucocyte adhesivity (see Sect. 3.1.2.2).

### 3.3.3 The Ischemic Penumbra

The basis of hemodilution is the existence of a penumbra (Fig. 41). This zone was defined as an area in which CBF is no longer sufficient to maintain the nerve tissue function but is high enough to prevent the transformation to structural destruction [15]. By careful measurements of the regional cerebral blood flow the most frequent position of the penumbra in infarctions of the middle cerebral artery can be characterized [282, 283].

Therefore, a hyperemic zone may arise prior to the infarction due to the short courses and the good perfusion conditions, whereas the hypoperfused penumbra arises mostly after the infarction due to the unfavourable supply by collaterals. Position and size depend on the kind of infarction and on the degree and duration of the circulatory disturbance. If the whole blood flow of a brain area is

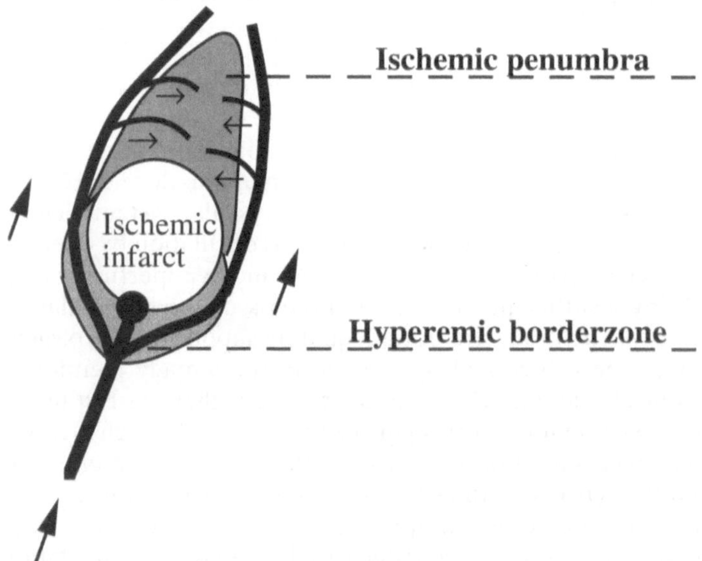


**Fig. 41.** The different perfusion zones in acute ischemic cerebral infarction after measuring the CBF in human beings. (Modified from [283])

interrupted without collateral supply, no great penumbra can be expected. In the case of an incomplete occlusion a partial recanalization arises or in the case of sufficient collaterals the penumbra may initially be significantly greater than the infarcted area itself, which persists for a longer period, and presents a good chance for treatment by hemodilution. This therapy should not only improve the oxygen supply but also accelerate the transportation of, for example, acid catabolites and mediators which lead to reperfusion damages. During the performance of hemodilution it must be remembered that autoregulation in the penumbra ceases due to the poor perfusion conditions [272, 281]. In this area the circulation depends mainly passively on *blood pressure and cardiac output* (CO) as well as PV in the disturbed microcirculation. This means that a simple lowering of the haematocrit level will not achieve an adequate perfusion but that additionally the CO will have to be raised by hemodilution (Sect. 3.3.5). This view is confirmed by two animal experiments with monkeys in which (at a constant Hct) the circulation in the infarcted area decisively depended on the CO, and CBF in the penumbra was improved sufficiently only by the hypervolemic and not by the isovolemic hemodilution [119, 170]. A further important clinical indication for the efficacy of hemodilution (in the case of a penumbra) is the successful use in the therapy of cerebral circulatory disturbances resulting from vasospasms during subarachnoid hemorrhage. In the United States, this hypervolemic, hypertensive treatment is an acknowledged form of treatment.

The third important issue is the question of how long the penumbra persists and what opportunities in time there are for the use of hemodilution or other measures. According to the results of animal experiments, a reversible disturbed function transforms into an irreversible structural destruction of the neural tissue at a CBF of 12–15 ml/min × 100 g or of 6–8 ml/min × 100 g after 2–3 or even 1 h [272]. If there is an occlusion of the middle cerebral artery in man, an infarction of the tissue is to be expected within 0.5–8 h [281]. PETexaminations showed that any influence on the development of the infarction by CBF can be exerted only within a period of 24 to 48 h [395]. The importance of a quick initiation of treatment can be derived from the experiences in myocardial infarctions in cases in which optimal treatment must be started within the first 3 hours.

### 3.3.4 Pathophysiological Basis of Hemodilution

Some 60% of all infarctions occur in the early morning. According to a survey of five stroke registers, an average of 25% of all ischemic cerebral infarctions are due to embolism [252]. Therefore, thrombotic occlusion of a vessel is the most frequent cause. Several factors apart from arteriosclerotic vascular changes contribute to the development of an infarction (Table 21).

The most important causes are hypovolemia during the morning hours with an increase in Hct and PV, a decrease in blood pressure and CO, and further

**Table 21.** Pathophysiologic risk factors of acute ischemic cerebral infarctions occurring in the morning

| | |
|---|---|
| CO | ↓ |
| Blood pressure | ↓ |
| Haematocrit | ↑ |
| Plasma viscosity | ↑ |
| Thrombocyte aggregation | ↑ |
| t-PA | ↓ |
| PAI | ↑ |

circadian rhythms such as a decrease in the activity of tissue plasminogen activators (t-PA) or an increase in plasminogen-activator inhibitor (PAI) activity and thrombocyte aggregation. Figure 42 presents the course of Hct, blood pressure, heart rate, and CO during the day and night hours. During the night the hemorheologically unfavourably high Hct values are combined with hemodynamically unfavourably low CO values. For this reason, the hemodilution treatment adjusted to the individual condition of the patient directly intervenes in the pathological mechanisms of an acute infarction at different places:

1. At first, hemodilution compensates hypovolemia and increases intravascular volume. This leads to an increase in CO by stabilization of the cerebral blood flow and an increase in the cardiac load. A schematic procedure in accordance with cardiac exercise tolerance is not possible. Especially in stroke patients with cardiac failure, the volume must be adjusted individually, and supported with positively inotropic substances.
2. With hemodilution a Hct optimal for the metabolism of the neural tissue is achieved. This reduces the whole blood viscosity, which in the macrocirculation depends especially on Hct and also improves cardiac output since peripheral resistance is decreased, and the venous return is facilitated.
3. Hemodilution decreases PV and SEA, thus also improving the microcirculation.
4. Depending on the special qualities of the plasma substitute chosen, other hemorheological parameters such as fibrinogen concentration, thrombocyte aggregation, leucocyte adhesivity or coagulation are also influenced.

Therefore, hemodilution aims not only at improving the cerebral $O_2$ supply but also, by an increase in perfusion at preventing further thromboses, at supporting recanalization and avoiding reperfusion damage.

By the rapid wash out of acid metabolism products and mediators, which tend to cause the reperfusion damage, hemodilution can positively influence the development of cerebral oedema. This is also decisive in the prognosis for cerebral infarction. [140]. Under intensive care conditions Goslinga et al. [85] quite impressively achieved an optimal hemodilution by influencing

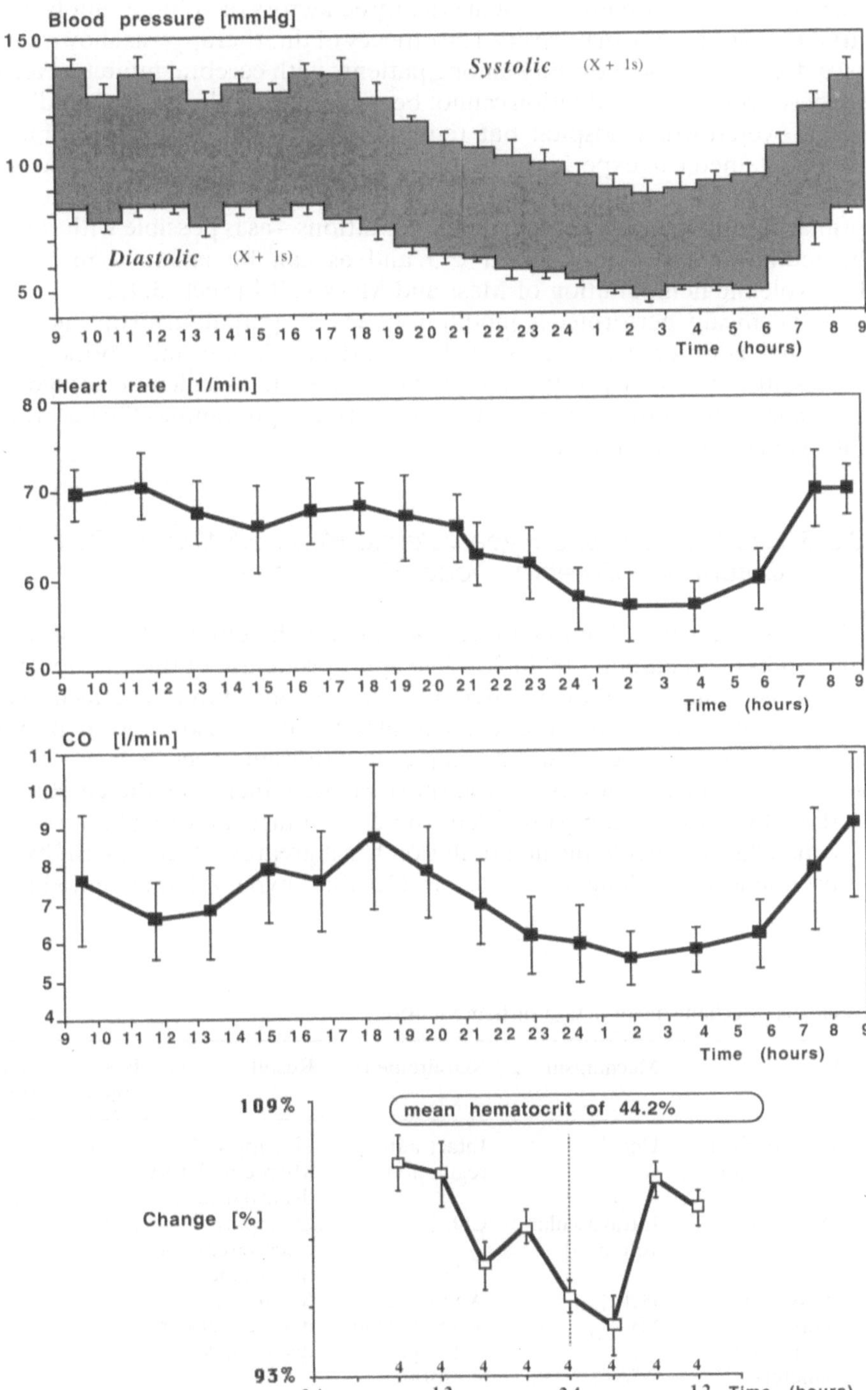


**Fig. 42.** Day and night variations in blood pressure (from [261]), heart rate, cardiac output (Haaß and Stoll) and Hct (from [333])

(adjusted to the individual patient) the three factors of volume supply, increase in CO, and reduction in viscosity. The efficacy of this therapy was shown clinically by a decrease in the mortality among patients with cerebral infarcts. According to these criteria, hemodilution cannot be performed in the general medical ward of an overcrowded hospital but requires special supervision combined with sufficient medical experience as characterizes the treatment of myocardial infarctions. Hemodilution should not lead to deterioration in the already primarily unfavourable hemodynamic conditions – as is possible with isovolemic hemodilution by a decrease in CO and as can be assumed in the partly hypovolemic hemodilution of Mast and Marx [250] (Sect. 3.4.2).

A specifically performed hemodilution puts the patient in an optimal position for other additional treatment such as anticoagulation and fibrinolysis. This represents the basis for further medication such as calcium antagonists or substances preventing reperfusion damage. It also guarantees the best transport into vulnerable brain areas.

### *3.3.5 Effect of Iso- and Hypervolemic Hemodilution on Cardiac Output and Cerebral Blood Flow in the Penumbra*

Three mechanisms of action are responsible for the effects of hemodilution on the cerebral circulation (Table 22). The appropriate use of this therapy depends on the iso- and hypervolemic hemodilution having different effects on these mechanisms. Therefore, the clinical effects of an iso- and hypervolemic hemodilution treatment can be completely different (Sect. 3.4.2):

- Reduction in Hct or oxygen transport capacity increases the cerebral blood flow by vasodilation (provided there is intact autoregulation). In this constellation isovolemic hemodilution has a greater effect on CBF by a more pronounced and longer decrease in Hct than hypervolemic hemodilution.

**Table 22.** Mechanisms of action of hemodilution

| Effect | Mechanism | Requirement | Result | Iso-volemic | Hyper-volemic |
|---|---|---|---|---|---|
| Flow velocity ↑ by vasodilation | Hct ↓ | Intact autoregulation | $O_2$ supply ↑ Microcirculatory disturbance ↓ | +++ | ++ |
| Flow velocity ↑ by improved hemodynamics | Intravascular volume ↑ | CO ↑ | $O_2$ supply ↑ Microcirculatory disturbance ↓ | (+) | +++ |
| Flow velocity ↑ by improved hemorheological parameters | Hct ↓ SEA ↓ PV ↓ s-TA ↓ Leukocyte adhesivity ↓ | Appropriate action profile of the plasma substitute | Macro- and microcirculatory disturbance ↓ | ++ | ++ |

- The cerebral circulation is also improved by an increase in CO. For this purpose, hemodilution must increase the intravascular quantity of fluid and the cardiac filling volume. According to the following findings this can be achieved sufficiently only by hypervolemic and not by isovolemic hemodilution. This improvement in perfusion is independent of cerebral autoregulation.

The increase in CO is essential for improved circulation of the penumbra in acute cerebral infarction (Sect. 3.3.3). Therefore we examined the hemodynamic effect of different hemodilution schemes by continous non-invasive measurements of CO (Fig. 43). Only a rapid hypervolemic hemodilution, for example, with a "loading dose", increases the CO significantly. CO increased within 45–60 min by about 18.9% with an infusion of 500 ml 10% Haes 200/0.5. This effect was not maintained by the subsequent hypervolemic long-term infusion of 1000 ml 10% Haes 200/0.5, but CO remained increased by 10%, which is necessary for an effective treatment. Compared to this the isovolemic loading dose and the following long-term treatment are accompanied only by a slow increase in CO, which can be retarded considerably in order to achieve clinical success. The two kinds of infusion led to a similarly reduced Hct and did not show any considerable effect on heart rate or blood pressure.

For the evaluation of isovolemic hemodilution studies the effect of a not strictly isovolemically performed hemodilution is of particular importance. Administration of the loading dose decreases CO by about 17% or 30% in an extreme case if the phlebotomy is performed more quickly than the infusion of the plasma substitute. Due to hypovolemia the infusion scheme of Mast and Marx [250] also results in a decrease in CO by an average of more than 10% (Fig. 44). This negative hemodynamic effect was clearly clinically detected neither by the reaction of heart rate nor by that of blood pressure; thus it is not necessarily noticed by the investigating physician. This negative reaction of the circulatory system may have been the cause for the less good clinical outcome of hemodynamical deep white matter cerebral infarctions in the Scandinavian hemodilution study (Sect. 3.1.4.2). The close agreement of CO effects of iso- and hypervolemic hemodilution with measurements in the microcirculation of the nail bed show that the changes in CO have a direct effect on capillary areas. The isovolemic hemodilution of the Italian Study [147] did not have any considerable effect on CO (Fig. 45). Thus, a decisive improvement of the circulation in the cerebral penumbra cannot be expected (Sect. 3.4.2).

CO is affected differently by iso- and hypervolemic hemodilution. A sufficiently acute increase in CO can be achieved only by hypervolemic hemodilution. According to animal experiments and clinical examinations, an increase in CO is necessary to improve the circulatory disturbance of the penumbra by hemodilution.

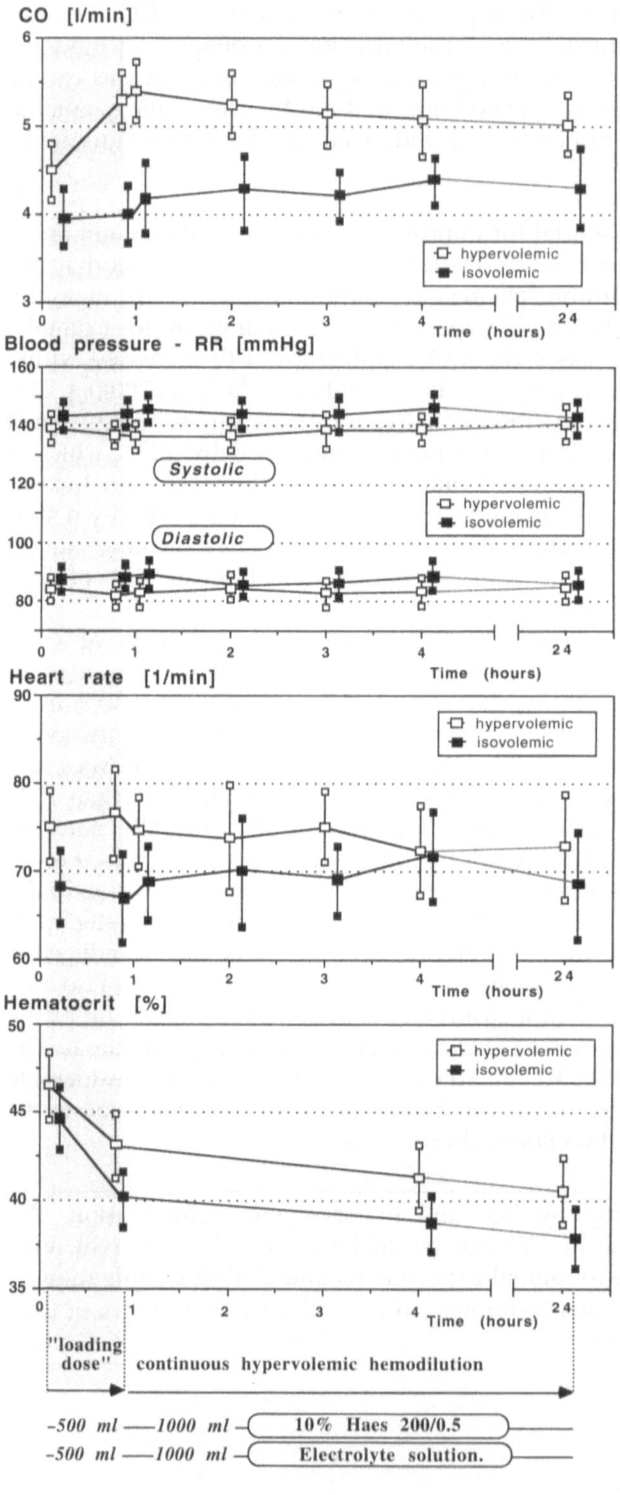

**Fig. 43.** Effect of hemodilution in the form of an iso- and hypervolemic "loading dose" and a hypervolemic long-term treatment on cardiac output (*CO*), blood pressure, heart rate, and Hct

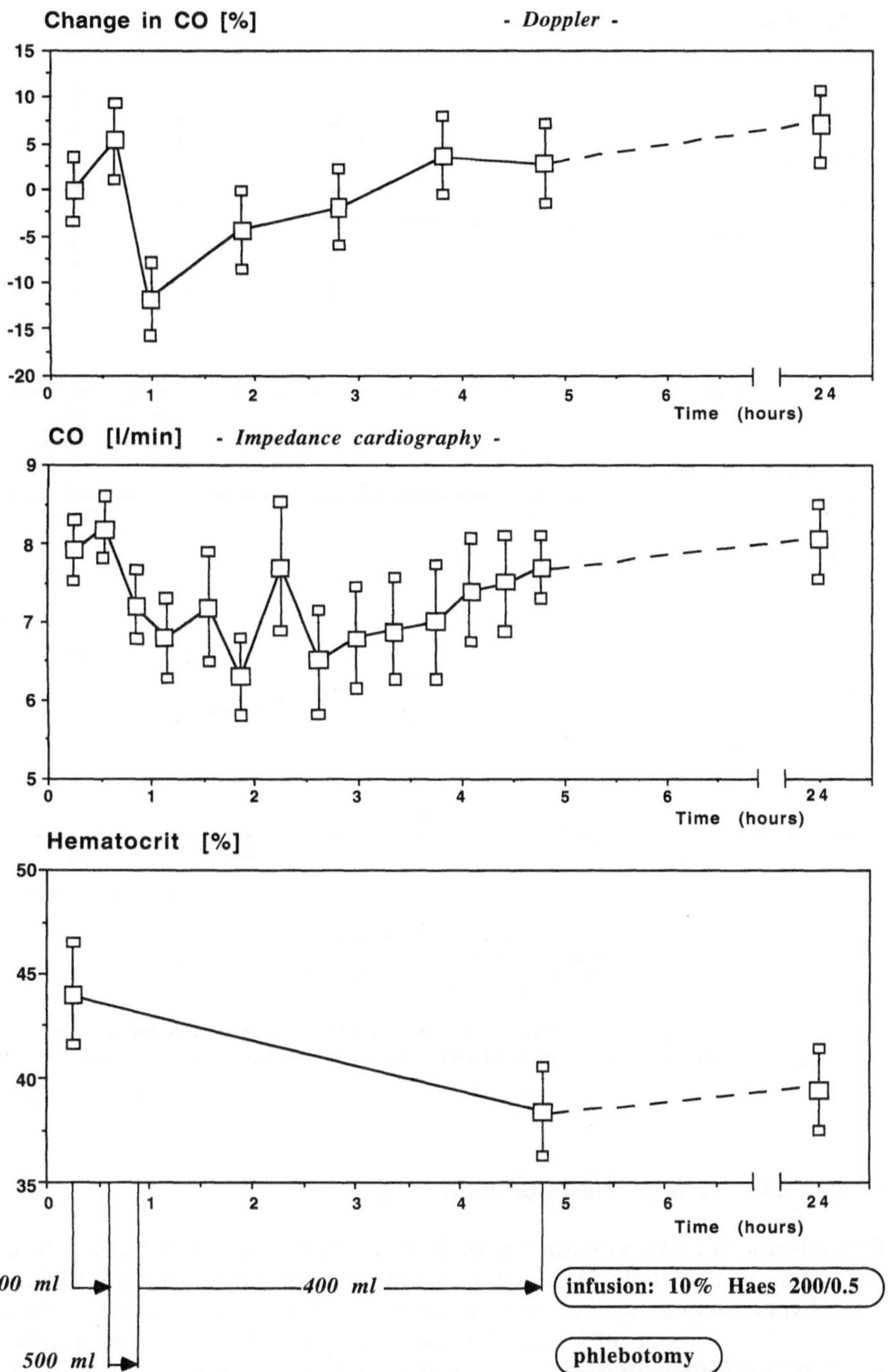


**Fig. 44.** Decrease in the cardiac output (*CO*) during a temporarily non-isovolemically hemodilution performed according to the infusion scheme by Mast and Marx [250]

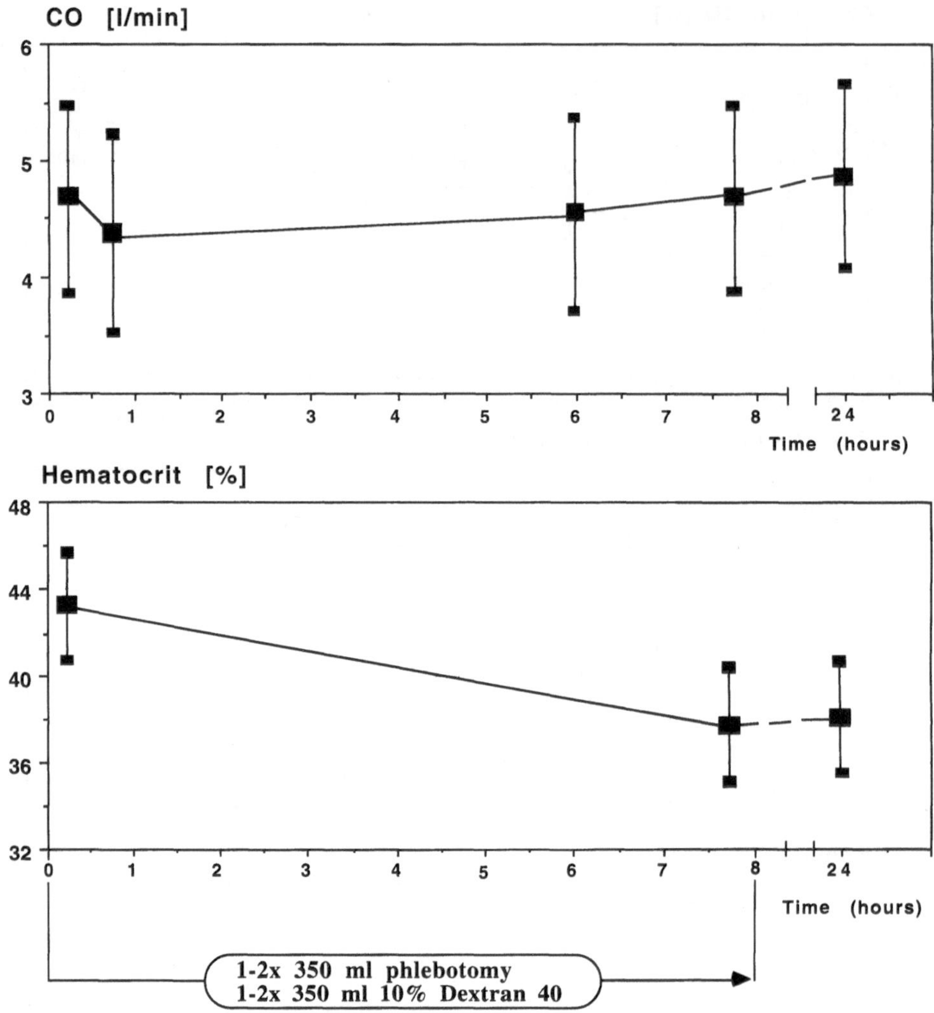


**Fig. 45.** Time course of cardiac output (*CO*) and Hct during isovolemic hemodilution according to the infusion scheme of the Italian Hemodilution Study [147]

### *3.3.6 Indications for Hemodilution*

The indications and requirements for hemodilution in cerebrovascular strokes are summarized in Table 23. In acute ischemic cerebral infarction a sufficiently early hypervolemic hemodilution orientated to cardiac exercise tolerance reduces Hct to about 40% and also increases CO. Therefore, hypervolemic hemodilution is the initial treatment in an acute ischemic cerebral infarction and may be supplemented by additional therapies or substituted by antikoagulation or fibrinolysis during the further course depending on the indication (Table 23).

**Table 23.** Indications for hemodilution

| Clinical picture | Optimal Hct and PV values | Type of hemodilution | Period |
|---|---|---|---|
| Acute ischemic infarction with penumbra | Hct = 40% (37%–42%) | Hypervolemic after cardiac load capacity CO ↑ > 10% | Within 0–12 h, over 6–10 days |
| Circulatory disturbance after SAH (with inactive or without aneurysm) | Hct = 40% (37%–42%) | Hypervolemic slow infusion, low dose | After clinical symptoms |
| Polycythemia | Hct = 45% | Isovolemic | After Hct |
| Dehydration | Hct = 40%–42% | Hypervolemic | After Hct |
| Haemoconcentration | Hct = 45% | Isovolemic and/or hypervolemic | After Hct and plasma volume |
| Hyperviscosity (e.g., in SAE, dyspro-tein-aemia, hyper-tension, diabetes melli-tus) | PV< 1.3 mPas | Isovolemic or bag plasmapheresis | After PV |

While in ischemic cerebral infarction treatment starts with a rapid infusion as a loading dose, in SAH a large volume load should not be given to avoid an increase in intracranial pressure (Sect. 3.4.6). Nonacute cerebrovascular strokes associated with haemoconcentration or polycythemia can be treated isovolemically as in prophylactic treatment if there is no volume deficiency, and hypovolemia is avoided during phlebotomy. Isovolemic hemodilution, or, better, bag plasmapheresis, is a prophylactic measure if PV is increased due to various causes.

## 3.4 Hemodilution in Acute Ischemic Cerebral Infarctions

### 3.4.1 Optimal Hematocrit

The discussion about optimal Hct is still in progress. For the understanding of hemodilution it is decisive that the optimal Hct is not a rigid parameter but depends also on cerebral blood flow velocity, vascular conditions, CO, blood pressure, and hemorheological factors.

In animal experiments [199] it was demonstrated impressively that even in healthy animals a Hct value which is too high or too low can lead to deterioration in the cerebral metabolism. This leads to decreased ATP and increased lactate concentration (Fig. 46). Due to the considerable compensation range of healthy brain, energy and glucose metabolism remain normal with Hct values of 30%–49%. The dependence on optimal Hct increases considerably if there are hypertension-induced vascular changes in animals. In these cases Hct of only about 40% guarantees good cerebral function. In addition, optimal Hct depends on hemodynamics, that is, on the cardiovascular system, blood pressure, and CO. Due to the particular conditions in the cardiovascular system of dogs the decrease in Hct from 40% to 30% and to 10% is accompanied by an increase in CO of 50% or even 120%. This increase in CO compensates the decrease in the $O_2$-transporting erythrocytes and leads to a very low optimal Hct of 30%–33% [358]. In normal persons and especially in patients suffering from vascular and cardiac diseases such a hemodynamic effect cannot be expected. Thus one cannot apply these values to human beings. Due to different findings (apart from peculiarities concerning the blood, heart, and vessels) an optimal Hct of 40% must rather be assumed in patients with cerebral infarcts. This value corresponds well with the results concerning coronoary heart desease. The optimal Hct range is particularly limited if the autoregulation, such as in the penumbra, is disturbed. Since the hemodynamic effect of isovolemic hemodilution is weak, that is, the reduction in Hct is not compensated by an improved CO, the low target Hct in the Scandinavian and Italian hemodilution studies must be regarded as too low. Only in the case of invasively controlled and improved hemodynamics can a considerably lowered Hct also be sufficient. This was demonstrated by the positive clinical findings of Goslinga et al. [85, 86] under intensive care conditions.

In this context the question arises of whether in the reperfusion phase an optimal high Hct alone or an optimal rapid perfusion is more important for diminishing damage by acid metabolism products and membrane-damaging mediators. A slight reduction below 40% in favour of an improved circulation is justifiable. Compared to this, poor vascular and cardiac circulatory conditions shift the value upwards. In patients with polycythemia and haemoconcentration a value of 45% is recommended. Furthermore, in the discussion about the optimal Hct one should not disregard that Hct is considerably higher in the large vessels than in the small vessels of the microcirculation, and that Hct changes in the large vessels do not have a linear effect on the Hct of the microcirculation.

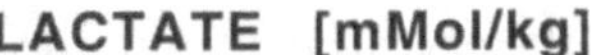


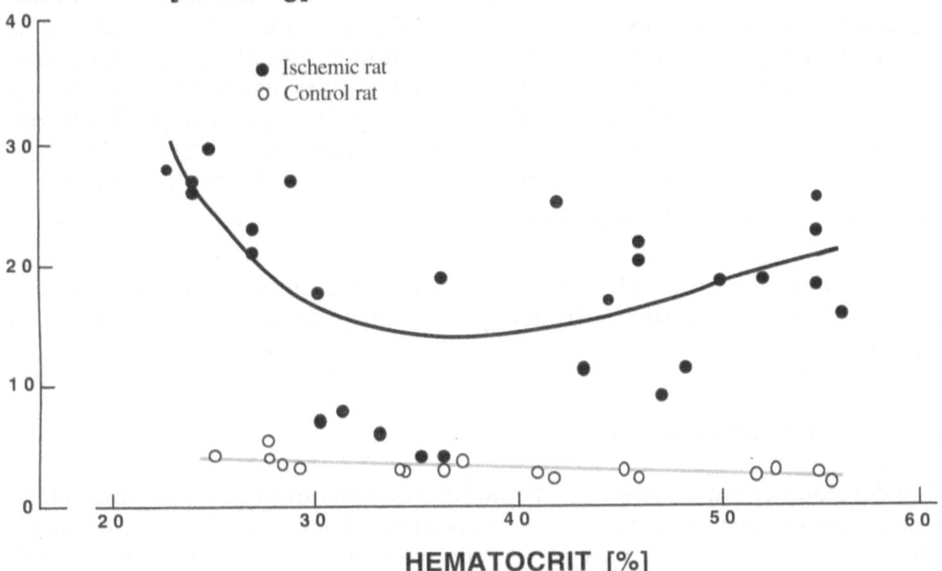


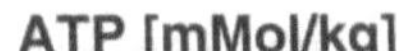


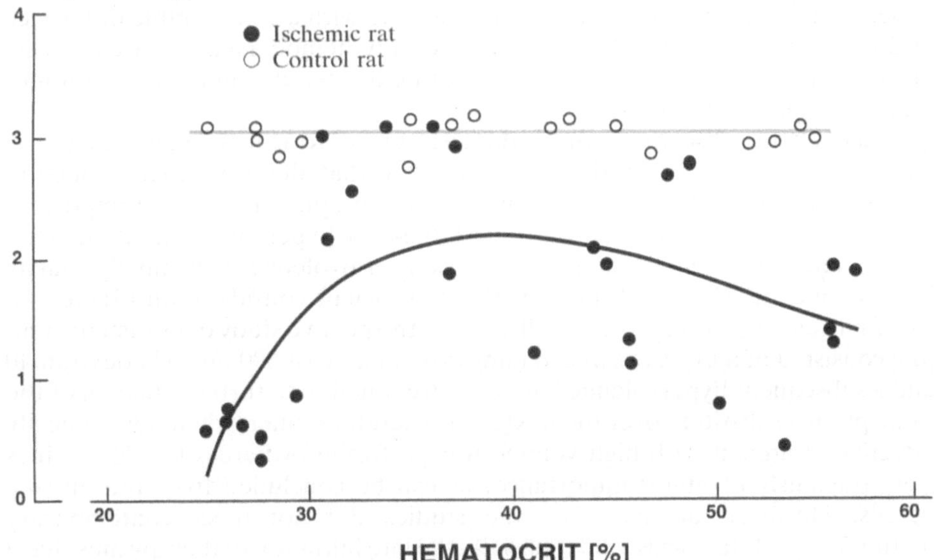


**Fig. 46.** Effect of Hct on ATP and lactate concentration in the brain of healthy or spontaneously hypertensive rats. (From [198])

By the so-called "plasma-skimming" of the plasma and the erythrocytes they are separated into two streams and therefore are differently affected by increase in whole blood viscosity (that is, Hct) and by hemodilution. SPECT examinations in stroke patients as well as direct measurements of the plasma and erythrocyte stream in the microcirculation of the nail bed fold [315] (see Chaps. 2, 4)show that a reduction in Hct by hemodilution leaves the Hct of the microcirculation in healthy brain tissue almost unchanged and reduces the Hct in the microcirculation of the nail bed by only about half.

> The optimal level of Hct is not absolute but depends upon various hemodynamic factors such as from CO, blood pressure, viscosity, and vascular conditions.

### 3.4.2 Hemodilution Studies

The development of treatment by hemodilution in neurological cases cannot be completely understood without the psychological background. In our opinion, the complexity of this therapy is not fully met by simply listing the previous studies and counting how many cases showed a positive, negative, or no effect without considering important procedural differences such as the time of initiation of therapy or the type, such as hyper–, iso–, or hypovolemic hemodilution. This is especially true for the differentiation between iso- and hypervolemic hemodilution since we are dealing with a considerable difference in dosages with hemorheological and especially hemodynamic consequences. Such a difference in dosage would also not be disregarded in the evaluation of other therapeutic methods.

First of all, the observation that reduced Hct leads to an increase in CBF (Sect. 3.3.3) is suggestive. One of the consequences is that all forms of Hct reduction are regarded as an effective hemodilution. In our opinion, the most important development, namely, the change from a large-dose hypervolemic dilution in the first studies to a more and more strictly isovolemic and finally partly hypovolemic dilution, took place without sufficient consideration (Table 24). The first studies (until 1976), as well as the retrospective study of Gottstein et al. [88] consisted of a *hypervolemic* loading dose of at least 500 ml 10% dextran 40 and a subsequent hypervolemic long-term treatment of a further 1000 ml of the same plasma substitute over the next 24 h. Therefore, mainly hemodynamically effective treatment with high volume was performed whereas low Hct values were obviously of minor importance, as can be concluded from the missing details. However, at that time the studies did not meet contemporary methodological standards, and especially the late initiation of therapy must have diminished the therapeutic possibilities decisively. At least one study showed a positive clinical effect, and in another mortality was significantly reduced. In this evaluation, the positive effect of the study by Gottstein et al. (1976) [88] was not taken into consideration due to the retrospective nature of the analysis.

Strand et al. [351] changed the concept and a reduced Hb with a target value below 120 g/l was emphasized. Furthermore, an isovolemic loading dose was

**Table 24.** Hemodilution studies

| Authors | Kind of hemodilution (within the first 24 h) | Target HCT | Evaluation | Start of treatment | Duration of treatment | Clinical result |
|---|---|---|---|---|---|---|
| Gilroy et al. (1969) | Loading dose hypervolemic 500 ml dextran 40<br>Long-term treatment: 2 × 500 ml dextran 40/12 h | ? | Hypervolemic | 24–72 h | 3 days | Positive |
| Spudis et al. (1973) | Loading dose hypervolemic 500 ml dextran 40<br>Long-term treatment: 2 × 500 ml dextran 40/12 h | ? | Hypervolemic | <24 h | 3 days | No effect |
| Kaste et al. (1976) | Loading dose hypervolemic 500 ml dextran 40<br>Long-term treatment: 500 ml dextran 40 + dexamethasone | ? | Hypervolemic | 24–48 h | 3 days | No effect |
| Matthews et al. (1976) | Loading dose hypervolemic 500 ml dextran 40<br>Long-term treatment: 2 × 500 ml dextran 40/12 h | ? | Hypervolemic | <48 h | 3 days | Positive |
| Gottstein et al. (1976) (retrospective investigation) | Loading dose hypervolemic 500 ml dextran 40<br>Long-term treatment: 1 × 500 ml dextran 40/6–8 h | ? | Hypervolemic | | | Positive |
| Strand et al. (1984) | Loading dose isovolemic: 150–200 ml dextran 40<br>Long-term treatment: 1 × 300–350 ml dextran 40 | 37% | Slightly iso- and hypervolemic | <48 h | 7 days | Positive |
| Scandinavian Stroke Study Group (1987) | Loading dose isovolemic:<br>a) Hct > 42%: 500 ml dextran 40<br>b) Hct 38%–42%: 250 ml dextran 40 + 250 ml hypervolemically<br>Loading dose hypervolemic:<br>c) Hct< 38%; 500 ml dextran 40 | <38% | Strictly isovolemic<br>Iso- and hypervolemic<br>Seldom hypervolemic | <48 h | 5 days | No effect |
| Italian Acute Stroke Study Group (1988) | Loading dose isovolemic: after Hct< 38%: 500 ml dextran 40 | <35% | Strictly isovolemic | <12 h | 2 days | No effect |

**Table 24.** Continued

| Authors | Kind of hemodilution (within the first 24 h) | Target HCT | Evaluation | Start of treatment | Duration of treatment | Clinical result |
|---|---|---|---|---|---|---|
| Hemodilution in Stroke Study Group (1989) | Loading dose after Hct iso- or hypervolemic<br>Long-term treatment hypervolemic, max. 1500 ml Haes 250/0.45 hypervolemically | 30%–33% | Iso- and hypervolemic<br><br>Hypervolemic | <24 h | 3 days | Positive |
| Mast and Marx (1989) | Loading dose 100 ml Haes hypervolemically<br>Phlebotomy: 500 ml<br>Long-term treatment: 400 ml Haes/5 h isovolemically | 35% | Slightly hypervolemic<br>Long hypovolemic<br>After 5 h isovolemic | <48 h | | Negative |
| Goslinga, Amsterdam Stroke Study (1989) | Normovolemic, hypervolemic, albumin, electrolyte solution according to viscosity | 32% | Normovolemic<br>Hypervolemic | | | Positive |
| Koller et al. (1990) | Loading dose isovolemic: 500 ml dextran 40<br>Long-term treatment hypervolemic, 1000 ml dextran 40/24 h | 30%–35% | Iso-hypervolemic | | 3 days | Positive |
| Haaß et al. (1990, 1991) | Loading dose after Hct iso- or hypervolemic 500 ml Haes 200/05<br>Long-term treatment hypervolemic, 2 × 500 ml Haes 200/05 /6 h | | Iso- or hypervolemic<br><br>Hypervolemic | <24 h | 10 days | Positive |

introduced for the first time, and the infused plasma substitute volume was reduced to one-third compared to the previous studies in order to perform the therapy also in patients with heart failure. It must be regarded as an essential advantage of this study that the treatment team of this specialist hospital was particularly familiar with the medical care of cerebral stroke patients, which, for instance, could not be demanded of the subsequent multicenter study. In our opinion, the result of this study was so clearly positive that it cannot be questioned by the technical disadvantage of an open study.

The study of the Scandinavian Stroke Study Group [316] is described as a follow-up study, but it must be taken into account that the hemodilution was performed increasingly isovolemically. The isovolemic loading dose of

250–500 ml was set twice as high so that some patients received no hypervolemic long-term treatment within the first 24 h.

In the subgroup analysis the condition of the patients with the lowest Hct values was worse than that of the patients with elevated values. The important objection can be raised that on hemodilution treatment of acute ischemic cerebral infarctions only a reduction in Hct, with the possible danger of a simultaneously decreased CO by phlebotomy or at least without an improvement in hemodynamics, is not reliably effective. Also, the accompanying measurements of CBF carried out in 12 patients did not confirm the sufficient hemodynamic efficacy of this hemodilution method since an improved circulation of the brain area concerned was seen in only two patients who, in contrast to the ten remaining patients, improved clinically significantly. On the other hand, several study groups have demonstrated that hypervolemic hemodilution leads almost invariably to an increase in perfusion of the infarcted area [100].

In addition a third observation clearly shows the negative hemodynamic effect of this form of hemodilution. In the subgroup analysis it was seen, also in spite of certain statistical reservations [9], that there was a possible negative influence on deep white matter infarcts. Since these terminal infarcts did worse, as typical hemodynamic infarcts (Sect. 3.1.3), this would be a convincing indication that CO is reduced by the treatment. Thus, this mainly isovolemically adjusted therapy involved the danger of influencing the hemodynamic perfusion conditions negatively. This possibility was confirmed by our investigation of CO with isovolemic and hypervolemic hemodilution (Sect. 3.3.5) and by the investigation of the circulation in the nail bed capillaries by Jung et al. (Chaps. 2, 4).

The Italian study used strictly isovolemic hemodilution [147] with an especially low target Hct of below 35%. For this reason, the isovolemic treatment was repeated even up to three times. According to our measurements, this form of hemodilution does not improve CO at all, and the early performance of phlebotomy can provoke a decrease in CO each time, which could have been possible in single cases up to three times during the course of the Italian hemodilution study (Figs. 44, 45).

An almost opposite concept, including hypervolemic hemodilution directed to CO, was pursued by the Hemodilution in Stroke Study Group [94]. The arguments for and against have been discussed elsewhere [99, 100] so that only the three most important results are summarized here. According to this study, a successful hemodilution must be started within at least 12 h. Secondly, it should reduce Hct by more than 15%; thirdly, it should simultaneously increase CO by more than 10%. The study was broken off since due to the double-blind study design it was not known before that an unequal distribution had arisen by randomization. Consequently, about twice as many severely infarcted patients were included in the hemodilution group than in the control group. Therefore, proportionally more patients died in the hemodilution group. But on consideration of the clinical result of the first 3 days, including the same number of patients in each group so that the clinical evaluation is not falsified by the failure of seriously ill patients (43 of 45 hemodilution; 41 of 43 standard therapy), it is also clear that only hemodilution patients improved considerably whereas the neurological symptoms in the control group even showed a tendency toward deterioration. Depending on the sites of action, hemodilution improved the acute neurological symptoms, which in this study receded by 50% more than in the control group.

On the basis of the results of the Scandinavian study it is evident why the performance of hemodilution in the study of Mast and Marx [250] resulted in deterioration. As reported by the first author, 100 ml Haes was infused acutely according to the hemodilution scheme, and then a phlebotomy of at least 500 ml blood was performed. The other 400 ml Haes which is necessary for isovolemia was then infused slowly over the following 5 h. According to our examinations, CO can decrease significantly in special cases during this procedure (Fig. 44). In terms of this infusion scheme, this was due to a hypovolemia of longer duration. Since in many cerebral stroke patients a decreased intravascular and extracellular volume must be expected even primarily, this at first hypo- and only later isovolemic hemodilution could have – from a hemodynamic point of view – an unfavourable effect on the extremely vulnerable initial phase of a cerebral infarction. Thus, this study emphasizes the clinically relevant differences between a hypervolemic and a more or less strictly isovolemic hemodilution. Comparison of the schemes by the Scandinavian [316, 317] and the Italian studies [147] and those by Strand et al. [351] and Mast and Marx [250] suggest that intensification of the isovolemic component could be responsible for the lack of success of these forms of hemodilution. It should be noted that isovolemic hemodilution is risky for acute cerebral infarction, and due to the perfusion conditions in the penumbra hypervolemic hemodilution should be preferred (Sect. 3.1.3.5). Therefore, the indication for isovolemic hemodilution is restricted to non-acute cases of cerebrovascular circulatory disturbances such as polycythemia and secondary haemoconcentration (Sect. 3.3.6).

Our own recently completed double-blind, placebo-controlled hemodilution study consisted of an iso- or hypervolemic loading dose depending on the initial Hct level and this was followed by hypervolemic Haes long-term treatment. The greater regression in neurological symtoms in the hemodilution group by 50% confirmed the clinical efficacy of the therapy (Sect. 3.5). It is understandable that there was uncertainty after the Scandinavian and Italian studies despite serious technical objections to the latter. Consequently, an article against hemodilution [16] met with a certain response although here "the baby was thrown out with the bathwater," and important aspects of the importance of Hct, PV, SEA, and intracranial pressure with hemodilution were unjustifiably neglected [134, 326]. These discrepancies were explained in detail in three studies [99, 100, 106].

The scientific discussion provided the opportunity to think again about the value of consequent hemodilution since it was no longer possible to regard any infusion performed at any time as an effective therapy. Besides the studies of the Hemodilution in Stroke Study Group [94], Goslinga [85, 86], and Koller et al. [213], supplementary findings for a hemodynamically effective hemodilution can also be derived from clinical pilot studies and animal experiments (Table 25).

**Table 25.** Hemodilution with examination of cardiac output

| Patient studies | Plasma substitute | Volume | Hct | CO |
|---|---|---|---|---|
| Wood and Fleischer (1982) [400] | Albumin<br>Dextran | 2.5 l<br>2.0 l | 32% | –<br>– |
| Korosue et al. (1988) [215] | Fresh plasma | 400–1000 ml | 33% | +29% |
| Hemodilution in Stroke Study Group (1989) [94] | 10% Haes 250/0.45 | 500–1000 ml | <−15%<br>>−15% | <10%<br>>10% |
| *Animal studies* | | | | |
| Sundt and Walt (1967) cats [359] | Dextran | – | – | – |
| Keller et al. (1985) monkeys [170] | Dextran | 25 ml/cg | −15% | +280% |
| Wood et al. (1984) dogs [402] | Fresh plasma | 40% total vol. | 30%–35% | +71% |
| Tranmer et al. (1986) monkeys [371] | Haes | 50–100 ml after CO | 28% | +130% |

In summary, it can be said that hemodilution treatment in acute cerebral infarction shifted from hyper- to isovolemic dilution. Comparison of the very positive results of the well-planned study performed by Strand et al. [351] with the following isovolemic therapy studies and the Hemodilution in Stroke Study Group [94] as well as our own study shows that the success of this treatment depends on hypervolemic infusions. This is supported by pathophysiological examinations, according to which only hypervolemic and not isovolemic hemodilution can sufficiently improve CO and the disturbed perfusion in a penumbra with abolished autoregulation. Besides the increase in CO and decrease in Hct, early start of treatment is necessary for a successful outcome.

It seems imperative now that this hemodilution concept be tested with regard to its efficacy in a large clinical study to remove any remaining doubts.

### 3.4.3 Description of Dextran and Hydroxyethyl Starch Solutions

Colloidal plasma substitutes from dextran and hydroxyethyl starch consist of a mixture of molecules of varying sizes. The mean molecular weight of the initial solution is always given in daltons. Our own experiences with dextran 40 and Haes 200/0.5 demonstrated for the first time that the composition of these plasma substitutes changes decisively in vivo [108, 221]. Therefore, a new molecular mixture with a new mean molecular weight, which is important for biological effects, is produced by elimination and metabolism. For a better characterization of the plasma substitutes not only the in vitro parameters but also the in vivo parameters must be given (see Sect. 3.4.4). First of all, the

**Table 26.** Characterization of the dextran and hydroxyethyl starch solutions

| | |
|---|---|
| *Characteristics of dextran solutions* | |
| Concentration | 6%, 10% |
| Mean molecular weight | 40 000, 60 000, 75 000 |
| *Characteristics of hydroxyethyl starch solutions* | |
| Concentration | 6%, 10% |
| Mean molecular weight | 40 000, 200 000, 450 000 |
| Degree of substitution | 0.5, 0.62, 0.7 |
| Kind of substitution | $C_2$ hydroxyethylation<br>$C_6$ hydroxyethylation |

concentration of the plasma substitute is indicated by the manufacturer, for instance, 6% or 10% (Table 26).

Not only the concentration itself is of importance but also whether it is a well-balanced oncotic or a hyperoncotic solution. This depends on how much free water can be bound additionally by the solution. The 10% dextran 40 solution binds an additional 100% of its volume; the same can be said of 10% Haes 200/0.62, and 10% Haes 200/0.5 achieves an increase by 50% [206] (Fig. 47).

In order to use the whole volume effect and to achieve optimal hemorheological conditions (Sect. 3.4.5.5) an appropriate additional quantity of fluid in the form of an electrolyte solution must be infused together with the plasma substitute since the patients are generally dehydrated, and free water is not available. This additional quantity of fluid is not necessary with 6% Haes 200/0.5. The 6% solutions therefore simplify the performance of the infusion treatment, but the volume effect is weaker.

The mean molecular weight (MW) is given in daltons. Since dextran 40 is hardly metabolized, the size of the molecule is decisive for the renal output and

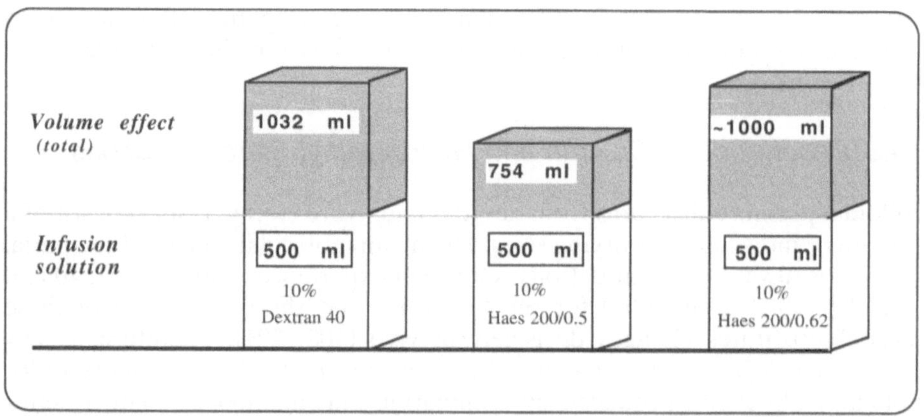


**Fig. 47.** Volume effect of 10% dextran 40, 10% Haes 200/0.5, and 10% Haes 200/0.62. (From [206])

the location of the dextran particles in the body. In contrast, the hydroxyethyl starch molecules are split by amylases. The size of the initial starch molecules, i.e., the mean initial MW given on the infusion solutions, is of minor importance for the decomposition velocity. The degree and kind of substitution is important. The higher the hydroxyethylation and the $C_2/C_6$ hydroxyethylation proportion, the slower the starch is metabolized.

### *3.4.4 Metabolism and Elimination of Plasma substitutes and the Consequences for an In Vivo Effect*

Dextran and hydroxyethyl starch solutions contain molecules of different sizes. The MW distributions of 10% dextran 40, 10% Haes 200/0.5, and 10% Haes 200/0.62 are given in Fig. 48. After the infusion they are metabolized differently, renally eliminated, or stored in the reticuloendothelial system, which changes their in vivo composition. With dextran 40 the renal output is dominant. The small molecules passing the kidney are eliminated, and the large ones accumulate during the course of long-term treatment [108, 221]. As a result, dextran 40 with a mean initial molecular weight of 52 kDa is no longer in the blood, but dextran molecules with a MW of 102 kDa are. The increase in large dextran molecules, which can barely leave the circulation, is responsible for the pharmacokinetic, hemorheological, hemostatic, and hemodynamic behavior (Table 27).

The slow elimination of the dextran molecules leads to a significantly long-lasting volume effect. In contrast to the small dextran molecules, the large ones increase the SEA because they are able to bind the erythrocytes due to their length. Since the large molecules are enhanced in the course of long-term treatment, the dextran concentration in the blood and the PV increase (Sect. 3.4.5.3). The coagulation parameters are shifted in the direction of hemorrhagic diathesis, and thrombocyte aggregation is reduced (Sect. 3.4.5.4).

**Table 27.** Survey of the mean in vitro and in vivo molecular weights (within 9 or 10 days of infusion) of 10% dextran 40, 10% Haes 200/0.5, and 10% Haes 200/0.62 and the consequences for the hemodynamic, hemorheological, and hemostatic parameters

| | 10% Dextran 10 | 10% Haes 200/0.62 | 10% Heas 200/0.5 |
|---|---|---|---|
| Mean molecolar weight<br>In vitro (infusion solution)<br>In vivo (9–10 days) | 52 000<br>102 000 | 270 000<br>120 000 | 200 000<br>37 000 |
| Hematocrit in vivo | ↓↓ | ↓↓ | ↓ |
| Erythrocyte aggregation in vivo | ↑↑ | ↑↓ | ↓ |
| Plasma viscosity in vivo | ↑↑ | ↑↑ | ↓ |
| Thrombocyte aggregation in vivo | ↓ | (↓) | ∅ |
| Partial thromboplastin time in vivo | ↑↑ | ↑↑ | ∅ |
| Factor VIII/vWF complex in vivo | ↓↓ | ↓↓ | ∅ |

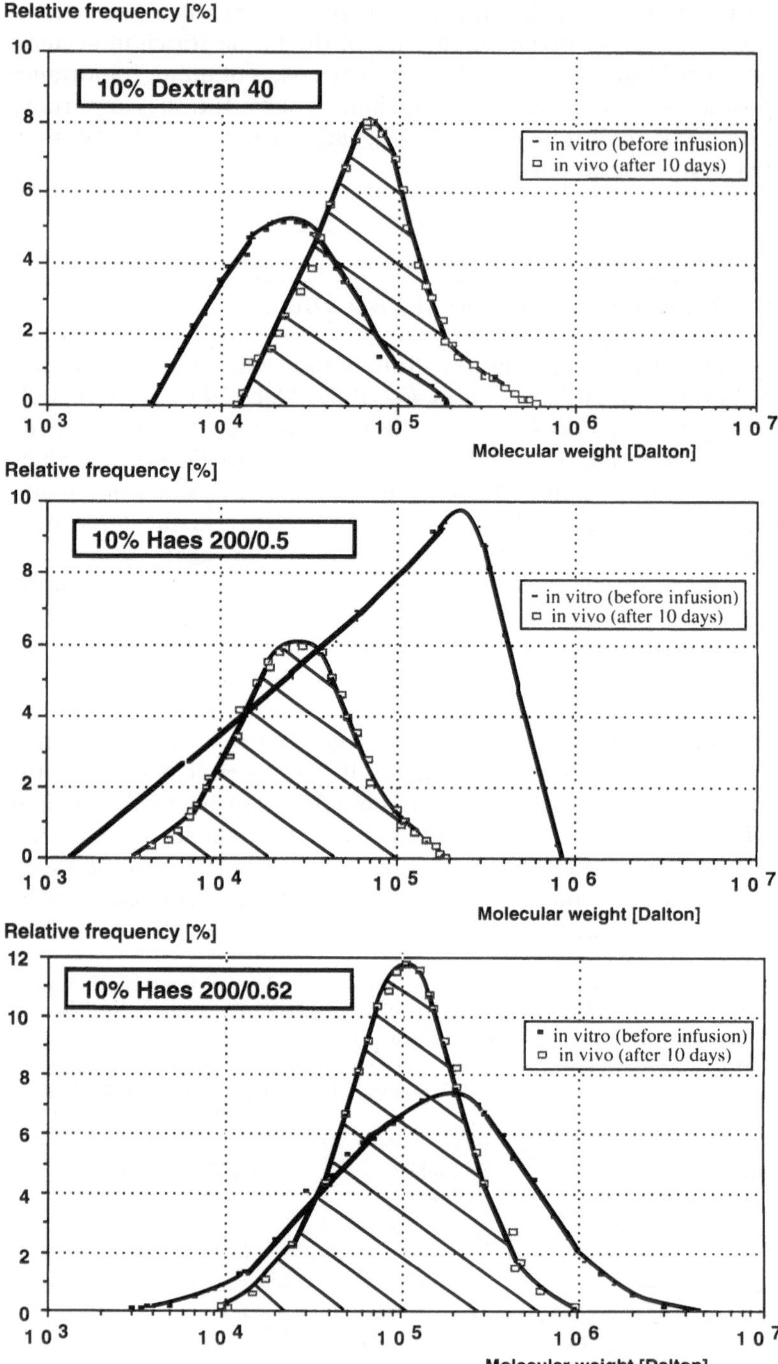


**Fig. 48.** Molecular weight distribution of 10% dextran 40, 10% Haes 200/0.5, and 10% Haes 200/0.62 in the initial solutions (in vitro) and in the blood after long-term treatment (in vivo)

To slow the catabolism of the starch it is hydroxyethylated. Haes 200/0.5 has a diffuse asymmetric MW distribution. In vivo it is rapidly split so that only low-MW starch molecules (37 kDa) are responsible for the in vivo effects. The half-life and thus the duration of the Hct-reducing effect is shorter than that of dextran 40.

Of the starch solutions that we have tested Haes 200/0.5 reduces SEA and PV most clearly without exerting a negative effect on coagulation values. Haes 200/0.62 has an average symmetric molecular weight distribution of 270 kDa (Fig. 48). It is split more slowly, and some large molecules are hardly decomposed, which results in a mean MW 120 kDa. The volume effect, taken from the Hct, is accordingly pronounced and long-lasting. The SEA can increase by a quick and decrease by a slow infusion. The PV increases due to the accumulation of large molecules in the course of long-term treatment (Sect. 3.4.5.3). The factor VIII complex is also influenced and leads to an increase in partial thromboplastin time (PTT).

## 3.4.5 *Hemorheological and Hemostatic Effects of Dextran 40 and Hydroxyethyl Starch Solutions*

For the clinician it often is difficult to form a general idea about the different effects of various substances from single findings. This is even more difficult in the case of plasma substitutes since their qualities change in vivo and depend on the duration and velocity of the infusion (Sect. 3.4.4). Therefore, the effects of 10% Haes 200/0.5, 10% dextran 40, and 10% Haes 200/0.62 are described below in terms of the loading dose and long-term treatment. The three infusion schemes are not completely identical but do not differ in general with the exception that the dose in the long-term treatment with 10% Haes 200/0.62 is 500 ml once during the first four days.

In principle, the treatment consists of a loading dose which was generally performed iso- or hypervolemically depending on the Hct value. A long-term treatment with a high dose over 4 days (except with Haes 200/0.62) and a reduced dose over 5 or 6 days follows.

**Loading dose**

Hct ≥ 42%: 450 ml phlebotomy
Hct 40%–42%: 300 ml phlebotomy

Simultaneous infusion of 500 ml of the respective plasma substitute and in addition 500 ml of an electrolyte solution (Elomel)

**Long-term treatment**

10% Haes 200/0.5 (Haes steril 10%)

1st– 4th days: 2×500 ml 10% Haes 200/0.5 each time within 12 h; 2×500 ml electrolyte solution each time within 12 h

5th–10th days: 1×500 ml 10% Haes 200/0.5 each time within 12 h; 1×500 ml electrolyte solution each time within 12 h

10% dextran 40 (dextran 40 electrolyte free)

1st–4th days: 2×500 ml dextran 40 each time within 6 h after each dextran infusion each time 1×500 ml electrolyte solution within 6 h

5th–10th days: 1×500 ml 10% dextran 40 after each dextran infusion 1×500 ml electrolyte solution

10% Haes 200/0.62 (Elohaest)

1st– 9th days: 1×500 ml Haes 200/0.62 within 12 h in addition 1×500 ml electrolyte solution

Concerning further details refer to the original studies [108, 111].

### 3.4.5.1 Hematocrit

As described in Sect. 3.4.4, it is not the hemorheological in vitro qualities of the dextran and starch solutions that are decisive for the biological effects but the qualities of the different plasma substitute compositions which are produced in the blood. The effect on Hct depends mainly on volume binding and plasma half-life (Fig. 49). Haes 200/0.62 has the greatest of these and due to its long half-life also has the most constant Hct-reducing effect, followed by 10% Haes 200/0.5 and 10% dextran 40. Haes 200/0.5 has the advantage of not accumulating. It has the shortest effect, and repeated infusions are necessary to produce a lasting Hct reduction. The volume effect of 10% Haes 200/0.62 is so great that rather than 500 ml per day, half of this volume would be sufficient for a long-term hemodilution treatment in cerebral infarction. The dose reduction would also reduce the hemodynamic effect but diminish the undesired increase in PV.

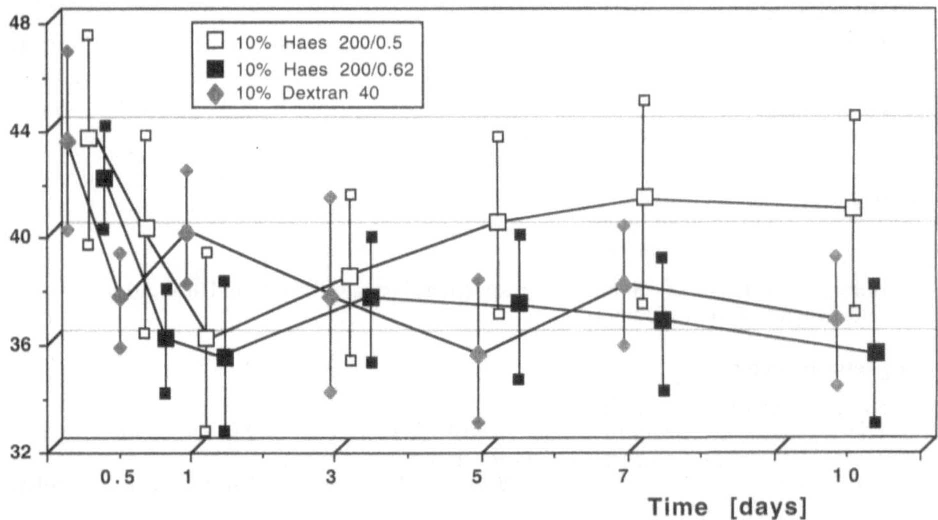


**Fig. 49.** Effect on Hct of long-term infusion treatment with 10% Haes 200/0.5, 10% Haes 200/0.62, and 10% dextran 40

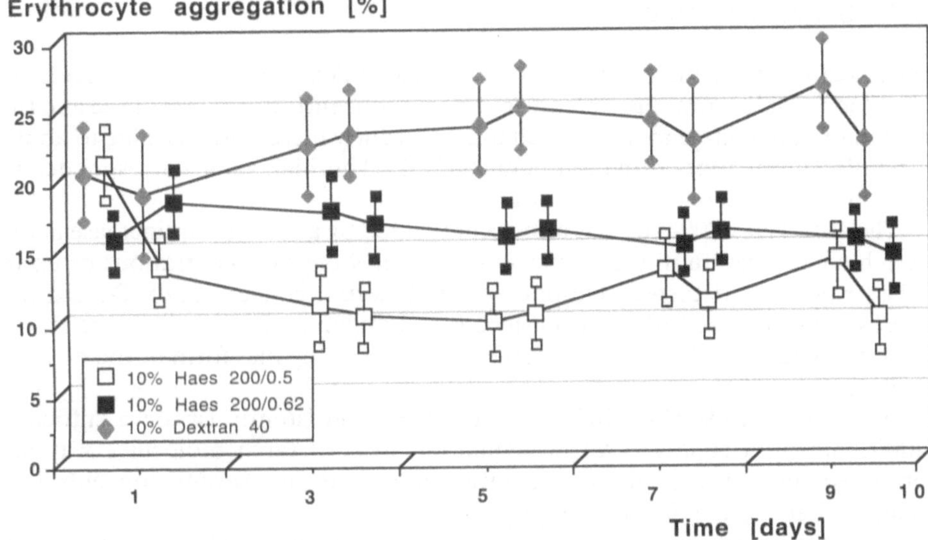


**Fig. 50.** Effect on SEA by long-term infusion treatment with 10% Haes 200/0.5, 10% Haes 200/0.62, and 10% dextran 40

### 3.4.5.2 Erythrocyte Aggregation

SEA clearly reflects the different biological effects of the dextran and starch solutions (Fig. 50). The dextran effect on SEA depends on infusion velocity, infused quantity, and duration of treatment. Since dextran 40 was formerly examined only in short-term infusions of 30–60 min, the small molecules dominate and lead to a decrease in SEA. This effect is quickly reversed in the case of a prolonged infusion period, and the large molecules increase SEA continuously during long-term treatment. Each single infusion led to an increase in SEA by 4%. After a 5-day infusion of 500 ml twice a day, SEA increased by 25%.

The highest SEA reduction was observed with Haes 200/0.5 during both short-term infusion and long-term treatment. A single infusion reduced SEA by 15% and the 5-day infusion treatment by 53%. Therefore, the disaggregating effect of the small molecules reduces SEA optimally.

The 10% Haes 200/0.62 increased SEA during the loading dose by 15%, but then reduced it during the 5-day long-term infusion by 8%.

Rapid infusion increased SEA via large molecules whereas during long-term infusion a sufficient number of starch molecules broken up by the α-amlyases were available to guarantee a fall in SEA.

### 3.4.5.3 Plasma Viscosity

PV is a direct measure for the number and size of dextran or starch molecules in the blood. The continuous increase in dextran concentration in the blood and the accumulation of large molecules led to significantly increased PV value to above 1.6 mPas during long-term treatment (Fig. 51). This high value corresponded to a dextran serum concentration of above 20 g/l.

The 10% Haes 200/0.62 was also accompanied by a continuous increase in the starch concentration in the serum so that after 9 days concentrations of up to 20 g/l were also detected. Despite this high serum concentration PV did not increase as much as with dextran since the globular configuration of the starch molecules has a more favourable effect than the string like form of the dextran molecules.

In contrast, 10% Haes 200/0.5 reduced PV consistently (given a sufficient additional fluid supply). An accumulation of the starch molecules was not observed and during the whole infusion period the serum concentration remained at the low level of 10 g/l.

Short-term infusion in the context of the loading dose and long-term infusion over 9 or 10 days led to an increase in PV by 4% or 24% with 10% dextran 40 and by 7% or 18.5% with 10% Haes 200/0.62, whereas 10% Haes 200/0.5 reduced it by 1% or 9%, respectively.

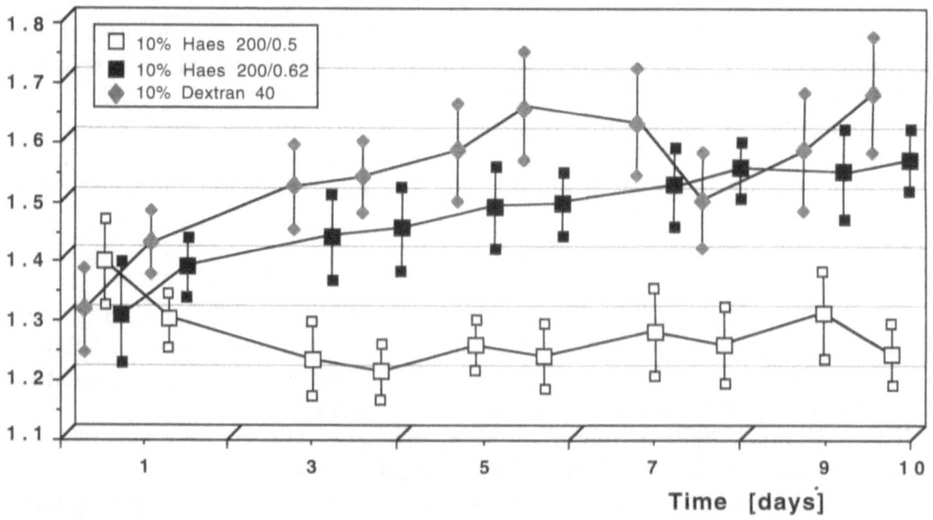


**Fig. 51.** Effect on PV by long-term infusion treatment with 10% Haes 200/0.5, 10% Haes 200/0.62, and 10% dextran 40

### 3.4.5.4 Thrombocyte Aggregation and Coagulation Parameters

With regard to thrombocyte aggregation there is a fundamental difference between dextran 40 and the substituted starch of middle grade. Whereas dextran 40 clearly inhibits the spontaneous and induced thrombocyte aggregation, 10% Haes 200/0.5 dues not have a considerable influence on the two thrombocyte function tests (Figs. 52, 53). Haes 200/0.62 takes a half-way position, i.e., a slightly reversible inhibition of the spontaneous aggregation was demonstrated.

A greater inhibition of thrombocyte aggregation (but weaker than with dextran) is found with administration of the high-MW and highly substituted starch as for example hetastarch 450/0.7. Thus, Haes 200/0.5 has the essential advantage of having no clinically relevant influence on this part of the coagulation cascade so that there need be no fear of hemorrhagic diathesis with a normal dosage and normal coagulation parameters. Therefore, this plasma substitute is suitable for the acute use.

In 1987 reports about severe cerebral hemorrhages during subarachnoid hemorrhage after the use of high-MW highly substituted hetastarch 450/0.7 were especially alarming [101]. Our examinations of the coagulation system showed that this is a volume- and starch-dependent effect. Hitherto, changes in blood coagulation after dextran 40 have been known. Figure 54 shows the effect of the three plasma substitutes on PTT. It is of particular importance that 10% Haes 200/0.5 does not influence this coagulation parameter apart from the dilution effect. In contrast to this, 10% dextran 40 and 10% Haes 200/0.62 led to a *dose-dependent PTT increase during long-term treatment*. These changes provoke no hemorrhage under normal conditions but could become dangerous in the case of disturbed coagulation, for example, during a subarachnoid hemorrhage. The use of Haes 200/0.62 or dextran 40 is not allowed in these cases. The essential cause of this disturbed coagulatin was revealed by additional examinations [110]. This was an effect on the factor VIII/von Willebrand factor complex, the three parameters of which are shown in Figure 55. The activity of factor VIII:c and the Willebrand ristocetin cofactor and the Willebrand factor antigen are reduced by more than 60% during the course of long-term treatment. This drop goes far beyond the dilution effect, is dose dependent, and is only slowly reversible, as is demonstrated by the course between the 9th and 13th days. This is a disturbance in the factor VIII/von Willebrand factor complex which is determined by the nature and degree of substitution of the hydroxyethylation and is provoked by the barely eliminable high-MW starch or dextran molecules. The accumulation of these large molecules in vivo is also decisive for provoking disturbances in coagulation. This shows why this pathological mechanism could not be clarified in vitro.

In the case of a previously existing tendency to hemorrhage dextran 40 and the highly-substituted mean- and high-MW starch solutions can provoke hemorrhagic complications by inhibition of the thrombocyte aggregation and impairment of the factor VIII/von Willebrand factor complex. This is a dose-dependent process which is provoked by the large accumulating dextran and hydroxyethyl starch molecules.

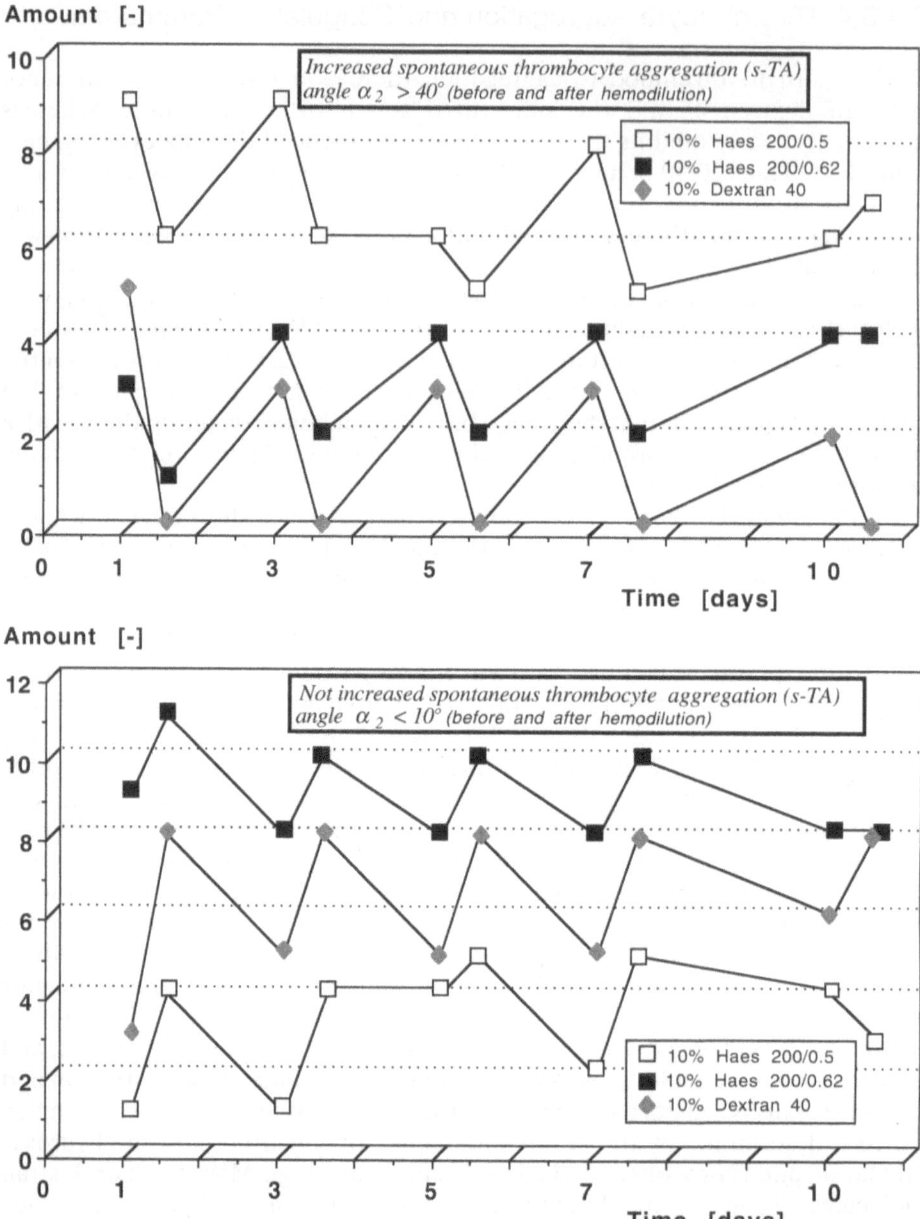


**Fig. 52.** Effect on spontaneous thrombocyte aggregation by long-term infusion treatment with 10% Haes 200/0.5, 10% Haes 200/0.62, and 10% dextran 40

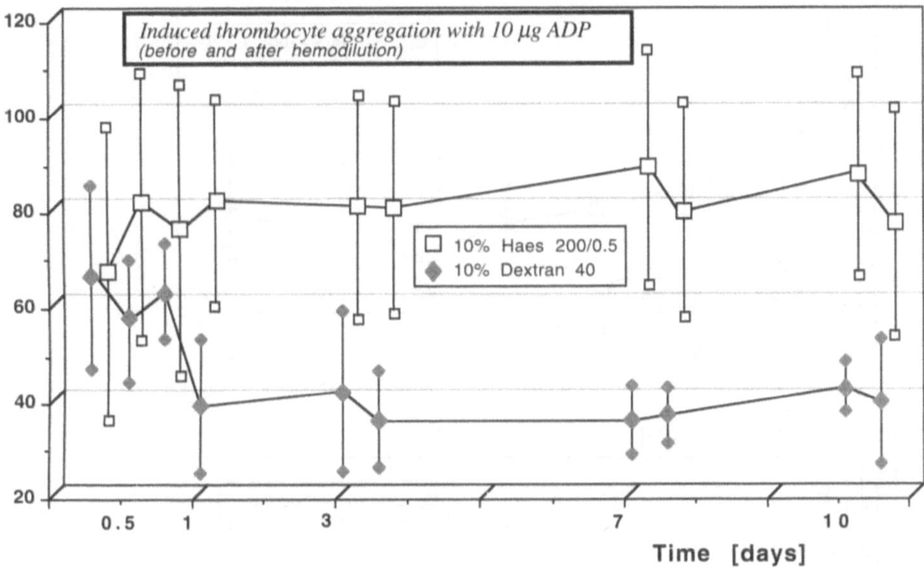


**Fig. 53.** Effect on induced thrombocyte aggregation with 10 µg ADP by long-term infusion treatment with 10% Haes 200/0.5, 10% Haes 200/0.62, and 10% dextran 40

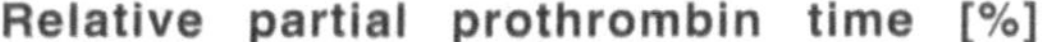

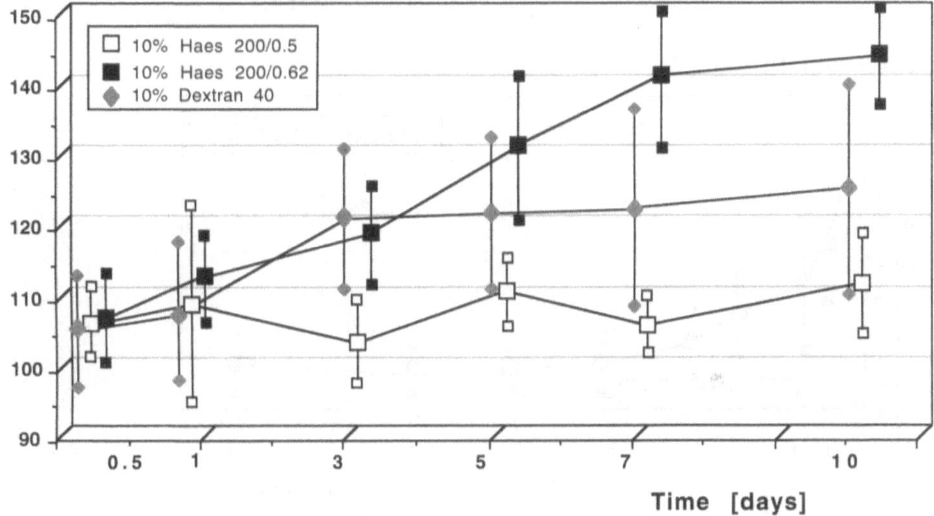


**Fig. 54.** Effect on relative partial prothrombin time by long-term infusion treatment with 10% Haes 200/0.5, 10% Haes 200/0.62, and 10% dextran 40

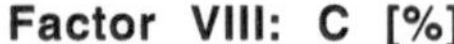


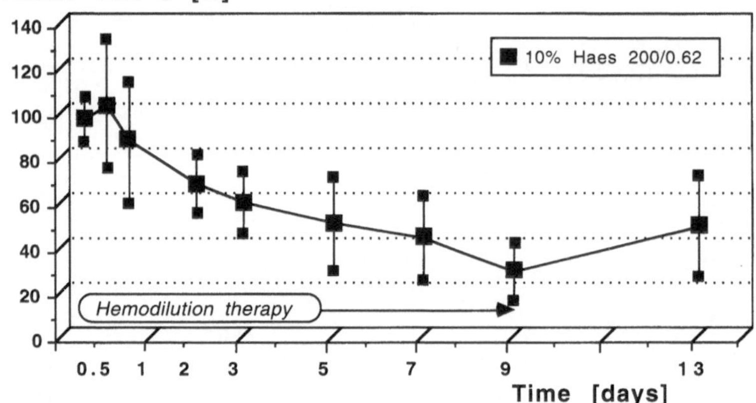


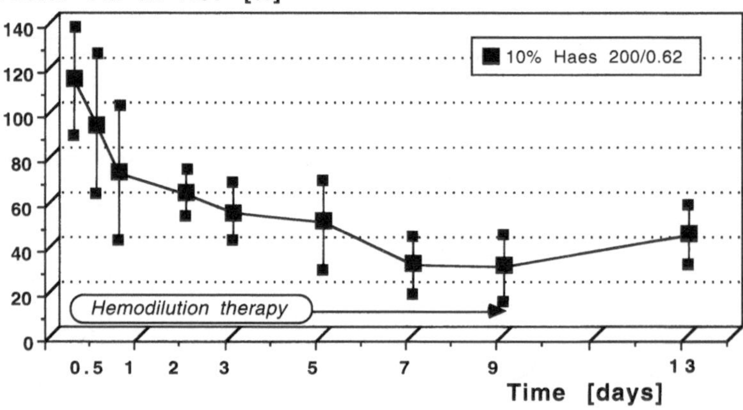


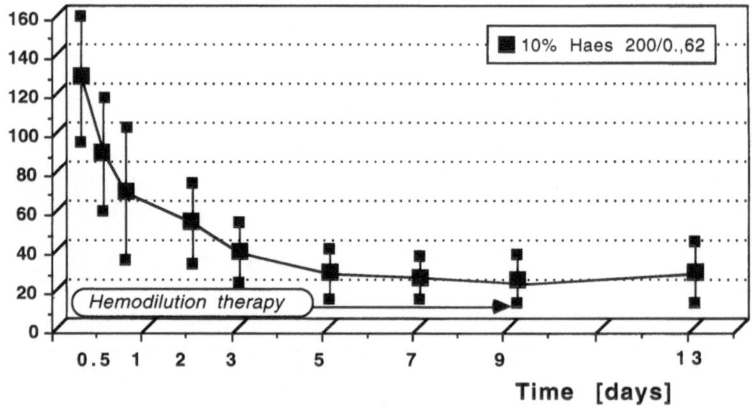


**Fig. 55.** Effect on the activity of factor VIII:C, the Willebrand ristocetin cofactor (*RCF*), and the Willebrand factor antigen (*Ag*) by long-term infusion treatment with 10% Haes 200/0.62

Concerning the moderately substituted mean-MW hydroxyethyl starch, neither coagulation changes were demonstrated to a clinically relevant extent. Thus, this substance is sufficiently safe.

#### 3.4.5.5 Special Hemorheological Problems of Hemodilution with Dextran and Hydroxyethyl Starch

The different in vitro and in vivo effects of dextran and hydroxyethyl starch solutions have confused clinicians unfamiliar with the pharmacological peculiarities. PV can increase if there is insufficient free water in the infusion of a hyperoncotic plasma substitute. Therefore we recommend infusing additionally the same quantity of an electrolyte solution, especially if 10% starch solution are used.

Furthermore, different hemorheological effects can occur following rapid and slow infusions (Sect. 3.4.4). Some authors have claimed to find contradictory effects of hemodilution on PV and SEA – due to their lack of knowledge about their relationships. This is due not to hemodilution itself but to the infusion method or the different biological reactions of the plasma substitutes used. Table 28 summarizes the essential points here.

**Table 28.** Hemorheological problems of hemodilution

| |
|---|
| Causes for the increase in PV and SEA during hemodilution |
| Substance-induced accumulation of large molecules |
| Therapy-induced insufficient free intravascular water |
| *Consequences* |
| Choice of plasma substitutes or their dose so that large molecules do not accumulate |
| Infusion of 10% Haes 200/0.5 with electrolyte solution |
| Infusion of 6% Haes 200/0.5 without electrolyte solution |

### *3.4.6 Hemodilution and Intracranial Pressure*

The results of the Hemodilution in Stroke Study Group [94] have raised the important question of the extent to which hemodilution increases intracranial pressure (ICP). First of all according to the study [401], cited by critics of hemodilution [16], even excessive hemodilution did not lead to a critical increase in ICP. In these experiments, ICP increased only from 6 to 11 mmHg even after a dextran volume infusion of at least 40% of the whole blood volume. This increase is not important when one considers that ICP requires treatment only at values above 20 mmHg. In addition, CBF increased by 40% in the brain area concerned despite this slight ICP increase.

Nevertheless, attention should be paid to the fact that any increase in intravascular and intracranial volume leads to increased ICP. Several authors have found that hemodilution with colloidal plasma substitutes such as dextran and Haes generally leads to less deterioration in ICP and cerebral oedema than treatment with electrolyte solutions. These findings are important for the evaluation of ICP changes with hemodilution (Table 29). ICP increased after NaCl administration by 21 mmHg whereas Haes 450/0.7 increased the pressure only by 2 mmHg [370]. Also, Ringer lactate infusion increased ICP and cerebral oedema of experimental infarctions whereas this was not observed under the same experimental conditions after hypervolemic dextran treatment [134]. In rabbits, the cerebral oedema of embolic cerebral infarctions did not deteriorate after use of low-MW Haes, but the survival probability of the animals improved. In 21 patients with cerebral infarction isovolemic hemodilution with fresh plasma increased CO by 29% and CBF by 30% on the affected side and by 17% on the unaffected side. ICP, however, was increased only from 10.6 to 12.3 mmHg. Therefore, not the ICP increase per se is decisive but the general influence on the cerebral circulation by hemodilution. Here, too, a differentiated and not a superficial delineation is necessary to understand the individual relationships.

**Table 29.** Hemodilution and intracranial pressure

| Authors | – Colloidal plasma substitutes<br>– Kind of hemodilution<br>– Species | Intracranial pressure |
|---|---|---|
| Wood et al. (1982) [400] | – Dextran<br>– 40% total volume increase<br>– Dogs | ICP by only 6 mmHg ↑ |
| Korosue et al. (1988) [215] | – Fresh plasma<br>– 400–1000 ml<br>– Humans | ICP increased only from 10.6 to 12.3 mmHg (16%) ↑ |
| Tu et al. (1988) [372] | – Low-MW dextran<br>– Isovolemic<br>– Dogs | ICP ↑ but less than in the control group |
| Heros and Corosue (1989) [134] | – Low-MW dextran<br>– Hypervolemic, Hct 30%–32%<br>– Dogs | ICP not increased, cerebral edema not aggravated |
| Tranmer et al. (1989) [370] | – Heta-HES 6%, 30 ml $kg^{-1}$ $h^{-1}$<br>– NaCl solution 30 ml $kg^{-1}$ $h^{-1}$<br>– Dogs | ICP by 2 mmHg ↑, ICP by 21 mmHg ↑ ↑ |
| Lyden et al. (1988) [246] | – Heta-HES 6%<br>– Electrolyte solution<br>– Rabbits | Compared with electrolyte solution cerebral edema not aggravated and survival probability even increased |
| Todd et al. (1985) [366] | – isotonic electrolyte solution<br>– Rabbits | ICP ↑ ↑<br>Cerebral edema ↑ ↑ |
| Heros and Korosue (1989) [134] | – Ringer lactate solution<br>– Dogs | ICP ↑ ↑ |

In this connection, a clinically convincing comparison results from the treatment of vasospasms in SAH which are frequently accompanied by a critical ICP increase since in these cases the hypervolemic or hypertensive therapy despite a high ICP influences the clinical condition favourably due to an improved cerebral circulation. Nevertheless, this treatment modality is also limited by the concomitant ICP increase and cannot be performed in an uncontrolled manner. The ICP increase in critical cases should not be under-valued, but the volume load must be adjusted to the development of the ICP. Therefore, in cases of acute cerebral infarction and considerable increase in ICP a loading dose in the form of a rapid infusion should be not given (Sect. 3.4.9.2). Furthermore plasma substitutes of middle grade MW without NaCl are to be preferred.

### *3.4.7 Start of Therapy and Acute Treatment of Ischemic Cerebral Infarctions*

The acute treatment of patients suffering cerebral infarction is started by the family or emergency physician. After diagnosis the question concerning cardiac load capacity, renal function, and ICP arises (Fig. 56). If there is no contrain-

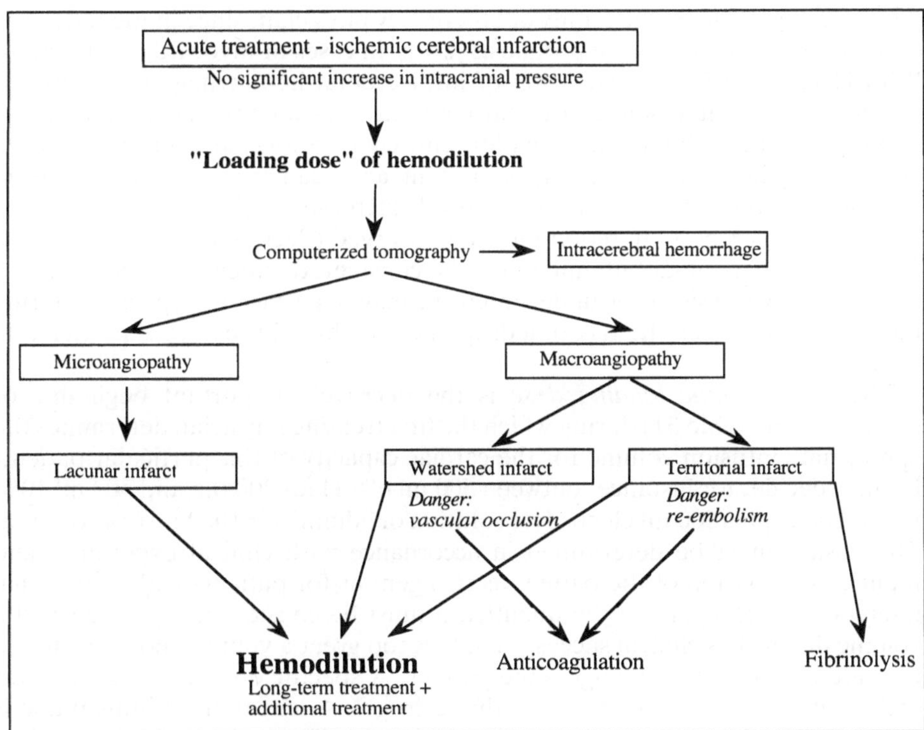


**Fig. 56.** Acute treatment of ischemic cerebral infarction (study schedule)

dication, hemodilution can be started in the form of the loading dose for quick volume substitution and improved cerebral blood flow.

Hospitalization follows, during which computer tomography is performed under continuation of long-term hemodilution treatment. It reveals an intracerebral hemorrhage and indicates a macro- or microangiopathy. During further clinical evalation it is decided how hemodilution is to be continued, or whether anticoagulation or fibrinolysis should be performed. During acute treatment, optimal lung, heart, and circulatory functions are of primary importance (Table 30).

*Optimal $O_2$* supply is guaranteed by an unobstructed respiratory system and possibly the administration of $O_2$ through a nasal tube. In the case of losing consciousness early intubation to assist additional cerebral oedema treatment should be performed. *Cardiac output* requires special attention since the circulation of the penumbra depends crucially on this due to the disturbed autoregulation. Because of the volume load by hemodilution rapid digitalization in proper dosage is indicated if there are no special contraindications. Moreover, hemodynamically detrimental dysrhythmias must be given priority treatment.

The *hemodynamics* are improved by the loading dose for the compensation of the often existing volume deficiency (Table 31). Since CO should be elevated to increase blood flow in the penumbra, only hypervolemic and not isovolemic hemodilution must be given (Sect. 3.3.5). This should be started as early as possible, if possible by the family or emergency physician, since immediate start of treatment here affects the prognosis just as in cases of myocardial infarction. With Haes 200/0.5 prior exclusion of intracerebral hemorrhage by computed tomography is not essential (as earlier with dextran 40) due to the minor influence on thrombocyte aggregation and coagulation parameters. Thus, an enormous gain in time is possible, but in accordance with clinical criteria contraindications such as a pronounced increase in ICP in ischemic or hemorrhagic cerebral infarction must be observed (Sect. 3.4.9.2). In addition, the use of dopamine-dobutamine must be considered under the supervision of an emergency physician or under intensive care supervision, especially during the night hours when the risk of a drop in CO or blood pressure is particularly high.

The *hypervolemic loading dose* is the decisively important beginning of hemodilution (Table 31) during which the first treating physician determines the appropriate infusion volume for the cardiac capacity of this particular patient. He may decide, for instance, between 500 ml 6% Haes 200/0.5 and 500 ml 10% Haes 200/0.5 plus 500 ml electrolyte solution or administer 1000 ml 6% solution. The dosage must be determined in accordance with clinical experience and requires supervision of the patient as stringent as for patients with moycardial infarction. With regard to the quantity, it must be considered that too small a volume diminishes clinical success, and that too great a volume, not adjusted to the cardiac situation, endangers the patient. A specific dosage is necessary (as with antihypertensives or anti-arrhythmic drugs). A schematic treatment that is the same for all patients is not possible. This is justified only to obtain standard clinical examination records. We think that phlebotomy in an acute situation is

**Table 30.** Special acute measures during emergency treatment of acute ischemic cerebral infarction

*Optimal $O_2$ supply*

Keeping the respiratory system unobstructed
Possibly $O_2$ tube
Possibly early intubation

*Improvement in cardiac output*

Digitalization, intravenous rapid saturation
Treatment of hemodynamically detrimental dysrhythmia

*Improvement in hemodynamics*

Compensation of the volume deficiency and cardiac output by hypervolemic hemodilution
Possibly dopamine-dobutamine infusion

*Improvement in cerebral macro- and microcirculation*

Hypervolemic hemodilution with moderately substituted hydroxyethyl starch or albumin, adjusted to the cardiac load capacity
Optimal hematocrit at 40%, in cases of polycythemia and secondary hyperglobulinemia at 45%

*Control of blood pressure*

Optimal systolic blood pressure 140–180 mmHg
Caution: rapid and significant decrease in blood pressure! (only values > 180–200 mmHg must be treated)
Caution: diuretics due to the increase in Hct and PV!
Hypertension: volume administration, dopamine-dobutamine infusion

*Adjustment of blood pressure*

Optimal value below 120 mg/dl as otherwise this worsens the prognosis of cerebral infarctions

*Treatment of cerebral oedema*

Elevation of the upper part of the body
Putting the head straight
Administration of hyperosmotic substances: glycerol orally or intravenously, sorbitol intravenously
Not indicated: cortisone or quickly effective diuretics

*Inhibition of thrombocyte aggregation*

Only if an intracerebral hemorrhage is excluded: acetylsalicylic acid (500 mg intravenously)

*Thrombosis prophylaxis*

Low-dose heparinization ($3 \times 5000$ IU)

*Additional treatment*

Possibly: hemorheologically effective substances: naftidrofuryl, pentoxifylline
Possibly: calcium antagonist nimodipine
Anticoagulation in cases of high-risk of further embolism
Fibrinolysis only after strict indication

**Table 31.** Hemodilution scheme in acute ischemic cerebral infarction

1st day:

Acute rapid infusion loading dose: 500 ml 6% or 10% Haes 200/0.5 (low sodium) within 45–60 min (contraindication: acute increase in intracranial pressure; mild intracerebral bleeding is not a contraindication)

Long-term hemodilution treatment: 1 or 2 × 500 ml 6% or 10% Haes 200/0.5 (low-sodium) for 6–12 h each time

During the infusion of 10% Haes always add the same volume of electrolyte solution (low-sodium)

No interruption of the infusion treatment during the night

Volume load should be according to cardiac capacity

2nd day, possibly also 3rd day: 1 or 2 × 500 ml 6% or 10% Haes 200/0.5 (low-sodium) for 6–12 h each time

4th to 10th day: 1 × 500 ml 6% or 10% Haes 200/0.5 (low-sodium) for 6–12 h each time

Begin the treatment as soon as possible, possibly acute treatment by the family or emergency physician
Volume should be according to cardiac load capacity
Decrease Hct by about 12%–15%
If possible, increase CO
Decrease in Hct can become detrimental for CO, therefore acutely no phlebotomy
If Hct after 24 h > 45%, isovolemic hemodilution

Additional therapy:
Digitalization according to clinical findings
3 × 5000 IU heparin subcutaneously as prophylaxis
After exclusion of an intracerebral bleed: 1st to 3rd days: 1 × 500 mg acetylsalicylic acid intravenously; from 4th day on: 1 × 500 mg or 2 × 250 mg tablets

Cave at: cardiac volume load

Measurement of heart rate and blood pressure: are not allowed to increase
Auscultation of the lung: moist rale: breaking off (insufficiency of the left heart)
Creatinine determination twice per week: is not allowed to exceed 2.0 mg/dl with an initial value < 1.5 mg/dl

Cave at: hypovolemia in isovolemic hemodilution and decrease in CO

Infusion always started before phlebotomy at the other arm (two intravenous routes)
Phlebotomy at the other arm never faster than the infusion (two intravenous routes)

not useful due to the possibly decreased CO (Sect. 3.3.5). This would only be appropriate in addition to the hypervolemic loading dose at an extremely high Hct which was not sufficiently reduced by the loading dose. If possible, sodium chloride-free or -poor plasma substitutes should be used to avoid the development of cerebral oedema. Balanced, possibly potassium-rich electrolyte solutions instead of physiological sodium chloride solutions are useful. The "optimal Hct" is about 40%; somewhat lower values are tolerable. In cases of polycythemia and secondary haemoconcentration a level of about 45% is recommended. The contraindications are summarized in Table 32.

**Table 32.** Contraindications to acute hemodilution treatment

| |
|---|
| Decompensated heart failure |
| Acute myocardial infarction |
| Renal insufficiency (serum creatinine not allowed to exceed 2.0 mg/dl at an initial value of 1.5 mg/dl |
| Systolic blood pressure ≥ 200 mmHg |
| Hematocrit< 34% |
| Tendency to hemorrhage |
| Hypersensitivity toward hydroxyethyl starch |
| Significant increase in intracranial pressure |
| Considerable space-occupying intracerebral hemorrhage |

The control of *blood pressure* is of special importance since optimal perfusion of the penumbra depends directly on the blood pressure. Therefore, a quick reduction is not useful, and the often reactively slightly increased values should be tolerated. Systolic values between 140 and 180 mmHg are optimal. Values above 200/120 mmHg require a slight reduction. A decrease in blood pressure should be carried out only with the greatest care, in low doses, and with repeated administration of drugs to avoid provoking a significant drop in blood pressure. Since in elderly and hypertensive persons the cerebral autoregulation is shifted toward higher values, high blood pressure values are better tolerated, and due to the so-called "resetting" and the decrease in sensitivity of the baroreceptor reflex lower values lead to a cerebral hypoperfusion [217].

The strong dependence of the cerebral circulation on blood pressure in these cases is clear. This is further supported by the observation that early mobilization did not prove useful due to the possibility of a drop in the blood pressure and an increased danger of reinfarction. Therefore, the patient should not leave his bed during the first few days [253].

The *administration of diuretics* is not useful due to the frequent hypovolemia and generalized dehydration in the elderly because of reduced extracellular fluid (by 40%) caused by old age and increased Hct. It must be restricted to special indications such as acute pulmonary oedema.

*Low blood pressure values* make adequate treatment necessary. Combined with the administration of a suitable volume early dopamine-dobutamine therapy can be considered. But these possibilities have not yet been tried sufficiently during hemodilution.

According to clinical and animal experiments, the *blood sugar adjustment* to values below 120 mg% improves the prognosis in the cerebral infarction [112, 337]. High sugar values worsen cerebral oedema and have a negative effect due to an increase in lactate acidosis. Since reactively elevated values are frequent in cerebral stroke patients, the administration of insulin may become necessary for rapid reduction.

The *treatment of cerebral oedema* is discussed in detail in Sect. 3.4.9.2. In the acute case there are simple but very effective measures such as elevation of the upper part of the body to a position of 30°, straight position of the head for a better venous drainage, and rapid infusion of hyperosmotic substances.

Cortisone did not prove to be effective in cerebral infarctions, and the World Health Organization regards its use as "more harmful than good" in its report on cerebral infarction. Diuretics are also not indicated since they can worsen microcirculatory disturbances and thus threaten the development of cerebral oedema by increasing the Hct level.

The *inhibition of thrombocyte aggregation* can be considered only after exclusion of an intracerebral hemorrhage (Sect. 3.4.9.3).

Prophylactic anticoagulation using low-dose heparinization should be undertaken on broad indications. An intracerebral hemorrhage and even subarachnoid hemorrhage are not contraindications if high bolus administration is avoided.

## 3.4.8 Long-Term Hemodilution Treatment

The narrow therapeutic window in ischemic cerebral infarctions means that the best treatment is one which is undertaken within the first hours. The loading dose is follwed by a long-term treatment closely related to the cardiac capacity. Previously, the high-dose phase was 4 days. Since, according to PET examinations, the first 36–48 h is the crucial period, high-dose treatment today is continued for 2–3 days (Table 31). Depending on practicability, 6% or 10% starch solutions can be used, the latter together with an appropriate electrolyte solution. There is no strictly limited period for the subsequent therapy, but this is generally 6–10 days, with half the quantity in volume.

## 3.4.9 Additional Drug Treatment

### 3.4.9.1 Blood Pressure and Blood Sugar

For long-term treatment the same principles apply as for the acute phase (Sect. 3.4.7). Sufficient perfusion pressure and low blood sugar values are decisive.

### 3.4.9.2 Treatment of Increased Intracranial Pressure

As explained in Sect. 3.4.6, any increase in intravascular volume elevates ICP. However, several examinations show that the infusion of colloidal plasma substitutes such as hydroxyethyl starch influences the development of a cerebral oedema more favourably than the administration of electrolyte solutions alone. Consequently, increased ICP does not exclude hemodilution, but an improvement in the microcirculatory disturbance in the area of a cerebral oedema can be expected at an adjusted dosage. For this reason, a quick and considerable volume supply, for instance with the loading dose, should only not be performed if ICP is considerably increased. As mentioned above, treatment of vasospastic cerebral infarctions in subarachnoid hemorrhage demonstrates that a hypervolemic, hypertensive therapy can also be successful in the case of cerebral oedema with increased ICP. A life-threatening increase in ICP in which the loading dose should generally not be given occurs during considerable intracerebral hemorrhages or severe ischemic cerebral infarctions. These clinical pictures can be easily diagnosed due to symptoms such as oppressive headache, disturbed consciousness, psychomotor restlessness, visual axis deviation, mydriasis in the late stage, and bilateral positive Babinski signs. In contrast to the acutely not necessary distinguishing nature of the ischemic infarction versus small intracerebral hemorrhages or slight increases in ICP these clinical pictures cause no differential-diagnostic difficulties (Table 33).

**Table 33.** Clinical features of the intracranial increase in pessure

| |
|---|
| Headache |
| Depressed level of consciousness |
| Psychomotor restlessness |
| Nausea, vomiting |
| Mydriasis, only if ICP > 40 mmHg |
| Disturbed consciousness |

Apart from very young patients with considerable lesions, ICP in ischemic cerebral infarctions is not considerably increased during the first hours but develops to a maximum within the following 24–48 h.

The first measures in treatment are elevation of the upper part of the body into a position of 30° and a straight position of the head (Table 34). The next step is the use of hyperosmotic substances, among which glycerol is to be preferred due to its long period of action. Because of the smaller fluid load we prefer the pharmaceutically prepared highly concentrated oral form. In contrast to parenteral infusion, no hemolysis can occur during oral adminstration. Prior to the first oral administration metoclopramide is injected intravenously for the purpose of preventing nausea or vomiting. Thirty minutes after the oral glycerol bolus, absorption is tested by an osmolality determination since in about 5% of the patients a deficient enteral uptake occurs [107]. Furthermore, the blood sugar must be carefully monitored since it may rise during this therapy and increase the osmolality. Possibly, the value must be kept below 120 mg% with insulin. At the same dose level in grams the period of action of glycerol is about twice as long as that of sorbitol or mannitol. The intravenous infusion of 10% glycerol should not last longer than 4 h as otherwise no osmolality gradient is achieved due to the rapid degradation, and the glycerol nourishes the patient but is useless for the treatment of ICP.

Serum osmolality is not allowed to increase above 340 mosmol/l in order to avoid hyperosmotic coma. It is at least unclear if not nonsensical to talk about a "target osmolality" which should be achieved since no definite osmolality value is decisive for its effect but only the osmolality gradient between plasma and the cerebral extracellular space. Generally speaking, the osmolality should be kept at the lowest possible level. A steady increase in osmolality by sorbitol or glycerol involves the danger of a penetration of the substances into neural

**Table 34.** The treatment of cerebral oedema in stroke

Elevation (30°)
Putting the head straight
Hyperosmotic substances

Glycerol orally: 50 g; 40%–45% solution
Glycerol intravenously: 10% solution, 500 ml 2–4 h; caution: blood sugar, hemolysis!
Sorbitol intravenously: 50 g; 40% solution, shorter effect
Mannitol intravenously: 50 g, 20% solution; caution: haemoconcentration!
Oral glycerol bolus therapy

Low dosage: 1 or 2 × 50 g glycerol
Mean dosage: 3 or 4 × 50 g glycerol
High dosage: 4 or 5 × 50 g glycerol
(50 g glycerol = 125 ml 40% solution for oral use)

(Prior to the first oral administration of glycerol, metoclopramide, 1 ampule intravenously, e.g., Paspertin, to avoid nausea and vomiting)

Treatment of increased intracranial pressure

Pressure values (ICP) > 20 mmHg: require treatment
Pressure values (ICP) ~ 30 mmHg: 2–4 × 50 g glycerol
Pressure values (ICP) 30–40 mmHg: 4 × 50 g glycerol alternating with 4 × 50 g sorbitol
Pressure values (ICP)< 25 mmHg: 1 × 50 g glycerol (~ 1 × 4–8 h active period), 1 × 50 g sorbitol (~ 2–3 h active period)
Pressure values (ICP) > 35 mmHg: 1 × 50 g glycerol (~ 3.5–4 h active period), 1 × 50 g sorbitol (~ 1.5 h active period)
(50 g glycerol = 125 ml 40% solution for oral use; 50 g sorbitol = 125 ml 40% solution for intravenous administration

General comments
Avoidance of serum osmolality > 340 mosmol/l
Avoidance of blood sugar concentration > 120 mg/dl

Intubation, mechanical respiration ($pCO_2$ = 25–30 mmHg)
Tromethamine intravenously, 1 or 2 mmol/kg BW, in 10 or 25 min
Caution: respiratory depression!

In ischemic cerebral infarctions
No cortisone
No fast-acting diuretics

tissue and thereby creating a "rebound" effect. Therefore, short bolus administrations of 50 g are to be preferred.

If the ICP increases considerably, early intubation and mechanical respiration with slight hyperventilation is necessary ($pCO_2$ 25–30 mmHg). THAM has also proven to be an ICP-reducing agent, but it can lead to respiratory depression so that its use must be restricted to patients who are already or can be supplied with oxygen.

There are not sufficient data concerning the efficacy of cortisone in the treatment of ischemic cerebral infarctions in man, in contrast to other indications and animal experiments.

Due to haemoconcentration therapy with rapid-acting diuretics for ICP reduction is considered to be not useful.

Mannitol thickens the blood after an initial hemodilution caused by osmosis. This is due to increased diuresis so that the cerebral blood flown is then disturbed after an acute temporary improvement as CBF measurements have shown (Table 34).

#### 3.4.9.3 Acetylsalicylic Acid, Low-Dose Heparinization, and Hemorheological Substances

Acetylsalicylic acid (ASA) is firmly established in secondary prophylaxis after cardiac or cerebral infarction [102]. The ISIS-II study investigating myocardial infarctions demonstrated that ASA increases the percentage of finally recanalized coronary arteries even during acute treatment. Two similiar observations have shown that ASA also improves the prognosis of the acute course in cerebral infarction [95]. Therefore, we administer ASA immediately after exclusion of intracranial hemorrhage by computed tomography in the form of a rapid parenteral infusion over 3 days for a faster and more effective onset of action. The rapid infusion of ASA is necessary since this substance is not stable and changes from the dissolved state into salicylic acid after a period of more than 30 min, which is ineffective for this range of indications.

Low-dose heparinization is always indicated in bed-ridden patients with paresis for thrombosis prophylaxis. Since in patients with disturbed coagulation and thrombocyte dysfunctions hemorrhagic complications can appear with the combination of heparin and ASA, observation is necessary [406]. During our 10 years of experience with this combination we have observed no corresponding complication. For safety we do not administer ASA with anticoagulation (Sect. 3.6.2).

The hemorheological substances naftidrofuryl and pentoxifylline improve erythrocyte aggregation. However, to what extent they improve prognosis through their hemorheological effect and if they have an additional influence on the cerebral metabolism in acute cerebral infarction has not yet been demonstrated beyond doubt [118, 289, 327]. This may result from difficulties concerning the examination technique since efficacy was proven for other indications such as PAVD. According to our examinations, Tebonin, which increases CBF upon acute administration [130], develops this effect by a reduction in Hct. There is not sufficient clinical experience with regard to its efficacy in cases of cerebral infarction.

A subject scarcely considered clinically is the inhibition of leucocyte adhesivity for the reduction of reperfusion damage, which is very important judging by animal experiments in myocardial infarction [323]. Clinically available substances are piracetam [135] and ASA.

## 3.5 Clinical Results of a Double-Blind, Placebo-Controlled, Randomized Iso- and Hypervolemic Hemodilution Study

A. Haass, I. Decker, G. Hamann, M. Stoll, and U. Kässer

A study recently completed by us demonstrated the greater efficacy of hemodilution therapy compared to infusion treatment with electrolyte solution [104].

### 3.5.1 Patients and Methods

The study included 45 patients with acute cerebral infarction in the area of the middle cerebral artery. The therapy was started within 12–24 h after the acute stroke. Patients whose symptoms were only moderate or showed a tendency to recede prior to randomization were excluded. The final outcome was judged by the neurological deficit and the degree of handicap.

Randomization allocated 26 patients to the Haes and 19 to the placebo group. The statistical evaluation was conducted with all patients and so-called matched pairs determined by a computer with respect to the best correspondence in age, risk factors, and degree of original neurological deficit.

The hemodilution consisted of a loading dose and hypervolemic long-term treatment. The loading dose, depending on the Hct value, was iso- or hypervolemic. Haes 500 ml was infused, and no phlebotomy was performed at Hct under 40%, a phlebotomy of 300 ml at Hct of 40%–42% or one of 500 ml at Hct over 42%. Then, 500 ml 10% Haes 200/0.5 with 500 ml of an electrolyte solution were infused twice in the first 4 days (spread over the day always within 6 h). Half the volume was infused during the following 6 days. The placebo group received the same volume as an electrolyte solution.

A standardized neurological score was determined on the 1st day prior to therapy and then on the 3rd, 8th, 15th, and 90th days. This included disturbances of consciousness and orientation as well as speech disturbances and especially the degree of the paresis in the arms and legs. The Karnofsky index was also determined on the 1st, 15th, and 90th days. Examinations by computed tomography were carried out before and after hemodilution to exclude intracerebral hemorrhages and to characterize the type of infarction.

### 3.5.2 Results

The initial values for neurological deficit and the Karnofsky index were almost identical in the 19 matched pairs. The time course of the curve demonstrates that the hemodilution group improved more rapidly than the placebo group especially in the first few days (Fig. 57). This more favourable effect in the hemodilution group was confirmed up to the 90th day. Within 15 days the hemodilution group improved by 3.7 points and the placebo group only by 2.4 points so that the regression of clinical symptoms in the hemodilution group was approximately 50% greater than in the placebo group. According to the test order schedule by Bross for matched pairs the difference was significant at the

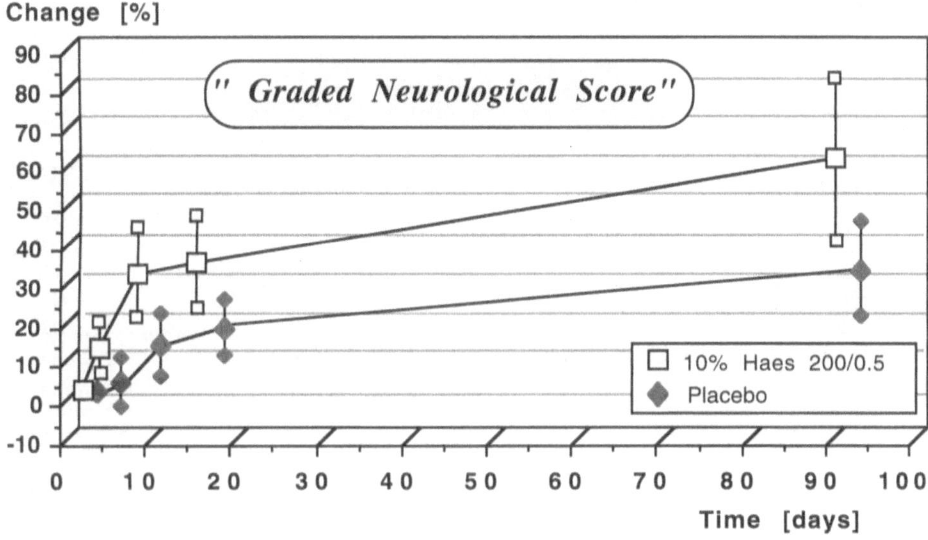


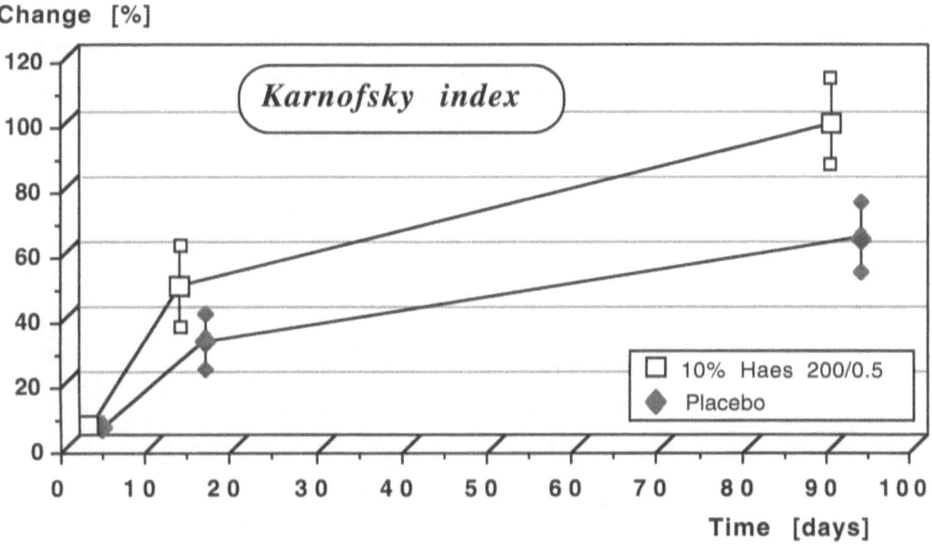


**Fig. 57.** Change in neurological score after acute ischemic cerebral infarction during hemodilution treatment with 10% Haes 200/0.5 or placebo treatment with electrolyte solution and on a control examination after 90 days. Neurological symptoms and signs were recorded by a standardized neurological score and the Karnofsky index

5% level after the 8th day. The course of the Karnofsky index showed the same development, i.e., the hemodilution group improved by 10 points more than the control group. It is especially important for the clinical course that the favourable prognosis for the hemodilution group still was demonstrable even at the control examination after 90 days.

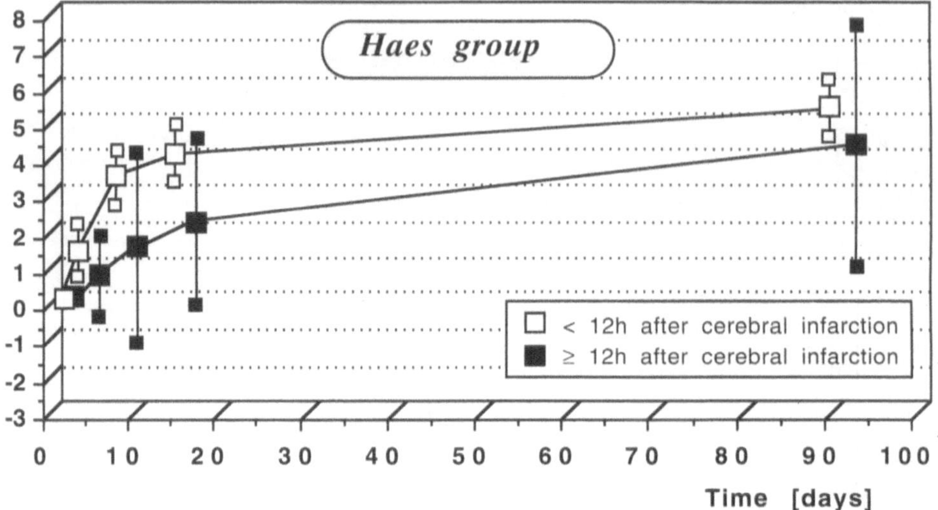


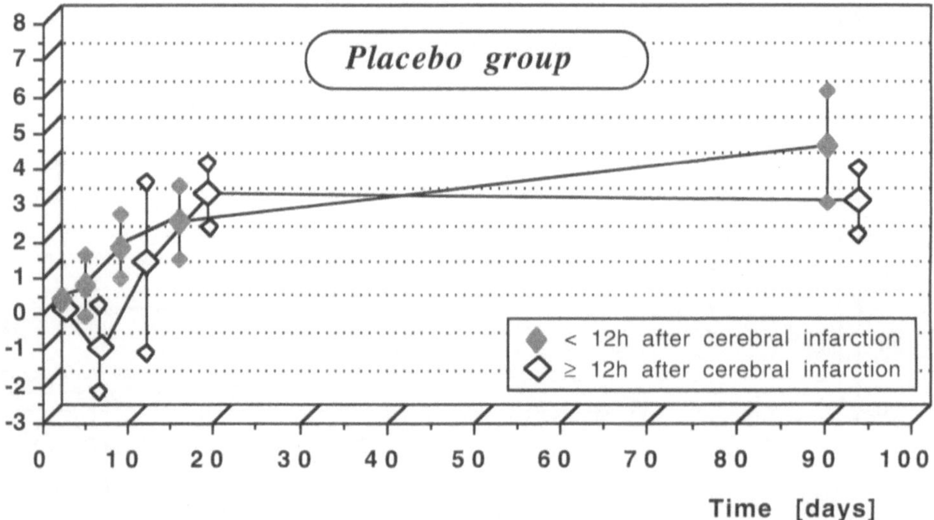


**Fig. 58.** Influence of hemodilution with 10% Haes 200/0.5 or infusion treatment with electrolyte solution which was started within 12 h or within 12–24 h after the acute occurrence of ischemic stroke on the neurological score.

The study confirms the necessity of early initiation of treatment. Increased improvement was detected only in those patients in whom hemodilution was started within 12 h after the cerebral infarction (Fig. 58). The clinical course of the patients with delayed hemodilution was comparable to that in the two placebo groups.

The dependence of the hemodilution effect on a sufficient reduction in Hct was also reflected by the curves (Fig. 59). Only the patients in whom Hct was

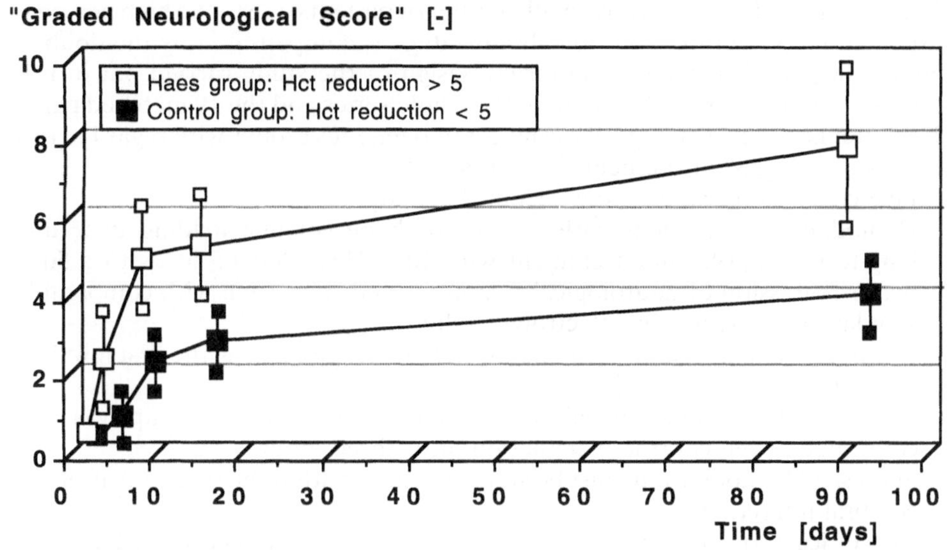

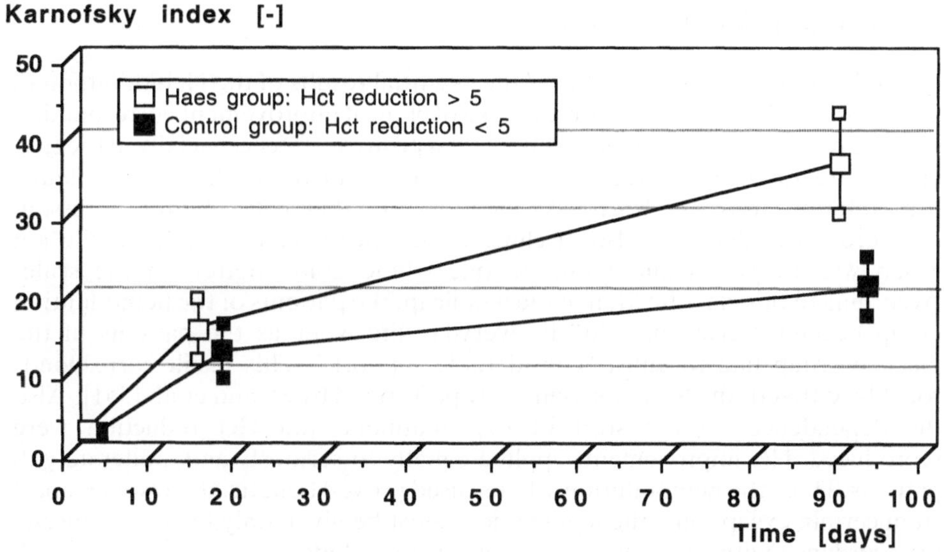

**Fig. 59.** Time course of neurological score after acute ischemic cerebral infarction on hemodilution treatment with 10% Haes 200/0.5 which led to a reduction in Hct by > percentage point, and in a control group with a reduction by < percentage point. Neurological findings were recorded by a standardized neurological score and the Karnofsky index

reduced by 5 percentage points or by 10% showed a better outcome than the patients with a smaller reduction or with the standard treatment.

Two patients died in the hemodilution group. In the placebo group one patient died, and one suffered severe reinfarction.

### *3.5.3 Discussion*

The study included a relatively small number of patients due to the high personal expenditure. In our opinion, this disadvantage is compensated by the double-blind, placebo-controlled, randomized design of the study carried out in two centers. The results were based upon the whole series and the 19 matched pairs. The latter had the advantage of forming homogeneous groups with regard to risk factors and degree of the neurological deficit.

Five conclusions can be drawn from the study:

- Hemodilution treatment with an iso- to hypervolemic loading dose and long-term hypervolemic treatment with 10% Haes 200/0.5 leads to a 50% better regression of neurological symptoms and signs than with comparable standard treatment using electrolyte solutions.
- The improvement caused by hemodilution developed during the first few days of treatment.
- The more favourable clinical course of the hemodilution group was also confirmed at the control examination after three months.
- Successful hemodilution must be started at least within the first 12 h after the cerebral infarction.
- The efficacy of hemodilution is accompanied by a reduction in Hct by 5 percentage points or by about 10%.

This hemodilution study confirms the essential results of the Hemodilution in Stroke Study Group [94]. The time course of clinical improvement corresponded with the expectation that hemodilution has a positive effect especially in the first days of treatment and with the course of curves in the earlier hypervolemic hemodilution study. The Karnofsky index showed that a 50% better regression of neurological deficit is also of clinical relevance because the hemodilution group was 10 points and therefore one whole grade better on the scale. According to this classification of the handicap, the patients of the hemodilution group needed "occasional aid" in everyday life whereas the patients of the placebo group had to enlist "considerable support." This result corresponds roughly to that of the Scandinavian study performed by Strand et al. [351]. Also the dependence on the start of the treatment and Hct reduction were reproduced. The improvements applied equally to seriously and moderately ill patients. Thus, the hemodilution scheme used proved beneficial; however, apart from certain exceptions, the loading dose must be given only hypervolemically in accordance with the present state of our knowledge.

## 3.6 Other Special Therapeutic Methods

A. Haass, M. Stoll, and J. Treib

Important and well-tested alternatives for hemodilution treatment are not yet available except with several special indications. Successful fibrinolysis improves the clinical "outcome" dramatically, but even on a generous indication only 15% of all cerebral infarction patients can receive such therapy due to the existing restrictions [280]. Anticoagulation can reduce only the reembolism rate, and according to earlier examinations it does not influence the course itself. The initially somewhat exaggerated expectations for calcium antagonists gave way to a certain disillusionment after the European and American nimodipine study since a statistically significant improvement was achieved only in the case of a very early initiation. This must be confirmed by another, larger study. These conditions show the slow development. In addition, a single treatment principle cannot be equally effective for all cerebral infarctions.

### 3.6.1 Fibrinolysis

Fibrinolysis requires special personal and instrument expenditure so that it is performed only in several centers (especially the local catheter lysis with streptokinase or urokinase). Therefore, systemic fibrinolysis, which is still in its early stage with thrombus-specific thrombolytics, is of special interest. A proven indication exists in the case of a life-threatening partial thrombosis in the vertebrobasilar circulation (Table 35). There are so far no general experiences for the carotid or middle cerebral artery circulation available. Microcir-

**Table 35.** General and specific contraindications of fibrinolysis in ischemic cerebral infarctions

| |
|---|
| *General contraindications* |
| Elderly, biological age |
| High-grade arteriosclerosis |
| Not adjusted hypertension (> 180 mmHg) |
| Gastrointestinal ulcers |
| Bleeding hemorrhoids |
| Intramuscular injections |
| Condition after acute surgery, accident or trauma |
| Severe liver or renal disease |
| Hemorrhagic diathesis |
| *Specific contraindications: infarction shown on computed tomography* |
| In the area of the middle cerebral artery |
| Clinical indications of the development of a large cerebral parenchymal necrosis |
| Infarction older than 4 h |
| In the circulation area of the vertebral and basilar arteries |
| Prolonged coma |

culatory disturbances are excluded due to the high risk of the treatment. Moreover, large and complete infarctions are not considered due to the danger of hemorrhage. It is extremely difficult to determine the period during which fibrinolysis could still be successful. The time interval can be several to 24 h in the vertebrobasilar circulation area if the patient is not comatose, and the clinical picture, for instance, in the case of a floating thrombus, is still changing considerably.

The limited time restriction in the middle cerebral artery circulation area is 4–6 h. We also exclude patients in whom a large infarction area with definite necrosis can be expected according to clinical symptoms such as early disturbed consciousness, visual axis deviation in the case of severe hemiparesis and -plegia, and early unilateral or bilateral Babinski signs. Also, patients in whom an infarction is apparent on computed tomography are not considered for this treatment.

For local catheter lysis we use urokinase 250 000 IU, infused within 30 min, and repeat the infusion after 30 min if the effect is not adequate (Table 36). Before and after lysis the therapy is controlled by digital subtraction angiography. The simultaneously started total heparinization to avoid rethrombosis is decisive for the further course. It is continued over 14 days until the end of reendothelization. It is started with a bolus of 2000 IU; then a maintenance dose

**Table 36.** Systemic and local fibrinolysis

Local fibrinolysis
- Streptokinase
- Urokinase ($250 \times 10^3$ IU, 30 min; one repetition)
- Indications: vertebrobasilar circulation area (internal carotid artery; middle cerebral artery)

Systemic fibrinolysis (with thrombus specific thrombolytics)
- Tissue plasminogen activator
- Urokinase, prourokinase ($250 \times 10^3$ IU bolus; $4.5 \times 10^6$ IU in 40 min)
- Advantage: uncomplicated use
- Disadvantage: still little proof

**Table 37.** Measures for improved therapeutic safety of anticoagulant treatment

Exclusion by computed tomography of intracranial hemorrhage.
Use *only* heparin and *not* coumarine derivates.
Continuous heparin infusion is safer than repeated bolus administrations.
Apply a new heparin solution every 6–12 h.
Avoid too-high a dose of the initial heparin bolus (loading dose).
Exact and close control of coagulation parameters.
*No* combination with thrombocyte aggregation inhibitors.
Blood pressure must be well controlled.
Elderly patients (> 60 or > 75 years) are more at risk.
Very large areas of infarction are at greater risk.

of 20 000–40 000 IU per 24 h or 350–500 IU kg per 24 h is given. The coagulation status must be controlled by the thrombin time (> 120 s) and the partial thromboplastin time (prolonged by 1.5–2 times).

We are presently gathering experience in pilot studies using urokinase-prourokinase for thrombus-specific thrombolysis after the very positive results of cardiologists with myocardial infarctions [113]. Preventive measures are listed in Table 37.

### 3.6.2 Anticoagulation

According to earlier studies, anticoagulation with coumarine derivates in cerebral infarction did not prove beneficial. A further obstacle to total heparinization as reinfarction prophylaxis was that embolic infarctions, at least anatomico-pathologically, are often accompanied by hemorrhagic transformation. Recently, several indications for total heparinization were proposed from CT scan studies. However, these still require examination in controlled studies (Table 38).

**Table 38.** Indications for antikoagulation in cerebrovascular accidents

| |
|---|
| Cardiac embolism |
| Cardiac infarction |
| Cardiac dysrhythmia |
| Valvular defect |
| Valvular replacement |
| Paradoxical embolism |
| Dissection of the internal carotid artery |
| High-grade extra- or intracranial stenosis |
| "Progressive stroke" |
| Thrombosis of a venous sinus |

It has been demonstrated that independently of the infarction size and depending on particular preventive measures the danger of hemorrhage which could threaten the patient is small. The critical points of this therapy are avoiding blood pressure peaks and sufficiently controlling of the heparin effect [98, 214].

**Table 39.** Clinical efficacy of calcium antagonists and other substances in ischemic cerebral infarctions

| | |
|---|---|
| Calcium antagonists | |
| Nimodipine (only if used early) | (+) (–) |
| Flunarizine) | ? |
| ACE inhibitors | ? |
| Prostacyclin | ? (–) |
| Naloxone | ? (–) |
| Glutamate antagonists | ? |

(+), Weak effect; ?, effect not yet proven; (–), negative effect.

### 3.6.3 Calcium Antagonists and Other Substances

The previous results with nimodipine after a PET examination give reason to expect a positive cerebral metabolic effect [138]. The result of an often quoted clinical cerebral infarction study still raises several questions since the reduced mortality was not achieved through treatment of the cerebral infarctions themselves but by a reduction in the number of pneumonia cases. Only moderately affected patients derived benefit whereas seriously and slightly affected patients showed none [78].

In any case, the treatment must be carried out very early, within the first 12 h, since according to several studies, including also the largest multicenter study, treatment with nimodipine has no effect within the first 48 h after infarction [263]. Its use within 12 h revealed a marginal improvement which was demonstrated by another study. According to this study, a dose higher than $4 \times 30$ mg/day can exert a negative effect (Table 39).

Clinical proof of the efficacy of flunarizine is still lacking. The positive clinical effect of ACE inhibitors is still questionable, whereas such effect can be disputed according to previous studies with prostacyclin and naloxone. With regard to glutamate antagonists and antioxidants there are only experimental data (Table 39).

According to clinical examinations, barbiturates, corticoids, and vasodilators are not useful in the treatment of acute ischemic cerebral infarctions [79].

# 4 Comparison of Iso- and Hypervolemic Hemodilution with Haes

## *4.1 Single Dilution in Healthy Individuals*

J. Koscielny, H. Förster, W. Kolepke, and F. Jung

### *4.1.1 Course of Infusion and Measurement*

The effect of iso- or hypervolemic hemodilution with 10% mean molecular weight hydroxyethyl starch solution 10% Haes 200/0.5 (Haes-steril 10%; Fresenius) on the circulation, oxygen transport capacity of the macro- and microcirculation, oxygen partial pressure in the skin and skeletal muscle, fluidity of blood, and several metabolic parameters were examined in a crossover study on ten healthy male volunteers (mean age 26 years, height 177 cm, body weight 74 kg). The comparison of individuals was chosen since carry-over effects with a single dose (wash-out phase 12 weeks) as well as changes due to the natural course of disease (which can occur in the investigations on patients) are not expected, and the great variability of the comparison of groups can be eliminated [373].

The following parameters were measured prior to the infusion: intramuscular oxygen partial pressure (oxygen partial pressure histogram of the tibialis anterior muscle), oxygen partial pressure on the conjunctiva of the left eye with closed eyelids, transcutaneous oxygen partial pressure of the left lower arm and on the dorsal aspect of the left foot, parameters of blood gas analysis, blood volume flow in the left common carotid artery, erythrocyte velocity under resting conditions in nail fold capillaries on the fourth finger of the left hand, subcutaneous blood flow with a laser Doppler system, fluidity of blood (hematocrit, plasma viscosity, erythrocyte aggregation, erythrocyte rigidity, spontaneous thrombocyte aggregation), blood picture, metabolic parameters (pH value of blood, lactate concentration and pyruvate concentration in plasma), blood pressure, heart rate, hydroxyethyl starch concentration and its molecular weight distribution. This was repeated 1, 3, 6, and 24 h after the end of the infusion.

Due to the multitude of data to be collected, the iso- and hypervolemic hemodilution were required two partial examinations. Isovolemic hemodilution was performed twice in the same participant at an interval of 3 months, and the respective parameters were measured. In the same examination design two hypervolemic examinations were performed after the two isovolemic hemodilution studies, again with the same subjects and a 3 month wash-out phase. The data presented here were thus gathered in four partial studies.

During the examination the subjects remained in the rooms of the Department for 8 h on the 1st day of the study and reported the next day at the same time for the 24-h examinations. These were started after a 1-h stay in the examination room to guarantee adaption of the peripheral circulation to room

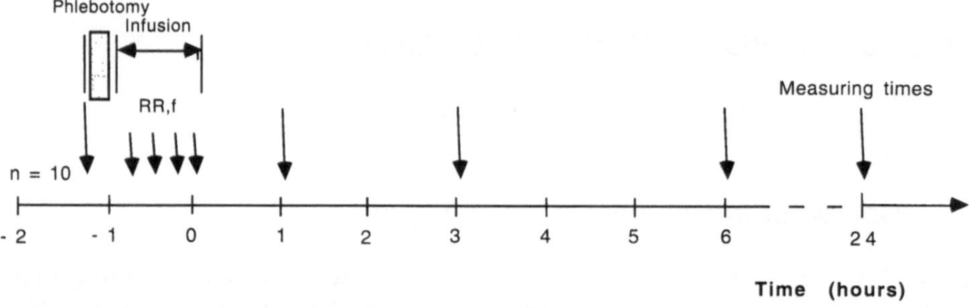


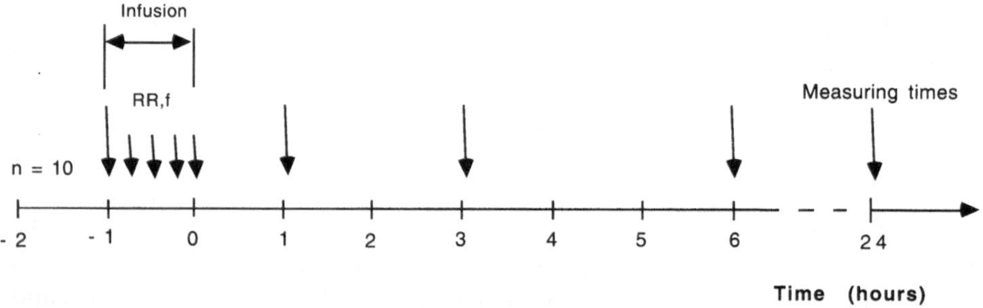


**Fig. 60.** Study design: iso- and hypervolemic hemodilution

temperature. The examinations were carried out at the same time in every subject to keep the circadian variations comparable [333].

On hypervolemic hemodilution 500 ml hydroxyethyl starch was infused in 60 min. On isovolemic hemodilution, first a phlebotomy of 500 ml blood about 15 min and afterwards an infusion of 500 ml hydroxyethyl starch for an infusion period of 60 min were carried out. During the infusion blood pressure and heart rate were checked at intervals of 15 min (Fig. 60).

### *4.1.2 Results*

At the beginning of the two hemodilution treatments the values did not differ significantly; thus the effect of the two forms of therapy was assessed under comparable circumstances [369]. Statistical comparison of associated samples (testing for the similarity before the two test phases) was done with the Wilcoxon test for paired differences in two samples [314]. Before the respective studies the changes in initial values on the specific parameters (except erythrocyte aggregation) ranged from 0% to 11% for individual subjects and from 0% to 4% for the overall group. Concerning erythrocyte aggregation the initial values differed before isovolemic and hypervolemic hemodilution by about 18.2% in the overall group. The extent of significant changes in all parameters determined was greater than the calculated relative errors.

The Kolmogoroff-Smirnow normal distribution test was used [220]. For normally distributed samples the statistics given are the mean + standard deviation and for skewed samples the median and percentiles (2.5 and 97.5 percentile).

For statistical comparison of dependent multiple samples the Friedman test was used, and to determine differences between groups the Wilcoxon test [314].

For normally distributed samples the mean and standard deviation are indicated in the tables; where indicated, however, the median and percentile limits (2.5 and 97.5 percentiles) are reported due to skewed samples. Where relevant to highlight the distinctions between isovolemic and hypervolemic hemodilution, the sets of corresponding figures are slightly shaded for the former and are unshaded for the latter.

### 4.1.2.1 Colloidal and Protein Chemistry Parameters

#### 4.1.2.1.1 Hydroxyethyl Starch Concentration

The mean hydroxyethyl starch concentration in serum showed (enzymatic hexokinase method and *o*-toluidine method) a significant decrease at the individual measuring points with both methods of measurement and after isovolemic and hypervolemic hemodilution (with regard to the 1-h value). Moreover, the hydroxyethyl starch concentrations after isovolemic hemodilution differed significantly in the group comparison from the hydroxyethyl starch concentrations after hypervolemic hemodilution (1, 3, 6, and 24 h after the infusion; Table 40, Fig. 61). At the 1-h measuring time the hydroxyethyl starch concentration after isovolemic hemodilution was 23.2% ($p<0.01$) higher than the concentration after hypervolemic hemodilution, 39.4% ($p<0.01$) at 3 h time, 22.8% ($p<0.01$) at 6 h, and 27.0% ($p<0.01$) at 24 h.

**Table 40.** Hydroxyethyl starch concentration after iso- or hypervolemic hemodilution

| Time (h) | Isovolemic Concentration (mg/dl) | Change (%) from 1-h value | Hypervolemic Concentration (mg/dl) | Change (%) from 1-h value | Difference (%) (iso-hyp) |
|---|---|---|---|---|---|
| Before | – | – | – | – | – |
| 1 | 935±120 | – | 759±104 | – | +23.2%* |
| 3 | 696±100 | −25.6%* | 491± 68 | −33.4%* | +39.4%* |
| 6 | 441± 68 | −52.8%* | 359± 54 | −52.7%* | +22.8%* |
| 24 | 148± 32 | −84.2%* | 108± 27 | −85.7%* | +27.0%* |

* p<0.01.

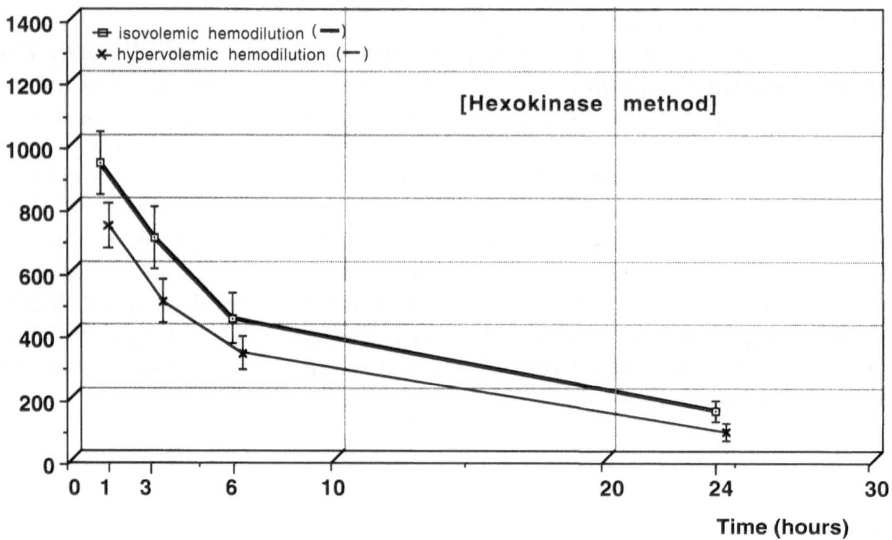


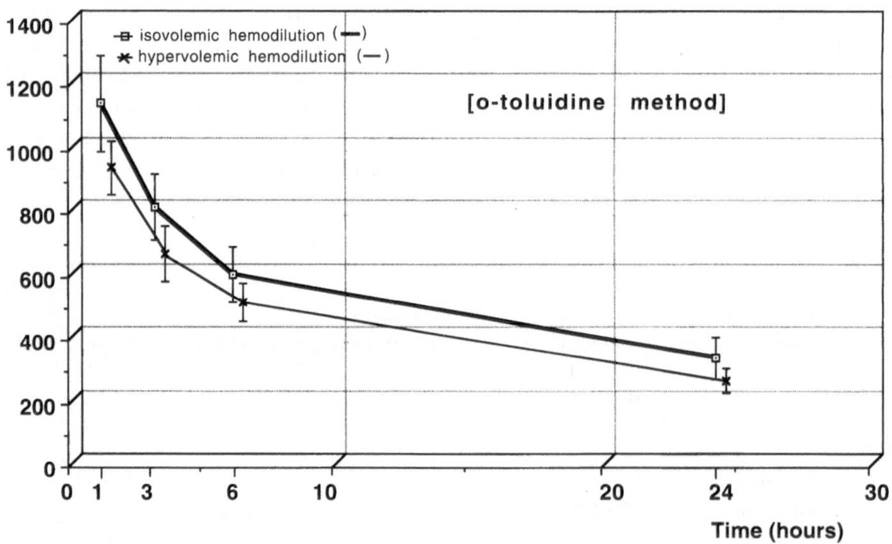


**Fig. 61.** Hydroxyethyl starch concentration 1, 3, 6, and 24 h after iso- or hypervolemic hemodilution. Significance level for all mean measuring points in time-series comparisons and in group comparisons, $< 1\%$

The results of the methods were confirmed by the fact that there were no starch molecules in serum before either hemodilution. The effect on the measured value by other saccharides is excluded.

#### 4.1.2.1.2 Molecular Weight Distribution

The molecular weight distributions after iso- and hypervolemic hemodilution shows an almost identical course, without significant differences. Hydroxyethyl starch molecules with a molecular weight below 3 kDa and above 4500 kDa were not found in the samples after the infusion. Table 41 and Fig. 62 show the course of mean molecular weight. Figures 63 and 64 indicate the relative proportions of the molecular weight groupings at individual measuring points before and after iso- or hypervolemic hemodilution. Figure 65 shows the hydroxyethyl starch concentration in terms of the molecular weight distribution before and after iso- or hypervolemic hemodilution.

**Table 41.** Mean molecular weight (MMw: daltons) before and after iso- or hypervolemic hemodilution

| Time (h) | Isovolemic MMw (Da) | Change (%) from initial value | Hypervolemic MMw (Da) | Change (%) from initial value |
|---|---|---|---|---|
| Before | 221 500±5 000 | – | 221 500±5 000 | – |
| 1 | 119 237±4 108 | –40.5%* | 118 046±4 079 | –41.0%* |
| 3 | 98 023±5 902 | –50.9%* | 99 433±5 553 | –51.0%* |
| 6 | 94 420±4 117 | –52.8%* | 95 341±4 475 | –52.5%* |
| 24 | 99 748±5 473 | –50.2%* | 98 555±4 498 | –50.7%* |

Because there are no significant differences in the group comparison (iso-hyp), the differences are not indicated in this table.
* $p<0.01$.

#### 4.1.2.1.3 α-Amylase Activity

Mean α-amylase activity in serum after isovolemic and after hypervolemic hemodilution showed a significant increase at all measuring points (1, 3, 6, and 24 h). In the group comparison there was a significant difference in α-amylase activities 1, 3, 6, and 24 h after iso- and hypervolemic hemodilution (Table 42, Fig. 66). After iso- and hypervolemic hemodilution enzyme activity increased significantly and remained significantly increased for up to 24 h. Furthermore, there was a tendency toward increase above the mean enzyme activity in serum; this was 7.8% higher 1 h after isovolemic hemodilution, 12.8% ($p<0.05$) higher at 3 h after, and 14.7% ($p<0.05$) higher at 6 h than the activity after hypervolemic hemodilution. Enzyme activities in serum of all subjects were within the reference range prior to hemodilution.

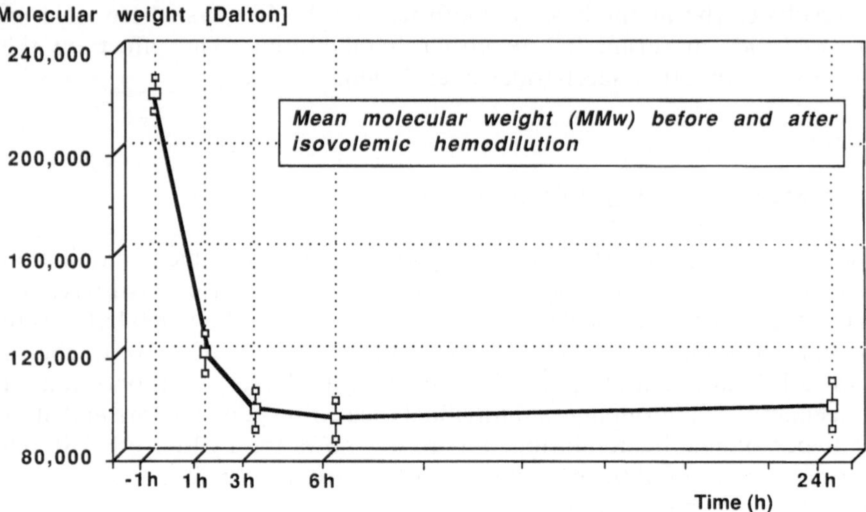


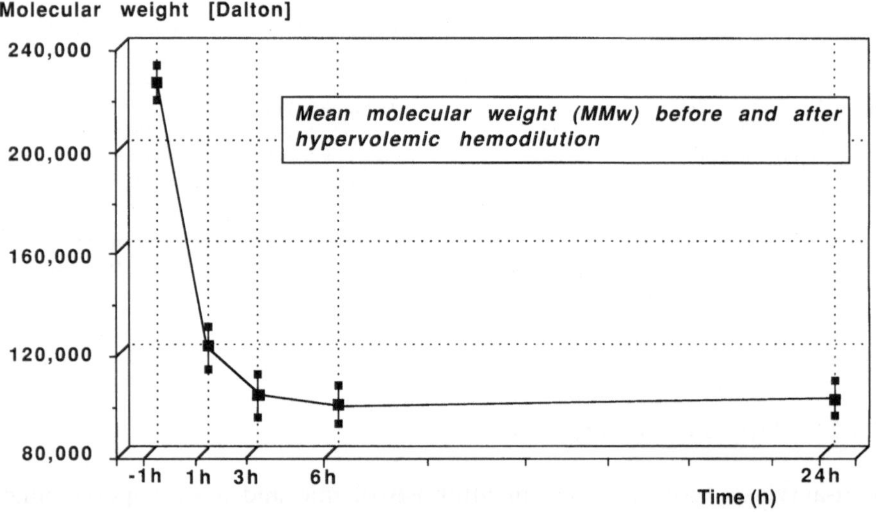


**Fig. 62.** Mean molecular weight of hydroxyethyl starch before and 1, 3, 6, and 24 h after iso- (*above*) or hypervolemic hemodilution (*below*)

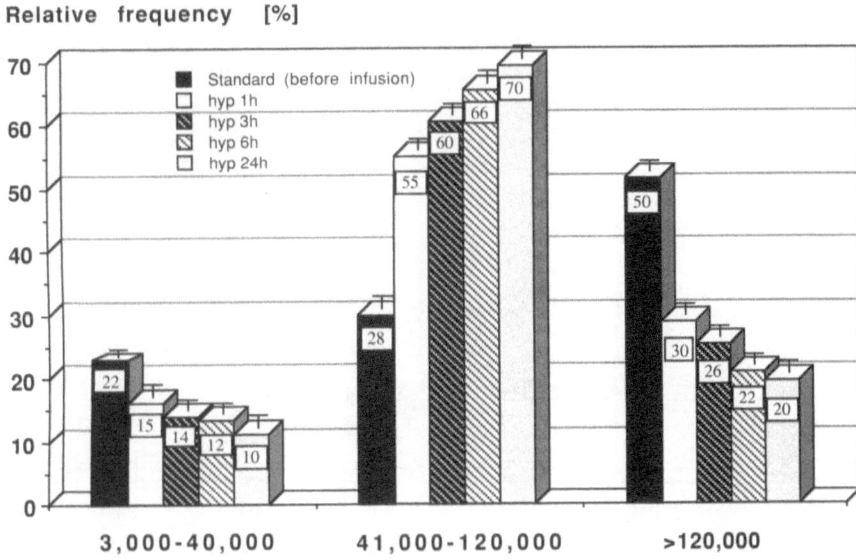


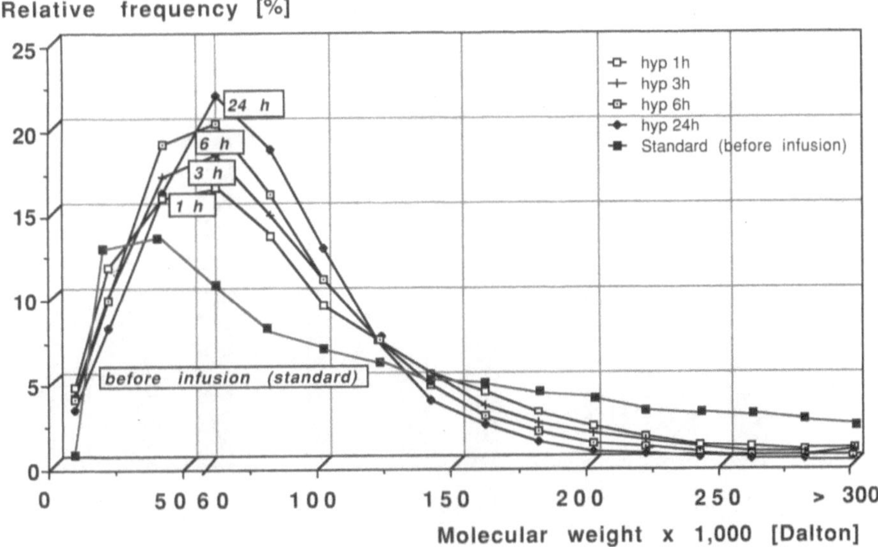


**Fig. 63.** Molecular weight distribution before and 1, 3, 6, and 24 h after isovolemic hemodilution

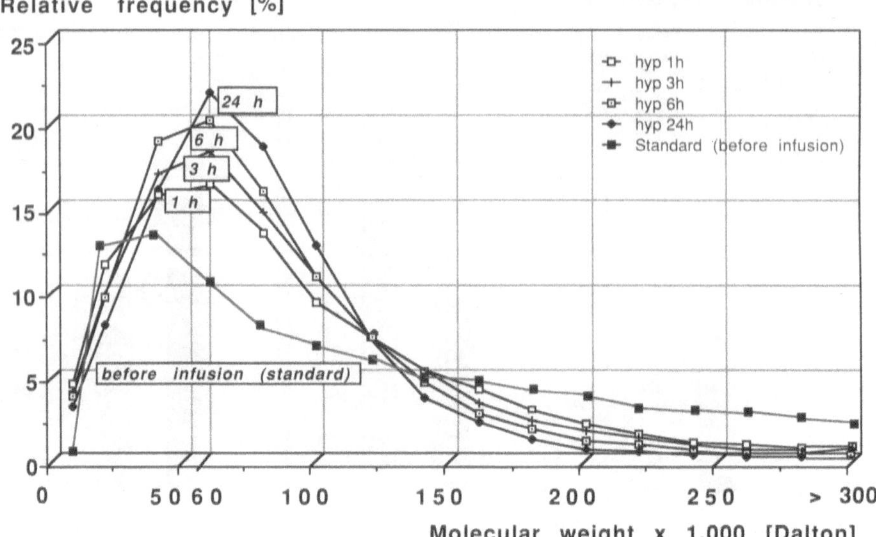


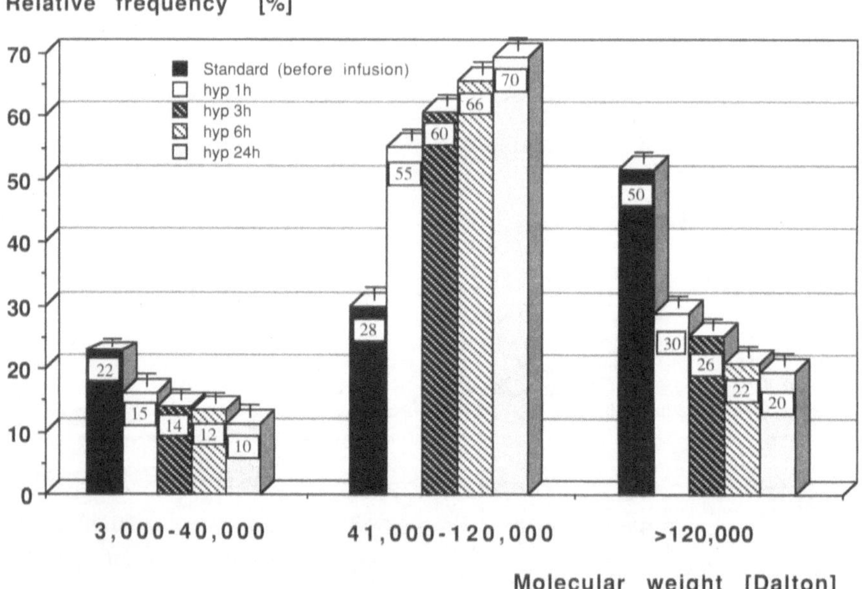


**Fig. 64.** Molecular weight distribution before and 1, 3, 6, and 24 h after hypervolemic hemodilution

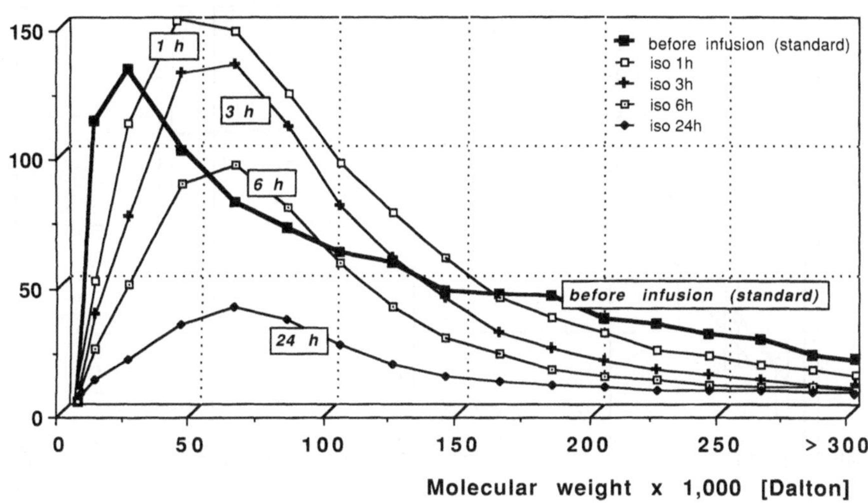


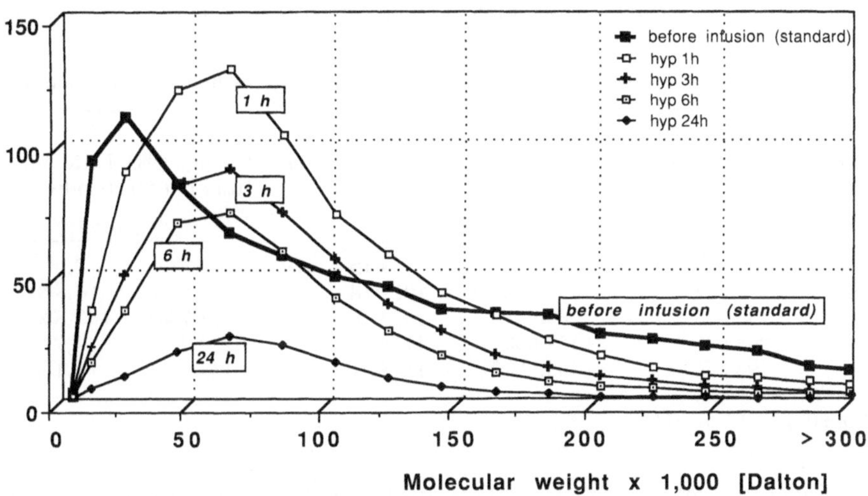


**Fig. 65.** Hydroxyethyl starch concentration by molecular weight before and 1, 3, 6, and 24 h after iso- (*above*) or hypervolemic hemodilution (*below*)

#### 4.1.2.1.4 Total Protein Concentration

Mean total protein concentration in serum decreased significantly after both dilution forms with regard to the initial value, which was within the reference range. This decrease was more distinct after isovolemic than after hypervolemic hemodilution (Table 43). After hypervolemic hemodilution the values were

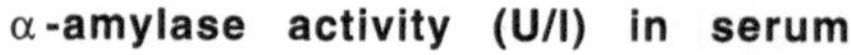


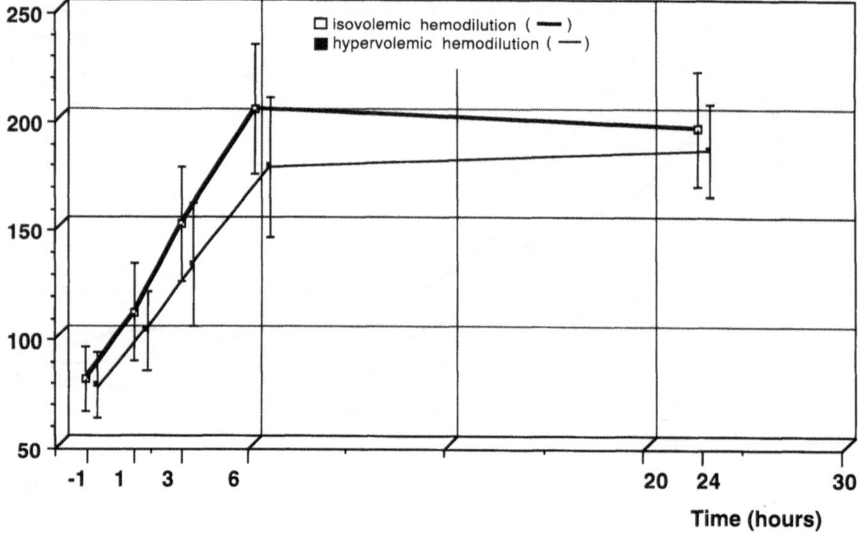


**Fig. 66.** α-Amylase activity in serum before and 1, 3, 6, and 24 h after iso- or hypervolemic hemodilution. Significance level for the mean measuring points in time-series comparisons and after iso- or hypervolemic hemodilution in group comparisons, < 1%

**Table 42.** α-Amylase activity (α-amyl.) before and after iso- or hypervolemic hemodilution

| Time (h) | Isovolemic α-amyl. (U/l) | Change (%) from initial value | Hypervolemic α-amyl. (U/l) | Change (%) from initital value | Difference (%) (iso-hyp) |
|---|---|---|---|---|---|
| Before | 79±15 | – | 77±15 | – | +2.5% |
| 1 | 110±22 | +39.2%* | 102±18 | +32.5%* | +7.8% |
| 6 | 150±26 | +89.9%* | 133±28 | +72.7%* | +12.8%** |
| 6 | 203±30 | +157.0%* | 177±32 | +129.9%* | +14.7%** |
| 24 | 194±26 | +145.6%* | 184±21 | +138.9%* | +5.1% |

* $p<0.01$; ** $p<0.05$.

significantly higher than the values after isovolemic hemodilution: by 12.4% ($p<0.01$) after 1 h, at 3 h by 10.3% ($p<0.01$), at 6 h by 8.3% ($p<0.01$), and at 24 h by 7.1% ($p<0.01$). Figure 67 shows the course of total protein concentration in serum before and after iso- or hypervolemic hemodilution.

#### 4.1.2.1.5 Albumin Concentration

After both hemodilution forms the mean albumin concentration in serum decreased significantly with regard to the initial value (Table 44). This was more

**Table 43.** Total protein concentration (protein) before and after iso- or hypervolemic hemodilution

| Time (h) | Isovolemic Protein (g/dl) | Change (%) from initial value | Hypervolemic Protein (g/dl)[a] | Change (%) from initial value | Difference (%) (iso-hyp) |
|---|---|---|---|---|---|
| Before | 8.39±0.49 | – | 8.45 (7.91/8.91) | – | −0.7% |
| 1 | 6.59±0.44 | −21.7%* | 7.41 (6.88/7.94) | −13.3%* | −12.4%* |
| 3 | 7.01±0.56 | −16.6%* | 7.73 (7.15/8.22) | −8.5%* | −10.3%* |
| 6 | 7.43±0.60 | −11.7%* | 8.05 (7.77/8.51) | −4.7%* | −8.3%* |
| 24 | 7.85±0.49 | −6.7%* | 8.25 (7.95/8.76) | −2.4%* | −7.1%* |

* $p<0.01$.
[a] (2.5/97.5 percentiles).

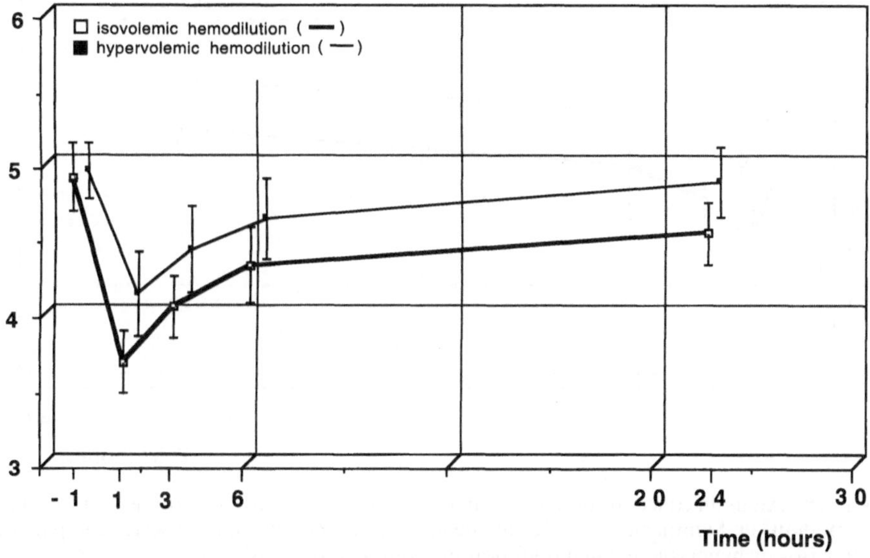


**Fig. 67.** Total protein concentration in serum before and 1, 3, 6, and 24 h after iso- or hypervolemic hemodilution. Significance level for all mean measuring points in time-series comparisons and after iso- or hypervolemic hemodilution in group comparisons, < 1%

pronounced after isovolemic than after hypervolemic hemodilution. Prior to hemodilution the concentration values in all subjects were within the reference range. Furthermore, after hypervolemic hemodilution the values were significantly higher compared to the values after isovolemic hemodilution (Fig. 68): by 12.6% ($p<0.01$) after 1 h, 9.1% ($p<0.01$) at 3 h, 7.8% ($p<0.01$) at 6 h, and 7.5% ($p<0.01$) at 24 h.

**Table 44.** Albumin concentration in serum (albumin) before and after iso- or hypervolemic hemodilution

| Time (h) | Isovolemic Albumin (g/dl) | Change (%) from initial value | Hypervolemic Albumin (g/dl) | Change (%) from initial value | Difference (%) (iso-hyp) |
|---|---|---|---|---|---|
| Before | 4.90±0.23 | – | 4.95±0.19 | – | −1.0% |
| 1 | 3.66±0.31 | −25.2%* | 4.13±0.28 | −16.7%* | −12.6%* |
| 3 | 4.03±0.33 | −17.7%* | 4.36±0.29 | −12.1%* | −9.1%* |
| 6 | 4.31±0.25 | −12.1%* | 4.64±0.33 | −6.4%* | −7.8%* |
| 24 | 4.53±0.21 | −7.6%* | 4.80±0.23 | −3.1%* | −7.5%* |

* $p<0.01$.

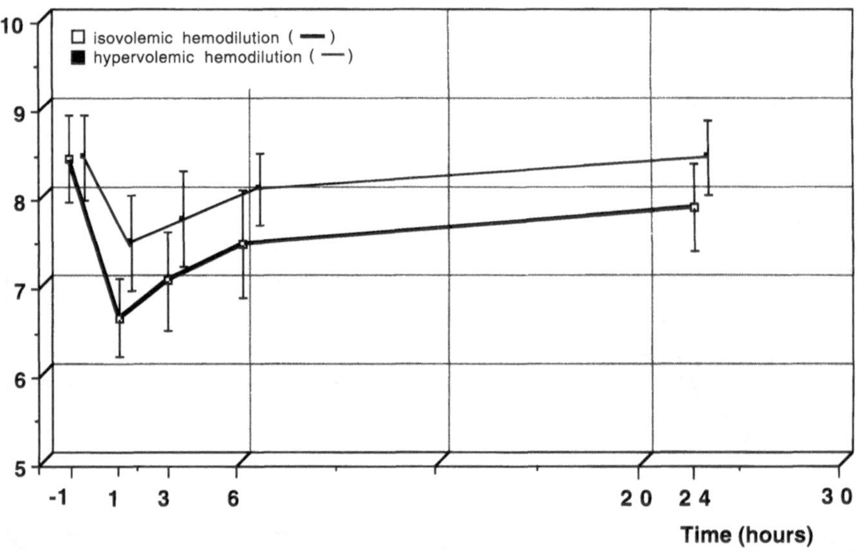


**Fig. 68.** Albumin concentration in serum before and 1, 3, 6, and 24 h after iso- or hypervolemic hemodilution. Significance level for all mean measuring points in time-series comparisons and after iso- or hypervolemic hemodilution in group comparisons.< 1%

Since the other protein fractions of the electrophoresis show identical courses with regard to concentration, only the albumin concentration is indicated as representative of the protein fractions.

### 4.1.2.2 Hemorheologic Parameters

The effect of iso- or hypervolemic hemodilution on the fluidity of blood is presented in Table 45 and Fig. 69. Systemic hematocrit (withdrawal of blood

**Table 45.** Systemic hematocrit (Hct) before and after iso- or hypervolemic hemodilution

| Time (h) | Isovolemic Hct (%) | Change (%) from initial value | Hypervolemic Hct (%) | Change (%) from initial value | Difference (%) (iso-hyp) |
|---|---|---|---|---|---|
| Before | 47.5±2.8 | – | 46.8±5.0 | – | +1.5% |
| 1 | 39.0±3.1 | −17.9%** | 41.4±3.5 | −11.5%** | −6.1%* |
| 3 | 41.0±3.9 | −13.7%* | 42.1±4.5 | −10.0%* | −2.7% |
| 6 | 41.8±3.7 | −12.0%* | 43.4±3.8 | −7.3%* | −3.9%* |
| 24 | 43.5±2.9 | −8.5%* | 44.7±3.7 | −4.5% | −2.8%* |

* $p<0.01$; ** $p<0.001$.

from the antecubital vein) decreased significantly after both hemodilution forms but after the isovolemic considerably more than after the hypervolemic (the hemoglobin concentration behaved similarly). For example, 1 h after the end of the infusion the hematocrit decreased by 17.9% ($p<0.001$) after isovolemic hemodilution and by 11.5% ($p<0.05$) after hypervolemic dilution. The differences declined in the late phase; 24 h after isovolemic hemodilution the decrease in hematocrit was 8.5% ($p<0.01$) and after hypervolemic hemodilution 4.5%.

One hour after the end of the infusion plasma viscosity after isovolemic hemodilution was lower than prior to the administration of hydroxyethyl starch. A slight but significant increase in plasma viscosity was observed after hypervolemic hemodilution (Table 46, Fig. 69). At 6 and 24 hours after isovolemic hemodilution plasma viscosity was significantly decreased compared to the initial value.

Erythrocyte aggregation was not significantly influenced by isovolemic hemodilution in this acute trial; however, 1 and 3 h after hypervolemic dilution a decrease appeared (Table 47, Fig. 69). In this connection it should be noted that

**Table 46.** Plasma viscosity (PV) before and after iso- or hypervolemic hemodilution

| Time (h) | Isovolemic PV (mPas) | Change (%) from initial value | Hypervolemic PV (mPas) | Change (%) from initial value | Difference (%) (iso-hyp) |
|---|---|---|---|---|---|
| Before | 1.29±0.04 | – | 1.28±0.04 | – | +0.8% |
| 1 | 1.24±0.03 | −3.9% | 1.30±0.05 | +1.6%** | −4.8%** |
| 3 | 1.25±0.04 | −3.1% | 1.26±0.04 | −1.6%* | −0.8% |
| 6 | 1.24±0.05 | −3.9%* | 1.26±0.05 | −1.6%** | −1.6% |
| 24 | 1.23±0.04 | −4.7%** | 1.26±0.05 | −1.6% | −2.4% |

* $p<0.01$; ** $p<0.05$.

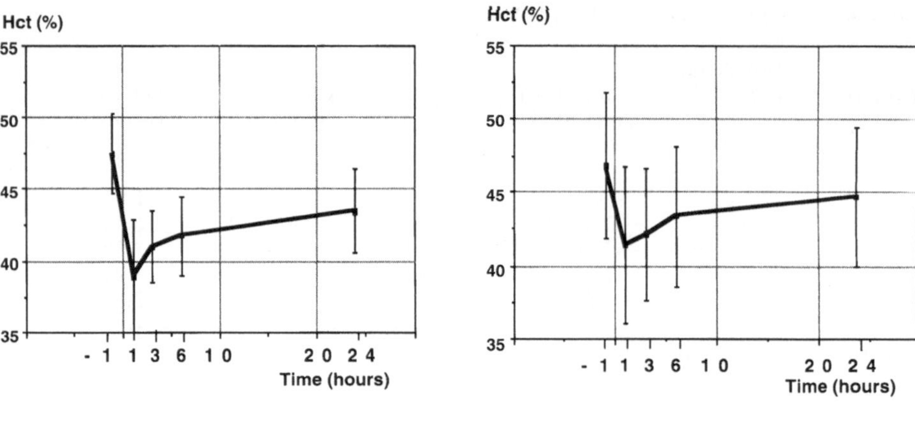


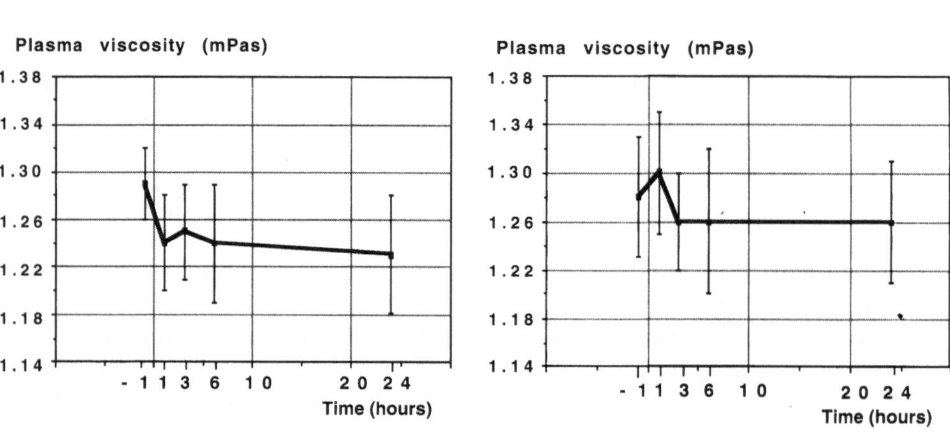


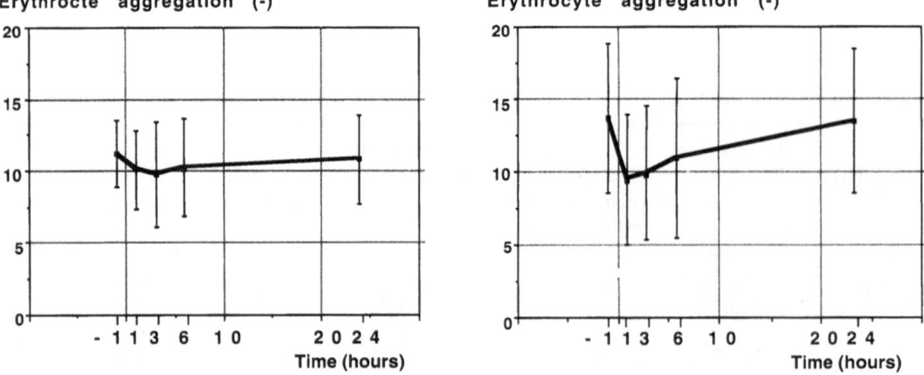


**Fig. 69.** Systemic hematocrit, plasma viscosity, and erythrocyte aggregation before and 1, 3, 6, and 24 h after iso- (*left*) or hypervolemic hemodilution (*right*)

**Table 47.** Erythrocyte aggregation (SEA) before and after iso- or hypervolemic hemodilution

| Time (h) | Isovolemic SEA (–)[a] | Change (%) from initial value | Hypervolemic SEA (–)[a] | Change (%) from initial value | Difference (%) (iso-hyp) |
|---|---|---|---|---|---|
| Before | 11.2 (8.0/14.2) | – | 13.7 (9.5/18.6) | – | –18.2%* |
| 1 | 10.1 (7.0/12.2) | –9.8% | 9.5 (5.0/14.8) | –30.7%* | +5.9% |
| 3 | 9.8 (6.0/13.7) | –12.5% | 9.9 (5.2/14.1) | –27.7%* | –1.0% |
| 6 | 10.2 (6.5/14.2) | –8.9% | 11.0 (5.6/17.2) | –19.7% | –7.8% |
| 24 | 10.8 (6.9/14.4) | –3.6% | 13.5 (8.2/18.9) | –1.5% | –25.0%* |

* $p<0.01$.
[a] Median (2.5/97.5 percentiles).

the initial values before isovolemic hemodilution were about 18.2% lower for the whole group than before hypervolemic hemodilution. Erythrocyte rigidity and spontaneous thrombocyte aggregation were not influenced significantly by the two forms of dilution.

In the following figures, the courses of the respective parameters are illustrated on the left side of the picture before and 1, 3, 6 and 24 h after isovolemic hemodilution (left background), and on the right side of the picture before and 1, 3, 6 and 24 h after hypervolemic hemodilution (right background).

### 4.1.2.3 Blood Picture Parameters

Mean corpuscular volume (MCV) and mean hemoglobin content (MCHC) remained constant after both forms of hemodilution at all measuring points: MCV between 88.9 and 89.6 µm and MCHC between 33.9 and 34.1 g/dl. This corresponds to the error range for the methods of measurement.

In contrast, the thrombocyte count changed significantly after both hemodilution forms (Table 48, Fig. 70). After hypervolemic hemodilution a less pronounced and shorter decrease was seen.

**Table 48.** Thrombocyte count (TC) before and after iso- or hypervolemic hemodilution

| Time (h) | Isovolemic TF ($\times 10^4/mm^3$) | Change (%) from initial value | Hypervolemic TF ($\times 10^4/mm^3$) | Change (%) from initial value | Difference (%) (iso-hyp) |
|---|---|---|---|---|---|
| Before | 25.5±3.5 | – | 25.3±3.3 | – | +0.8% |
| 1 | 20.4±3.4 | −19.9%* | 21.7±2.6 | −14.1%* | −6.4% |
| 3 | 22.0±3.5 | −13.9%* | 23.1±3.1 | −12.6%** | −5.0% |
| 6 | 23.2±3.1 | −9.0%** | 25.0±4.2 | −1.2% | −7.7%* |
| 24 | 25.6±3.1 | +0.4% | 25.4±3.7 | +0.4% | +0.8% |

* $p<0.01$; ** $p<0.05$.

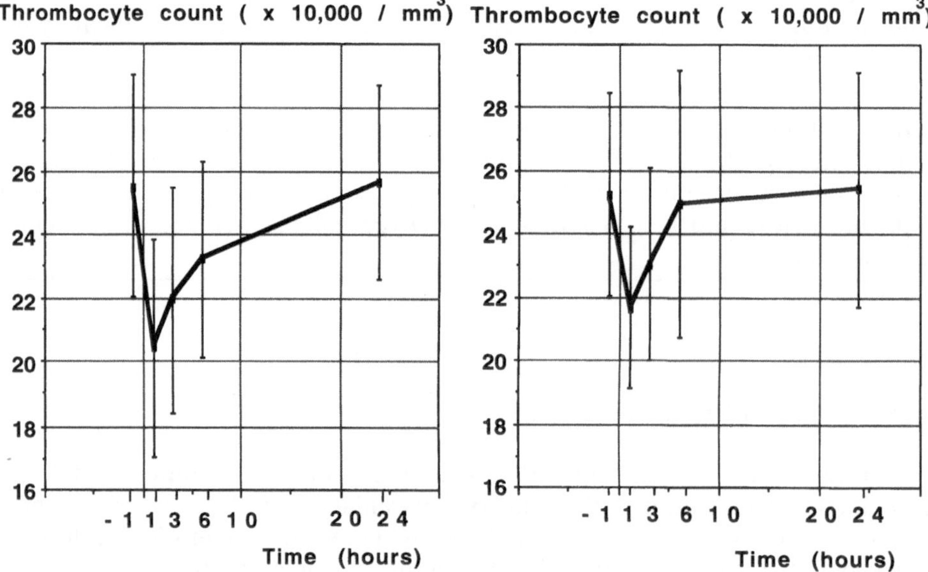


**Fig. 70.** Thrombocyte count before and 1, 3, 6, and 24 h after iso- (*left*) or hypervolemic hemodilution (*right*)

## 4.1.2.4 Blood Pressure and Heart Rate

Whereas blood pressure (Table 49) and heart rate (Table 50) remained almost constant after hypervolemic hemodilution, the former decreased significantly 1 h after isovolemic hemodilution (with regard to the initial heart rate). After 6 hours the initial value was achieved again. Blood pressure did not change significantly after either form of hemodilution (Fig. 71).

**Table 49.** Blood pressure (RR) before and after iso- or hypervolemic hemodilution

| Time (h) | | Isovolemic RR (mmHg) | Change (%) from initial value | Hypervolemic RR (mmHg) | Change (%) from initial value |
|---|---|---|---|---|---|
| Before | Systolic | 120±12 | – | 118± 7 | – |
| | Diastolic | 73± 8 | – | 76± 8 | – |
| 1 | Systolic | 114±11 | −5.0% | 116± 7 | −1.7% |
| | Diastolic | 70± 7 | −4.1% | 74±10 | −2.6% |
| 3 | Systolic | 117± 7 | −2.5% | 112±10 | −5.0% |
| | Diastolic | 73± 7 | ±0% | 75± 8 | −1.3% |
| 6 | Systolic | 120±10 | ±0% | 116± 7 | −1.7% |
| | Diastolic | 74± 8 | +1.4% | 74± 7 | −2.6% |
| 24 | Systolic | 121± 9 | +0.8% | 120± 9 | +1.7% |
| | Diastolic | 73± 8 | ±0% | 75± 8 | −1.3% |

Because there are no significant differences in the group comparison (iso-hyp), the differences are not indicated in this table.

**Table 50.** Heart rate (HR) before and after iso- or hypervolemic hemodilution

| Time (h) | Isovolemic HR (1/min) | Change (%) from initial value | Hypervolemic HR (1/min) | Change (%) from initial value | Difference (%) (iso-hyp) |
|---|---|---|---|---|---|
| Before | 74 (66/82) | – | 77 (64/92) | – | −4.1% |
| 1 | 64 (56/72) | −13.5%* | 71 (64/78) | −7.8% | −10.9%* |
| 3 | 67 (54/78) | −9.5% | 72 (64/82) | −6.5% | −7.5% |
| 6 | 72 (62/82) | −2.7% | 73 (64/84) | −5.2% | −1.4% |
| 24 | 75 (66/84) | +1.3% | 78 (66/90) | +1.3% | −4.0% |

* $p<0.05$.

### 4.1.2.5 Hemodynamic Parameters in the Macrocirculation

#### 4.1.2.5.1 Oxygen Saturation, Oxygen Partial Pressure, and Hemoglobin Concentration (Arterial)

Oxygen saturation decreased significantly after isovolemic hemodilution with regard to the initial value (Table 51, Fig. 72). At 6 h it increased again but did not achieve the initial value until 24 h. After hypervolemic hemodilution oxygen saturation remained constant.

The hemoglobin concentration of blood decreased significantly after both forms of hemodilution but, as with hematocrit, after isovolemic hemodilution more distinctly than after hypervolemic hemodilution (Table 52, Fig. 72).

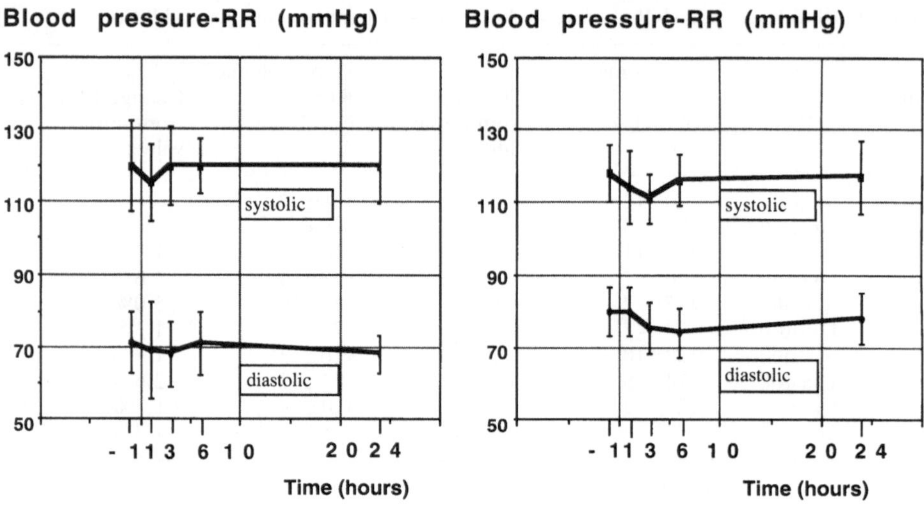


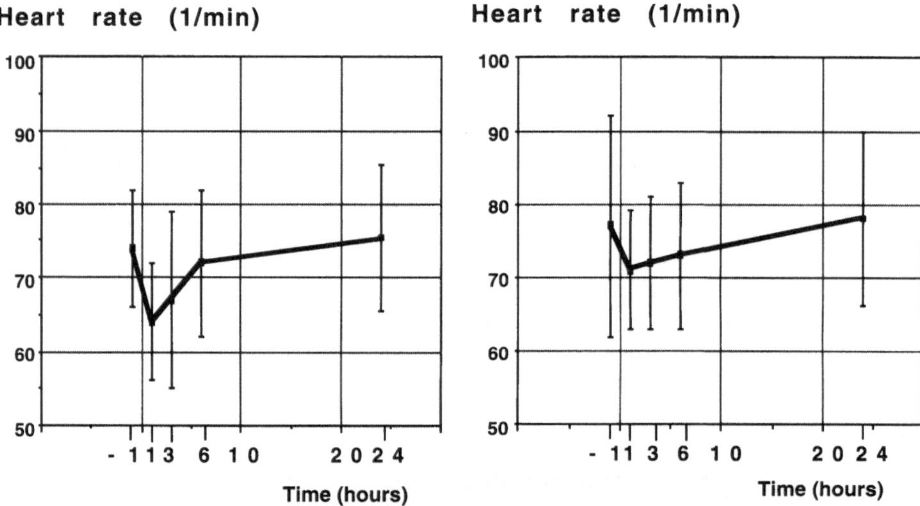


**Fig. 71.** Blood pressure and heart rate before and 1, 3, 6, and 24 h after iso- (*left*) or hypervolemic hemodilution (*right*)

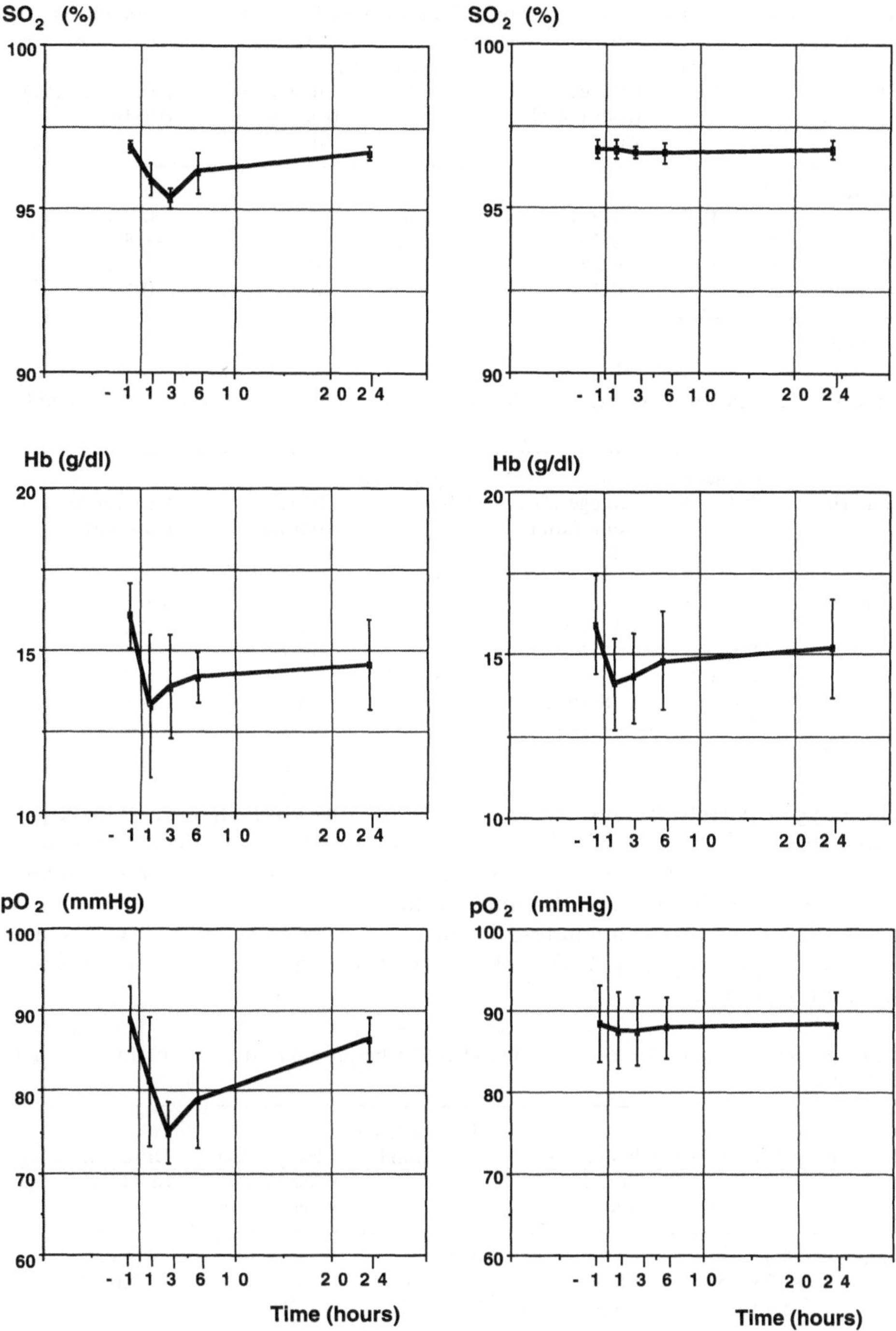


**Fig. 72.** Oxygen saturation ($SO_2$), hemoglobin concentration (*Hb*), and oxygen partial pressure ($pO_2$) in the arterial system before and 1, 3, 6, and 24 h after iso- (*left*) or hypervolemic hemodilution (*right*)

**Table 51.** Oxygen saturation ($SO_2$) before and after iso- or hypervolemic hemodilution

| Time (h) | Isovolemic $SO_2$ (%) | Change (%) from initial value | Hypervolemic $SO_2$ (%) | Change (%) from initial value | Difference (%) (iso-hyp) |
|---|---|---|---|---|---|
| Before | 96.9±0.2 | – | 96.8±0.3 | – | +0.1% |
| 1 | 95.9±0.5 | −1.0%* | 96.8±0.3 | 0% | −0.9%* |
| 3 | 95.3±0.3 | −1.7%* | 96.7±0.2 | −0.1% | −1.5%* |
| 6 | 96.1±0.6 | −0.8% | 96.7±0.3 | −0.1% | −0.6% |
| 24 | 96.7±0.2 | −0.2% | 96.8±0.3 | 0% | −0.1% |

* $p<0.01$.

**Table 52.** Hemoglobin concentration (Hb) before and after iso- or hypervolemic hemodilution

| Time (h) | Isovolemic Hb (g/dl) | Change (%) from initial value | Hypervolemic Hb (g/dl) | Change (%) from initial value | Difference (%) (iso-hyp) |
|---|---|---|---|---|---|
| Before | 16.1±1.0 | – | 15.9±1.5 | – | +1.2% |
| 1 | 13.3±2.2 | −17.4%* | 14.1±1.4 | −11.3%* | −6.0% |
| 3 | 13.9±1.6 | −13.7%* | 14.3±1.4 | −10.1%* | −2.9% |
| 6 | 14.2±0.8 | −11.8%* | 14.8±1.3 | −6.9% | −4.2% |
| 24 | 14.8±1.4 | −8.1%* | 15.3±1.5 | −3.8% | −3.5% |

* $p<0.01$.

The oxygen partial pressure in arterial blood was equivalent to the oxygen saturation (Table 53, Fig. 72). Whereas the $pO_2$ value showed a constant course after hypervolemic hemodilution, it decreased significantly after isovolemic hemodilution with regard to the initial value.

The changes in these parameters had an effect on oxygen content ($CaO_2$) and oxygen transport capacity ($OTC = BF \times (CaO_2)$; Fig. 73), according to Eqs. 1 and 2 in Sect. 5.7.

**Table 53.** Oxygen partial pressure in blood ($pO_2$) before and after iso- or hypervolemic hemodilution

| Time (h) | Isovolemic $pO_2$ (mmHg) | Change (%) from initial value | Hypervolemic $pO_2$ (mmHg) | Change (%) from initial value | Difference (%) (iso-hyp) |
|---|---|---|---|---|---|
| Before | 88.9±4.0 | – | 88.4±5.1 | – | +0.6% |
| 1 | 81.3±4.5 | −8.5%* | 87.5±4.6 | −1.0% | −7.6%* |
| 3 | 76.9±3.8 | −13.5%* | 87.4±4.2 | −1.2% | −13.5%* |
| 6 | 78.9±5.9 | −11.2% | 87.9±3.8 | −0.6% | −11.4%* |
| 24 | 87.4±2.7 | −1.7% | 88.2±4.1 | −0.2% | −0.9% |

* $p<0.01$.

#### 4.1.2.5.2 Blood Flow in the Left Common Carotid Artery, Oxygen Content, and Oxygen Transport Capacity in the Macrocirculation

After isovolemic hemodilution blood flow in the left common carotid artery remained almost constant (Table 54, Fig. 73). After hypervolemic dilution a significant increase (with regard to the initial value) was observed 1 h after the end of the infusion. At 3 h blood flow achieved the initial value.

**Table 54.** Blood flow in the left common carotid artery (BFAcc) [ml/min] before and after iso- or hypervolemic hemodilution

| Time (h) | Isovolemic BFAcc (ml/min) | Change (%) from initial value | Hypervolemic BFAcc (ml/min) | Change (%) from initial value | Difference (%) (iso-hyp) |
|---|---|---|---|---|---|
| Before | 294±56 | – | 284±51 | – | +3.4% |
| 1 | 296±40 | +0.7% | 349±38 | +22.9%* | −17.9%* |
| 3 | 272±44 | −7.4% | 298±43 | +4.9% | −5.9% |
| 6 | 275±45 | −6.4% | 292±51 | +2.8% | −6.2% |
| 24 | 281±33 | −4.4% | 289±48 | +1.8% | −2.8% |

* $p<0.01$.

The oxygen content [$CaO_2 = SO_2 \times Hb \times 1.34 + (\alpha \times 100/760) \times pO_2$ (ml $O_2$/100 ml blood)] of arterial blood decreased significantly after iso- and hypervolemic hemodilution (Table 55, Fig. 73).

According to Eq. 1 (see Sect. 5.7.1) the oxygen transport capacity (OTC) of the macrocirculation can be calculated from blood flow and oxygen content

**Table 55.** Oxygen content ($CaO_2$) in the macrocirculation before and after iso- or hypervolemic hemodilution

| Time (h) | Isovolemic $CaO_2$ (ml $O_2$/100 ml blood)[a] | Change (%) from initial value | Hypervolemic $CaO_2$ (ml $O_2$/100 ml blood)[a] | Change (%) from initial value | Difference (%) (iso-hyp) |
|---|---|---|---|---|---|
| Before | 21.2 (20.4/23.8) | – | 20.9 (20.7/21.4) | – | +1.4% |
| 1 | 17.3 (16.8/17.6) | −18.4%* | 18.6 (18.0/19.0) | −11.0%* | −7.5%* |
| 3 | 18.0 (17.4/18.8) | −15.1%* | 18.8 (18.2/19.4) | −10.0%* | −4.4%* |
| 6 | 18.5 (17.9/18.9) | −12.7%* | 19.5 (19.2/20.3) | −6.6% | −5.4%* |
| 24 | 19.5 (19.1/19.8) | −8.0% | 20.0 (19.7/20.5) | −4.3% | −2.5% |

* $p<0.01$.
[a] Median (2.5/97.5 percentile)

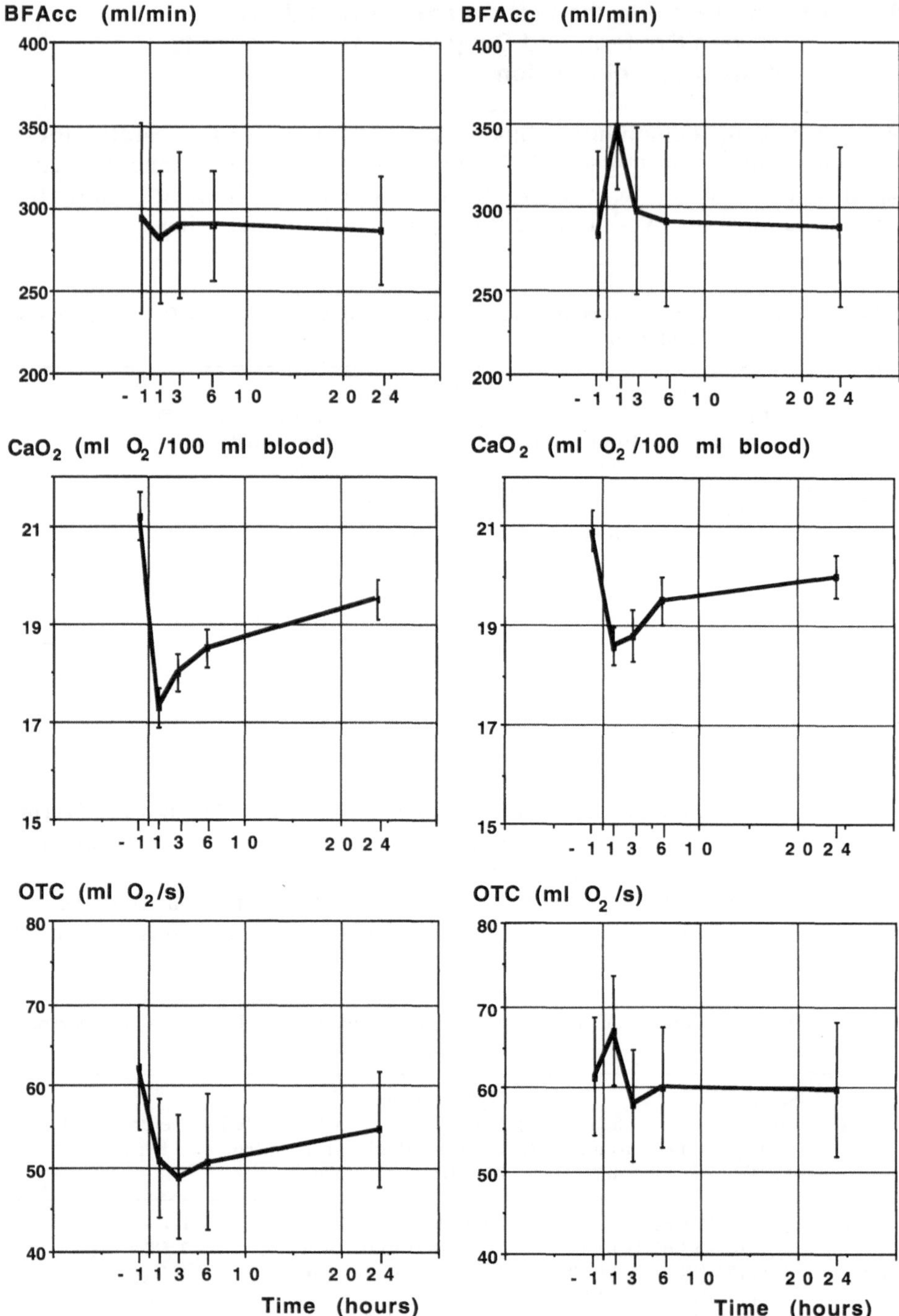


**Fig. 73.** Blood flow in the common carotid artery (*BFAcc*), oxygen content ($CaO_2$), and oxygen transport capacity (*OTC*) in the system of the major vessels before and 1, 3, 6, and 24 h after iso- (*left*) or hypervolemic hemodilution (*right*)

**Table 56.** Oxygen transport capacity (OTC) in the macrocirculation before and after iso- or hypervolemic hemodilution

| Time (h) | Isovolemic OTC (ml $O_2$/s)[a] | Change (%) from initial value | Hypervolemic OTC (ml $O_2$/s)[a] | Change (%) from initial value | Difference (%) (iso-hyp) |
|---|---|---|---|---|---|
| Before | 62.3 (55.0/70.1) | – | 61.4 (54.2/68.7) | – | 1.4% |
| 1 | 51.2 (45.0/58.4) | −17.8%* | 66.9 (60.1/75.8) | +10.0%* | −30.7%* |
| 3 | 49.0 (41.2/57.8) | −21.3%* | 58.0 (51.0/65.0) | −5.5% | −18.4%* |
| 6 | 50.9 (42.5/59.6) | −18.3%* | 60.1 (53.2/68.5) | −2.1% | −18.1%* |
| 24 | 56.8 (45.0/63.6) | −8.8% | 59.8 (52.2/68.8) | −2.6% | −5.3% |

* $p<0.01$.

[OTC = BFAcc × $CaO_2$ (ml $O_2$/s)]. Whereas OTC decreased significantly after isovolemic hemodilution, it increased significantly 1 h after hypervolemic hemodilution; afterwards it returned to the initial value (Table 56, Fig. 73).

## 4.1.2.6 Hemodynamic Parameters in the Microcirculation

### 4.1.2.6.1 Packing Density of Erythrocyte Columns

The differences in density between erythrocyte column and capillary environment before and 1 h after iso- or hypervolemic hemodilution, standardized by the measuring times (video pictures of the same erythrocyte columns at specific seconds for 1 min), revealed no significant changes according to Wilcoxon's test for matched pairs. The same results are also found at 3, 6, and 24 h (not shown) after both forms of hemodilution. Thus, a constant packing density of erythrocytes in the erythrocyte columns at all measuring times can be assumed (Sect. 5.8). Figures 74 and 75 show the differences in density in the same capillary areas of six subjects (not of all ten) before and 1 h after iso- or hypervolemic hemodilution. Here both hemodilution forms present the greatest dilution effect in the vasuclar system. The mean values given refer to the whole group and not to only the values in the figures.

### 4.1.2.6.2 Erythrocyte Column Diameter

Erythrocyte column diameters were not significantly affected by hemodilution. Table 57 shows the measuring data quantified by a computer (see Sect. 5.8).

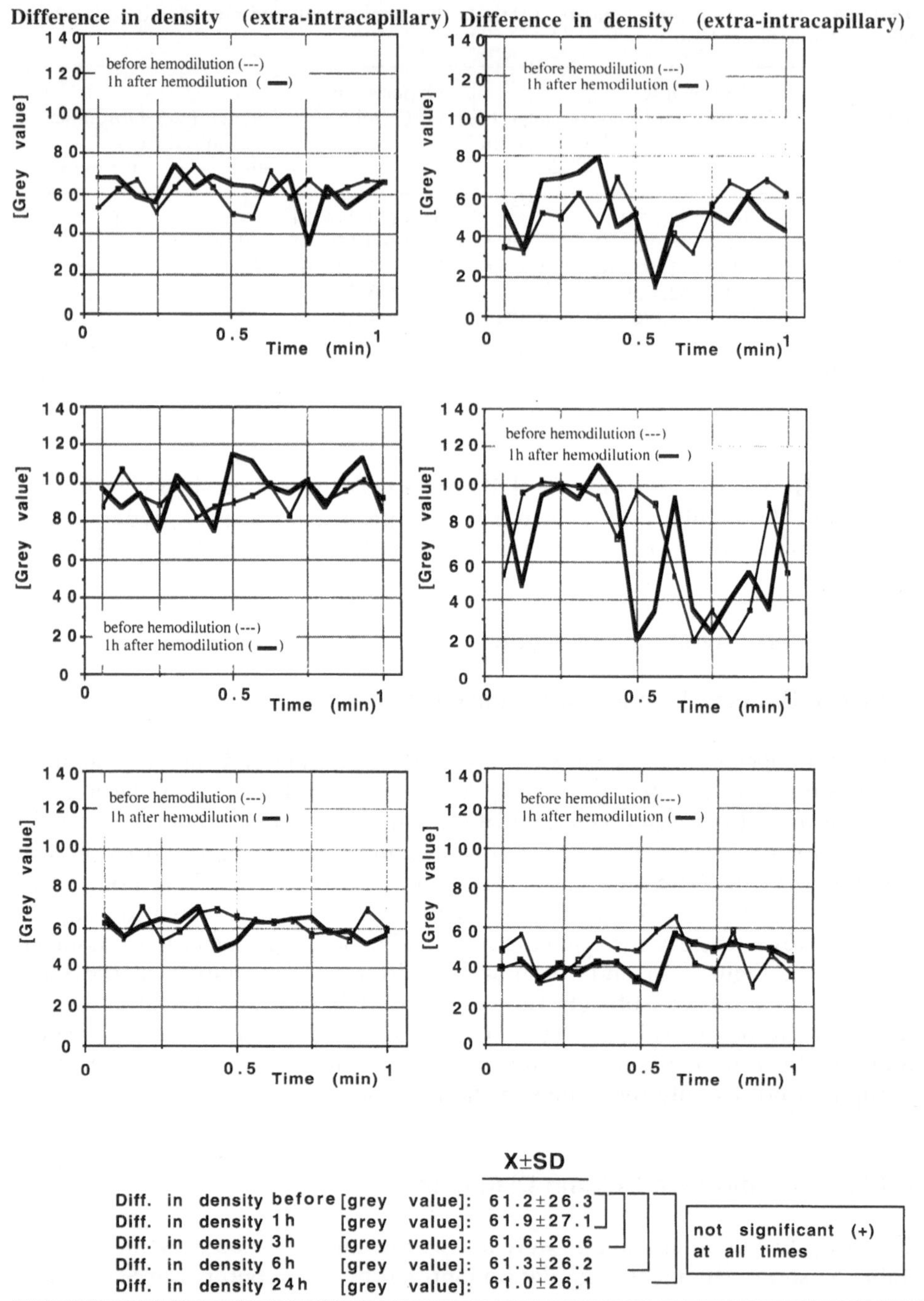


| | X±SD |
|---|---|
| Diff. in density before [grey value]: | 61.2±26.3 |
| Diff. in density 1 h [grey value]: | 61.9±27.1 |
| Diff. in density 3 h [grey value]: | 61.6±26.6 |
| Diff. in density 6 h [grey value]: | 61.3±26.2 |
| Diff. in density 24 h [grey value]: | 61.0±26.1 |

not significant (+) at all times

(+): Wilcoxon's test for pair differentiation

**Fig. 74.** Evaluation of the packing density (difference extra- versus intracapillary) of erythrocyte columns in the main capillaries and 1 h after isovolemic hemodilution with the optic difference in density (illustrated for six subjects). (+), Wilcoxon test for matched pairs

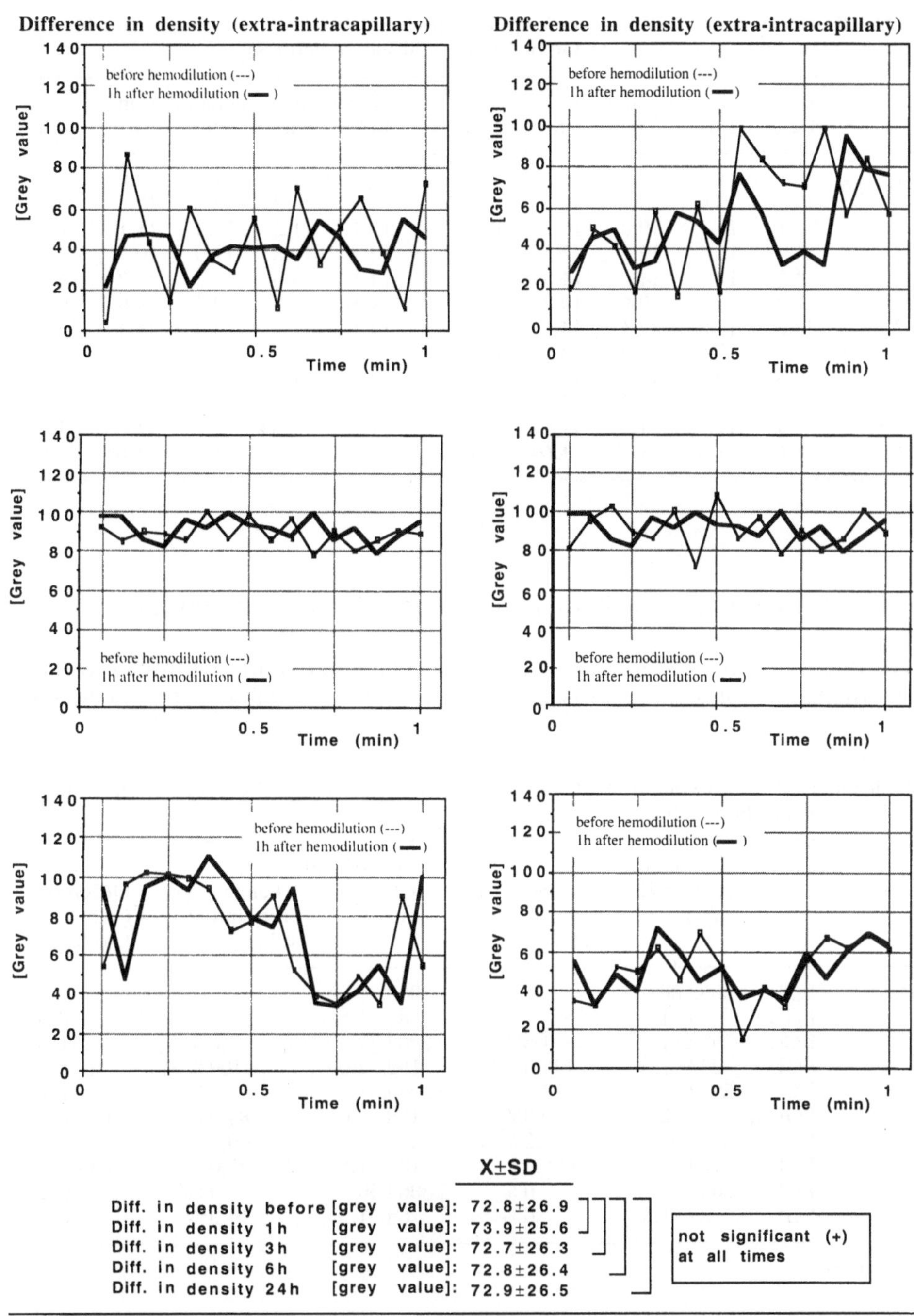


(+): Wilcoxon's test for pair differentiation

**Fig. 75.** Evaluation of the packing density (difference extra- versus intracapillary) of erythrocyte columns in the main capillaries and 1 h after hypervolemic hemodilution with the optic difference in density (illustrated for six subjects. ( I ), Wilcoxon test for matched pairs

**Table 57.** Erythrocyte column diameter [μm] before and after iso- or hypervolemic hemodilution (each single value, mean value of 60 different video pictures)

| | Isovolemic hemodilution | | | | | Hypervolemic hemodilution | | | | |
|---|---|---|---|---|---|---|---|---|---|---|
| | Before | 1 h | 3 h | 6 h | 24 h | Before | 1 h | 3 h | 6 h | 24 h |
| 1 | 10.8 | 11.0 | 11.0 | 10.8 | 10.9 | 10.9 | 11.0 | 11.2 | 10.8 | 10.9 |
| 2 | 10.3 | 10.0 | 10.4 | 10.3 | 10.3 | 10.5 | 10.3 | 10.6 | 10.5 | 10.5 |
| 3 | 11.1 | 10.4 | 10.8 | 10.7 | 10.9 | 11.1 | 11.2 | 11.4 | 11.1 | 11.2 |
| 4 | 12.4 | 12.3 | 12.2 | 12.5 | 12.5 | 10.7 | 10.8 | 11.0 | 10.7 | 10.8 |
| 5 | 14.2 | 14.4 | 14.5 | 14.5 | 14.2 | 14.1 | 14.3 | 14.2 | 14.2 | 14.2 |
| 6 | 9.9 | 10.4 | 9.6 | 10.2 | 9.9 | 9.8 | 9.7 | 9.7 | 9.9 | 9.9 |
| 7 | 14.3 | 14.2 | 14.4 | 14.2 | 14.2 | 14.1 | 14.2 | 14.4 | 14.1 | 14.2 |
| 8 | 13.6 | 13.4 | 13.6 | 13.5 | 13.6 | 13.9 | 14.0 | 13.8 | 13.8 | 13.8 |
| 9 | 10.8 | 10.9 | 11.2 | 10.8 | 10.9 | 10.9 | 11.0 | 11.0 | 10.8 | 10.9 |
| 10 | 12.1 | 12.3 | 12.2 | 12.2 | 12.2 | 12.3 | 12.3 | 12.2 | 12.4 | 12.4 |
| Mean | 11.95 | 11.93 | 11.99 | 11.97 | 11.96 | 11.83 | 11.88 | 11.95 | 11.83 | 11.88 |
| SD | 1.63 | 1.63 | 1.70 | 1.64 | 1.61 | 1.64 | 1.71 | 1.64 | 1.65 | 1.64 |

#### 4.1.2.6.3 Erythrocyte Column Length and Plasma Gap Length

The effect of hemodilution on mean plasma gap length and erythrocyte column length of all visible capillaries is presented in Table 58 and Fig. 76 (see Sect. 5.8).

**Table 58.** Erythrocyte column length (ECL) and plasma gap length (PGL) before and after iso- or hypervolemic hemodilution

| Time (h) | | Isovolemic ECL/PGL (μm) | Change (%) from initial value | Hypervolemic ECL/PGL (μm) | Change (%) from initial value | Difference (%) (iso-hyp) |
|---|---|---|---|---|---|---|
| Before | ECL | 306±30 | – | 306±29 | – | 0% |
| | PGL | 8± 1.5 | – | 8± 1.5 | – | 0% |
| 1 | ECL | 292±31 | −4.6%* | 298±31 | −2.6% | −2.1% |
| | PGL | 22± 3.0 | +175.0%* | 16± 2.0 | +100% | +27.3%* |
| 3 | ECL | 294±32 | −3.9%* | 299±31 | −2.2% | −1.7% |
| | PGL | 20± 2.5 | +150.0%* | 15± 2.0 | +88.0% | +25.0%* |
| 6 | ECL | 299±31 | −2.2% | 304±30 | −0.7% | −1.7% |
| | PGL | 15± 2.0 | +88.0% | 10+ 1.5 | +25.0% | +33.3%* |
| 24 | ECL | 306±30 | 0% | 306±30 | 0% | 0% |
| | PGL | 8± 1.5 | 0% | 8± 1.5 | 0% | 0% |

* $p<0.01$.

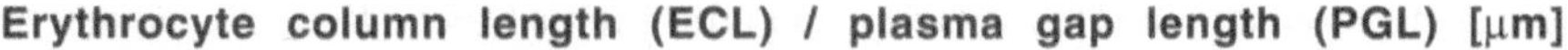


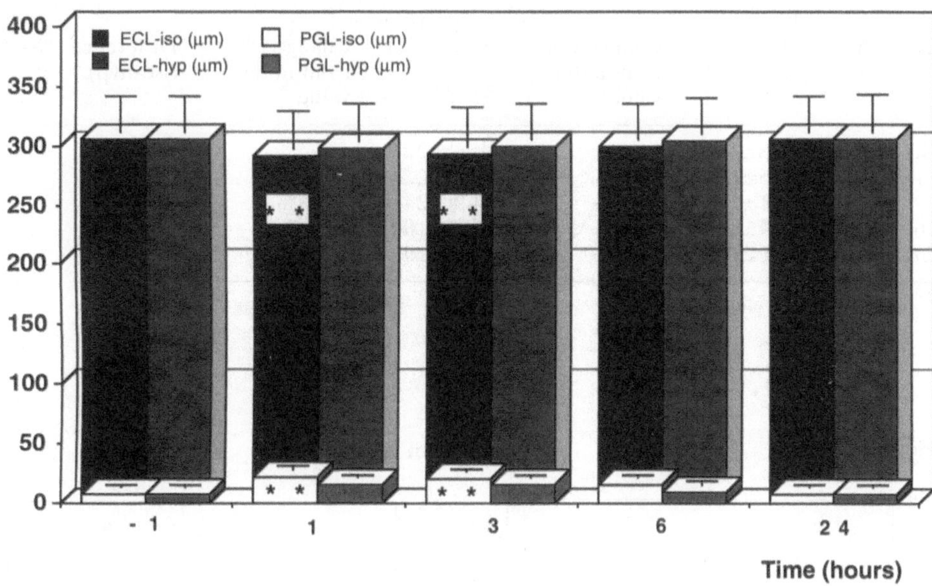


**Fig. 76.** Mean length of the visible erythrocyte columns (*ECL*) and plasma gaps (*PGL*) in the same capillary areas before and 1, 3, 6, and 24 h after iso- or hypervolemic hemodilution. **, $p<0.01$

Mean plasma gap length increased significantly after isovolemic hemodilution, while a tendency toward an increase appeared after hypervolemic hemodilution.

#### 4.1.2.6.4 Capillary Hematocrit

The initial value for capillary hematocrit is determined by systemic hematocrit (Sect. 5.8). Here, capillary hematocrit was 33% of systemic hematocrit [72, 238]. The difference between systemic hematocrit (Hct) and capillary hematocrit is explained by the Fahraeus-Lindqvist effect [58, 59] or by the screen effect ("red cell screening" or "plasma skimming" [72, 222]; hemoconcentration in the shunt preference canals, hemodilution in the nutritive main capillaries).

Table 59 and Fig. 77 show the course of capillary hematocrit. A significant increase in capillary hematocrit of the main capillaries was observed only after isovolemic hemodilution, but 1 h after the end of infusion the decrease was by 1.3 hematocrit points (8.2%), only half as pronounced as the decrease in macrocirculation, by 8.5 hematocrit points (17.9%). The decrease in capillary hematocrit was accompanied by an increase in plasma gaps [158].

**Table 59.** Capillary hematocrit ($Hct_{cap}$) before and after iso- or hypervolemic hemodilution

| Time (h) | Isovolemic $Hct_{cap}$(%) | Change (%) from initial value | Hypervolemic $Hct_{cap}$(%) | Change (%) from initial value | Difference (%) (iso-hyp) |
|---|---|---|---|---|---|
| Before | 15.8±1.4 | – | 15.4±2.5 | – | ±2.5% |
| 1 | 14.5±1.5 | −8.2%* | 14.9±2.2 | −3.3% | −2.8%* |
| 3 | 15.1±2.2 | −4.4% | 14.9±2.4 | −3.3% | −1.3% |
| 6 | 15.4±1.8 | −2.5% | 15.3±1.8 | −0.6% | −0.6% |
| 24 | 15.9±2.0 | +1.2% | 15.5±1.9 | +0.6% | +2.5% |

* $p<0.05$.

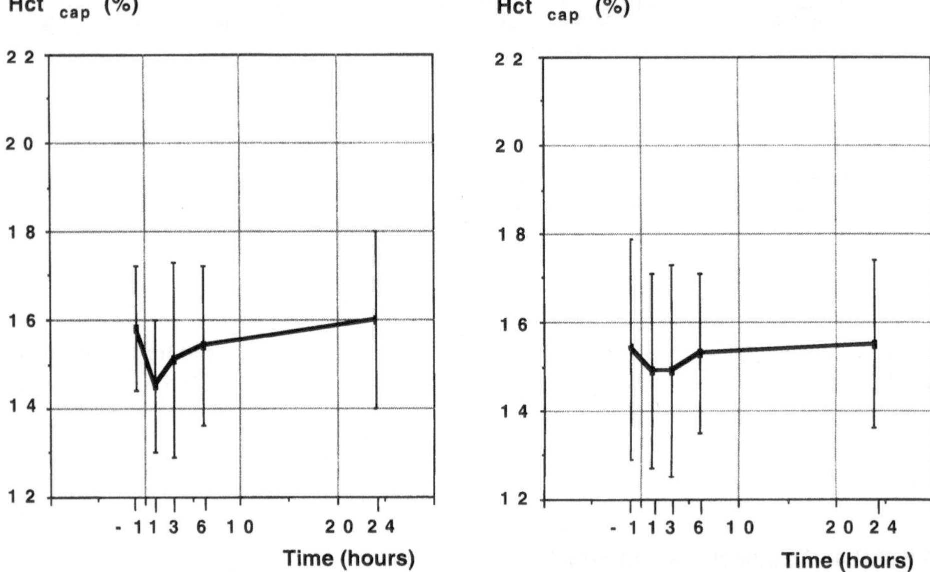


**Fig. 77.** Capillary hematocrit before and 1, 3, 6, and 24 h after iso- (*left*) or hypervolemic hemodilution (*right*)

#### 4.1.2.6.5 Capillary Hematocrit Change (at Different Initial Hematocrit Values)

Figure 78 illustrates the changes in the capillary hematocrit value with respect to the initial value (see Sect. 5.8).

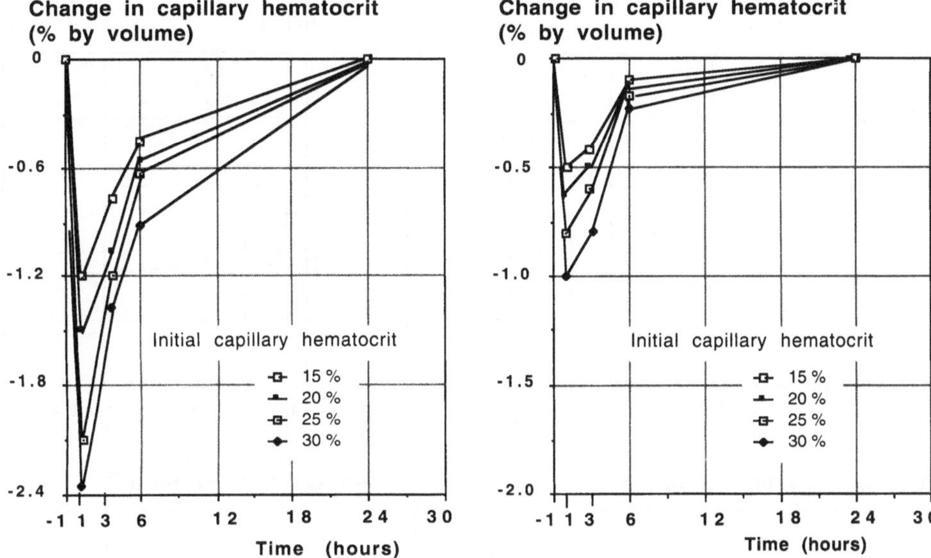


**Fig. 78.** Change in capillary hematocrit value (percentage by volume) dependent on the initial value before and 1, 3, 6, and 24 h after iso- (*left*) or hypervolemic hemodilution (*right*)

### 4.1.2.6.6 Blood Flow in the Capillaries, Oxygen Content, and Oxygen Transport Capacity in the Microcirculation

One hour after hypervolemic hemodilution there was a significant increase in capillary blood flow in the main capillaries, compared to a significant decrease after isovolemic hemodilution. Afterwards the mean capillary blood flow increases again to the initial value (Table 60, Fig. 79).

**Table 60.** Blood flow (BFcap) in the main capillaries before and after iso- or hypervolemic hemodilution

| Time (h) | Isovolemic BFcap ($10^{-9}$ ml/s) | Change (%) from initial value | Hypervolemic BFcap ($10^{-9}$ ml/s) | Change (%) from initial value | Difference (%) (iso-hyp) |
|---|---|---|---|---|---|
| Before | 32±11 | – | 34±14 | – | −6.2% |
| 1 | 22±13 | −29.0%* | 64±22 | +88.2%* | −190.9%* |
| 3 | 23±12 | −25.8%* | 40±18 | +17.6% | −73.9%* |
| 6 | 28±11 | −9.7% | 36±16 | +5.9% | −28.6%* |
| 24 | 33±13 | +6.5% | 33±12 | −2.9% | +0% |

* $p<0.01$.

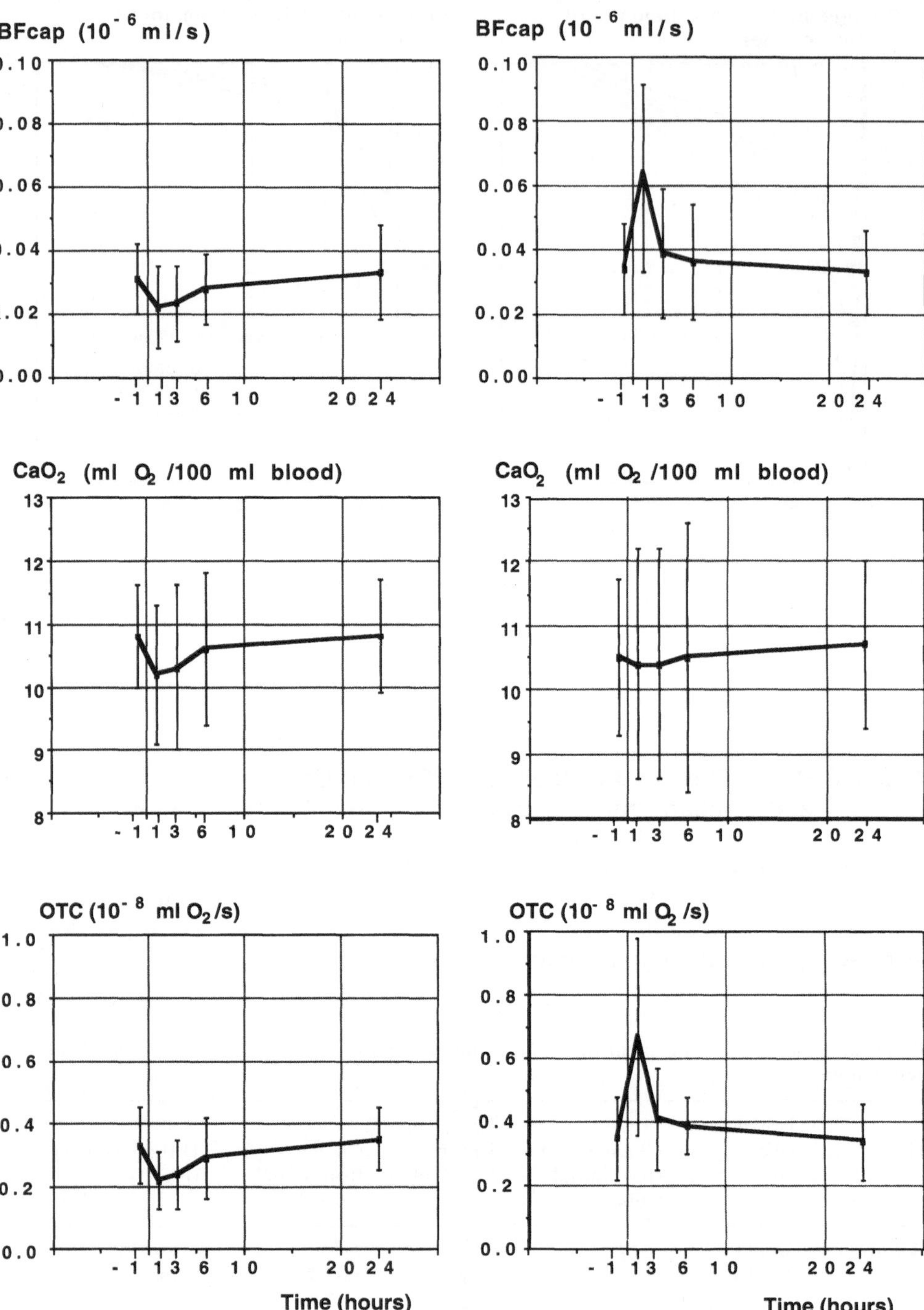


**Fig. 79.** Blood flow in the nutritive main capillaries (*BFcap*), oxygen content ($CaO_2$), and oxygen transport capacity (*OTC*) in the microcirculaton before and 1, 3, 6, and 24 h after iso- (*left*) or hypervolemic hemodilution (*right*)

**Table 61.** Oxygen content ($CaO_2$) in the microcirculation before and after iso- or hypervolemic hemodilution

| Time (h) | Isovolemic $CaO_2$ (ml $O_2$/ 100 ml blood) | Change (%) from initial value | Hypervolemic $CaO_2$ (ml $O_2$/ 100 ml blood) | Change (%) from initial value | Difference (%) (iso-hyp) |
|---|---|---|---|---|---|
| Before | 10.8±0.8 | – | 10.5±1.2 | – | +2.8% |
| 1 | 10.2±1.1 | −5.6%* | 10.4±1.8 | −0.9% | −2.0% |
| 3 | 10.3±1.3 | −4.6% | 10.4±1.8 | −0.9% | −0.9% |
| 6 | 10.6±1.2 | −1.9% | 10.5±1.1 | ±0% | +0.9% |
| 24 | 10.8±0.9 | ±0% | 10.7±1.3 | +1.9% | −0.9% |

* $p<0.01$.

**Table 62.** Oxygen transport capacity (OTC) in the microcirculation before and after iso- or hypervolemic hemodilution

| Time (h) | Isovolemic OTC ($10^{-8}$ ml $O_2$/s) | Change (%) from initial value | Hypervolemic OTC ($10^{-8}$ ml $O_2$/s) | Change (%) from initial value | Difference (%) (iso-hyp) |
|---|---|---|---|---|---|
| Before | 0.33±0.12 | – | 0.35±0.13 | – | −6.1% |
| 1 | 0.22±0.09 | −33.3% | 0.67±0.31 | +80.2% | −204.5% |
| 3 | 0.24±0.11 | −27.3% | 0.41±0.14 | +17.1% | −70.8% |
| 6 | 0.29±0.13 | −12.1% | 0.39±0.09 | +11.4% | −34.5% |
| 24 | 0.35±0.13 | +6.1% | 0.34±0.12 | −2.9% | +2.9% |

* $p<0.01$.

Oxygen content [$CaO_2 = SO_2 \times Hb \times 1.34 + (\alpha \times 100/760) \times pO_2$ (ml $O_2$/100 ml blood)] in the microcirculation showed an almost constant course after hypervolemic hemodilution, whereas it decreased significantly 1 h after isovolemic hemodilution and increased again gradually to the initial value (Tables 61, 62; Fig. 79). This led to a significant increase in the oxygen transport capacity [$OTC = BFcap \times CaO_2$ (ml $O_2$/s)] of capillary blood after hypervolemic hemodilution, and after isovolemic hemodilution to a decrease with regard to the initial value.

In order to calculate these parameters the values for oxygen partial pressure ($pO_2$) and oxygen saturation ($SO_2$) in arterial blood were used (see Fig. 72).

#### 4.1.2.6.7 Reactive Hyperemia

The duration of reactive hyperemia was significantly prolonged 1 and 3 h after isovolemic hemodilution ($p<0.05$); after hypervolemic hemodilution there was no significant change (Table 63, Fig. 80).

**Table 63.** Duration of reactive hyperemia (DrH) before and after iso- or hypervolemic hemodilution

| Time (h) | Isovolemic DrH (s)[a] | Change (%) from initial value | Hypervolemic DrH (s)[a] | Change (%) from initial value | Difference (%) (iso-hyp) |
|---|---|---|---|---|---|
| Before | 180 (140/200) | – | 184 (140/200) | – | −2.2% |
| 1 | 220 (160/240) | +22.2%* | 180 (120/220) | −2.1% | +18.2%* |
| 3 | 220 (140/240) | +22.2%* | 194 (160/240) | +5.4% | +11.8%* |
| 6 | 210 (150/240) | +16.7% | 190 (160/220) | +3.3% | +9.5%* |
| 24 | 180 (140/200) | +0% | 184 (150/220) | +0% | −2.2% |

* $p<0.01$.
[a] Median (2.5/97.5 percentiles)

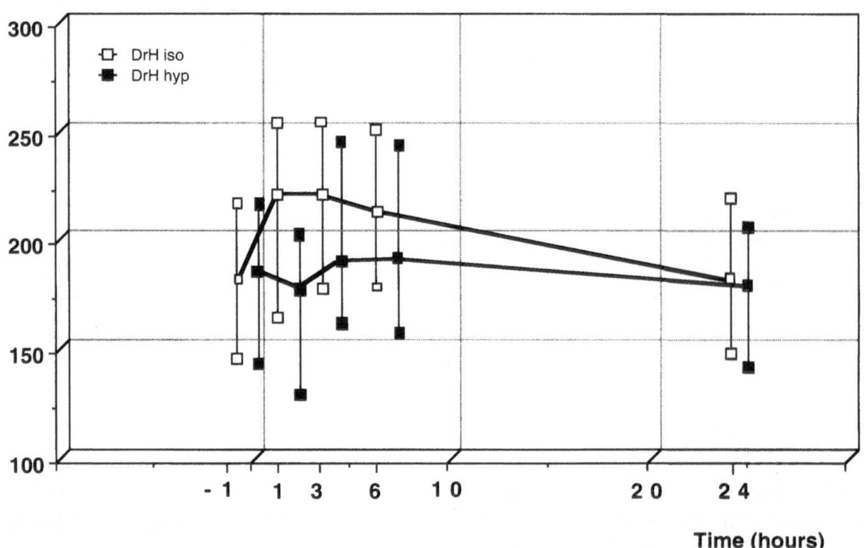


**Fig. 80.** Duration of reactive hyperemia before and 1, 3, 6, and 24 h after iso- or hypervolemic hemodilution (2.5 and 97.5 percentiles as limits with same symbols as the corresponding mean measuring points)

The difference between maximal flow velocity after stasis and resting velocity remained unchanged during all phases after both hemodilution variants (Tables 64, 65). Flow velocities at rest and maximal velocity after stasis decreased significantly after isovolemic hemodilution (1 h and 3 h) and increased after hypervolemic hemodilution (1 h; Fig. 81). Due to the fact that 1 h and 3 h after isovolemic hemodilution identical courses appeared, only one time is given.

**Table 64.** Resting erythrocyte velocity in the capillaries of the skin ($v_{rest}$) [mm/s] before and after iso- or hypervolemic hemodilution

| Time (h) | Isovolemic $v_{rest}$ (mm/s) | Change (%) from initial value | Hypervolemic $v_{rest}$ (mm/s) | Change (%) from initial value | Difference (%) (iso-hyp) |
|---|---|---|---|---|---|
| Before | 0.74±0.33 | – | 0.72±0.37 | – | +2.7% |
| 1 | 0.53±0.32 | −28.4%* | 1.44±0.68 | +100.0%* | −171.7%* |
| 3 | 0.53±0.32 | −28.4%* | 0.85±0.41 | +18.0% | −60.4%* |
| 6 | 0.70±0.29 | −5.4% | 0.78±0.42 | +8.3% | −11.4% |
| 24 | 0.75±0.36 | +1.4% | 0.76±0.42 | +5.5% | −1.3% |

* $p<0.01$.

**Table 65.** Maximal erythrocyte velocity in the capillaries of the skin after 3 min of ischemia ($v_{max}$) before and after iso- or hypervolemic hemodilution

| Time (h) | Sovolemic $v_{max}$ (mm/s) | Change (%) from initial value | Hypervolemic $v_{max}$ (mm/s) | Change (%) from initial value | Difference (%) (iso-hyp) |
|---|---|---|---|---|---|
| Before | 1.40±0.48 | – | 1.42±0.45 | – | −1.4% |
| 1 | 1.20±0.44 | −14.3%* | 2.10±1.00 | +47.9%* | −75.0%* |
| 3 | 1.20±0.44 | −14.3%* | 1.61±0.57 | +13.3% | −34.2%* |
| 6 | 1.30±0.49 | −7.2% | 1.50±0.48 | +5.6% | −15.3% |
| 24 | 1.42±0.48 | +1.4% | 1.44±0.51 | +1.4% | −1.4% |

* $p<0.01$.

### 4.1.2.7 Laser Doppler Flux

Corresponding to the blood flow in the common carotid artery, the laser Doppler flux decreased after isovolemic but increased after hypervolemic hemodilution (Table 66, Fig. 82). Afterwards the values returned to the initial values. The duration of reactive hyperemia determined with the laser Doppler flux as a response to ischemia of 3 min did not change with regard to the initial values after either hemodilution form.

### 4.1.2.8 Oxygen Partial Pressure in Skin and Muscle

#### 4.1.2.8.1 Transcutaneous and Conjunctival Oxygen Partial Pressure

The course of the transcutaneous oxygen partial pressure in the arm, foot, and eye after iso- or hypervolemic hemodilution is presented in Tables 67, 68, and 69.

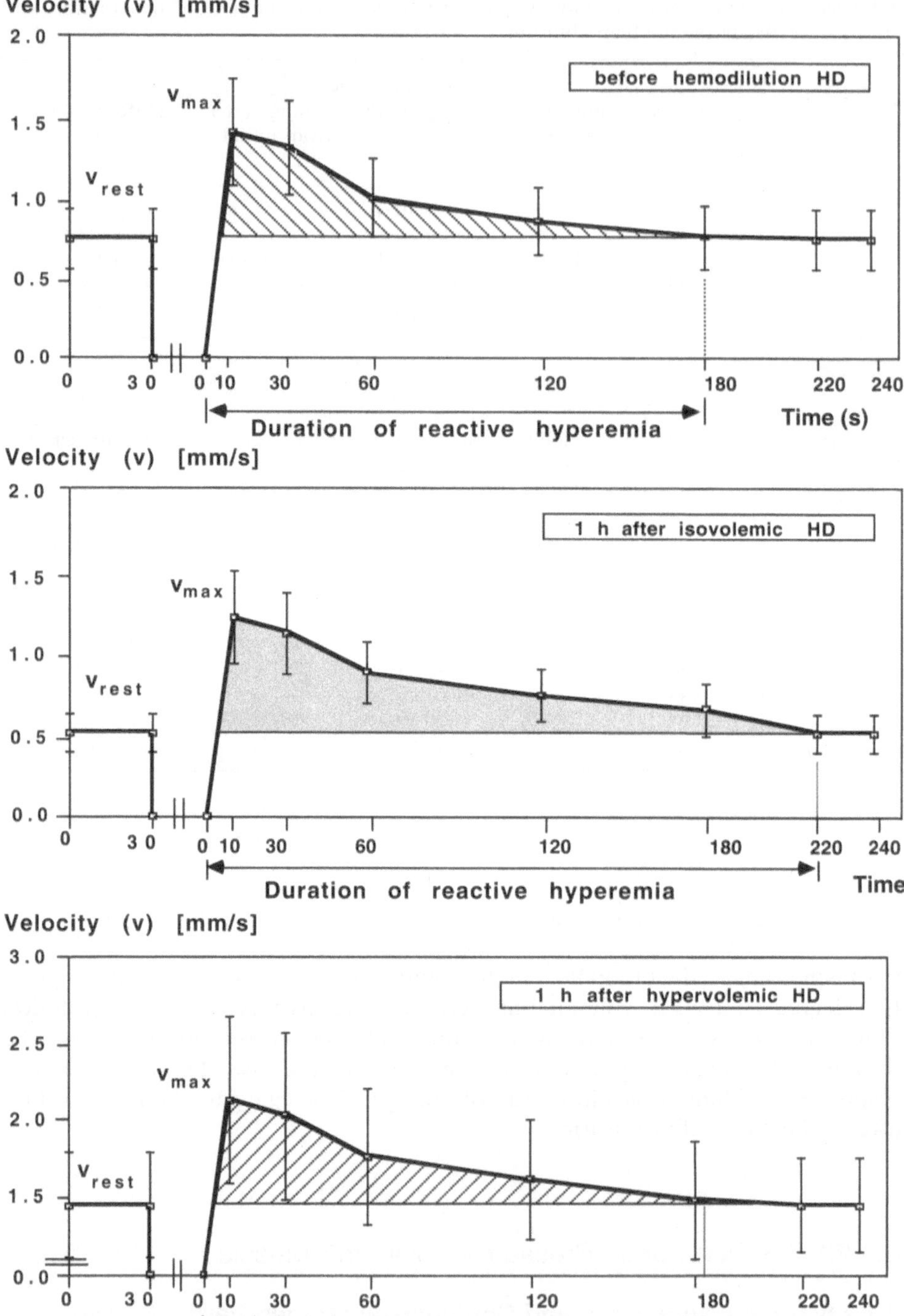


**Fig. 81.** Reactive hyperemia as a function of velocity and time before and 1 h after iso- or hypervolemic hemodilution

**Table 66.** Laser Doppler flux (LDF) before and after iso- or hypervolemic hemodilution

| Time (h) | Isovolemic LDF (PU)[a] | Change (%) from initial value | Hypervolemic LDF (PU)[a] | Change (%) from initial value | Difference (%) (iso-hyp) |
|---|---|---|---|---|---|
| Before | 25.5 (15.2/34.5) | – | 24.8 (14.0/33.0) | – | +2.7% |
| 1 | 16.1 ( 8.8/24.0) | −36.9%* | 28.9 (20.1/38.9) | +16.5%* | −79.5%* |
| 3 | 22.1 (10.0/30.9) | −13.3% | 28.2 (14.2/37.3) | +13.7% | −27.6%* |
| 6 | 23.3 (10.9/32.1) | −8.6% | 25.1 (16.3/34.4) | +1.2% | −7.8% |
| 24 | 26.6 (15.4/35.8) | +4.3% | 24.8 (14.2/34.0) | +0% | +6.8% |

* $p<0.01$.
[a] Median (2.5/97.5 percentiles)

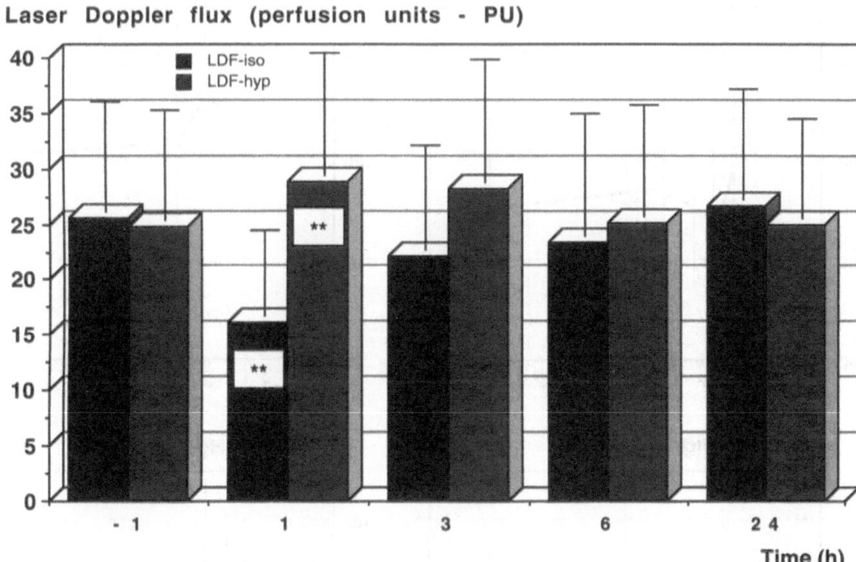


**Fig. 82.** Laser Doppler flux (*LDF*) in perfusion units (*PU*) before and 1, 3, 6, and 24 h after iso- and hypervolemic hemodilution. **, $p<0.01$

respectively (see also Fig. 83). Comparable to the course of capillary blood flow in the skin there was a significant increase in transcutaneous oxygen partial pressure ($pO_2$) in the foot after 3 h, transconjunctivally after 1 and 3 h. A tendency toward an increase was found in the transcutaneous oxygen pressure of

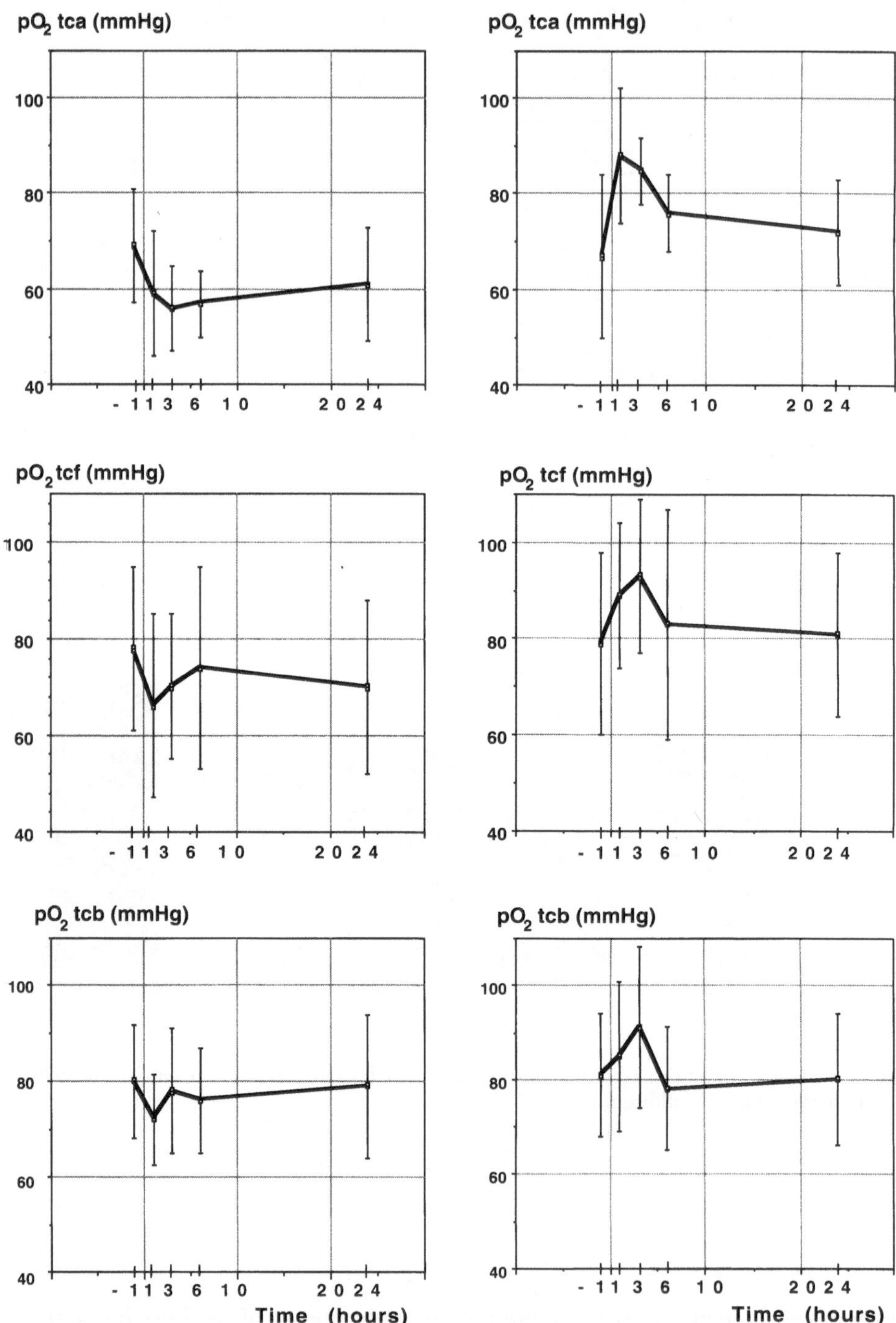


**Fig. 83.** Transcutaneous oxygen partial pressures at the arm (*$pO_2$-tca*), back of the foot (*$pO_2$-tcf*), and transconjunctival oxygen partial pressure (*$pO_2$-tcb*) before and 1, 3, 6, and 24 h after iso- (*left*) and hypervolemic hemodilution (*right*)

**Table 67.** Arm $pO_2$ (transcutaneous) before and after iso- or hypervolemic hemodilution

| Time (h) | Isovolemic Arm $pO_2$ (mmHg)[a] | Change (%) from initial value | Hypervolemic Arm $pO_2$ (mmHg)[a] | Change (%) from initial value | Difference (%) (iso-hyp) |
|---|---|---|---|---|---|
| Before | 69 (55/81) | – | 67 (48/ 83) | – | +2.9% |
| 1 | 59 (44/70) | −14.5% | 88 (73/104) | +31.3%* | −49.1%* |
| 3 | 56 (47/63) | −18.8%* | 85 (77/ 89) | +26.9% | −51.8%* |
| 6 | 58 (50/61) | −15.9% | 76 (66/ 84) | +13.4% | −31.0%* |
| 24 | 63 (51/75) | −8.7% | 72 (60/ 82) | +7.5% | −14.2% |

* $p<0.01$.<>

[a] Median (2.5/97.5 percentiles)

**Table 68.** Foot $pO_2$ (transcutaneous) before and after iso- or hypervolemic hemodilution

| Time (h) | Isovolemic Foot $pO_2$ (mmHg) | Change (%) from initial value | Hypervolemic Foot $pO_2$ (mmHg) | Change (%) from initial value | Difference (%) (iso-hyp) |
|---|---|---|---|---|---|
| Before | 78±17 | – | 79±19 | – | −1.3% |
| 1 | 66±19 | −15.4%* | 89±15 | +12.7% | −34.8%* |
| 3 | 70±15 | −10.3%* | 93±16 | +17.7%* | −32.8%* |
| 6 | 76±22 | −2.6% | 83±24 | +5.1% | −9.2% |
| 24 | 74±18 | −5.1% | 81±17 | +2.5% | −9.5% |

* $p<0.01$.

**Table 69.** Eye $pO_2$ (transconjunctival) before and after iso- or hypervolemic hemodilution

| Time (h) | Isovolemic Eye $pO_2$ (mmHg) | Change (%) from initial value | Hypervolemic Eye $pO_2$ (mmHg) | Change (%) from initial value | Difference (%) (iso-hyp) |
|---|---|---|---|---|---|
| Before | 80±12 | – | 81±13 | – | −1.3% |
| 1 | 72±10 | −10% | 85±16 | +5.0% | −18.1%* |
| 3 | 78±13 | −2.5% | 91±19 | +12.3% | −16.7%* |
| 6 | 76±11 | −5% | 78±13 | −3.7% | −2.6% |
| 24 | 79±15 | −1.3% | 80±14 | −1.2% | −1.3% |

* $p<0.01$.

the arm. Afterwards all $pO_2$ values decreased again and achieved the initial values after 24 h. After isovolemic hemodilution there is a significant decrease with regard to the initial value at the arm and foot. Also here the initial values reappeared after 24 h. The transconjunctival oxygen partial pressure shows no statistically significant changes after isovolemic hemodilution.

#### 4.1.2.8.2 Intramuscular $pO_2$ in the Tibialis Anterior Muscle

Intramuscular oxygen behaves differently (Table 70, Fig. 84). One hour after the end of isovolemic hemodilution a decrease in oxygen partial pressure appeared; during the further course there was a tendency toward an increase, and a significant increase was observed after 24 h. On hypervolemic hemodilution there was a steady increase (or shift to the right) in the intramuscular oxygen histogram. Intramuscular oxygen partial pressure values for hypervolemic hemodilution were significantly ($p<0.01$) higher than for isovolemic hemodilution 24 h after the end of the infusion.

**Table 70.** Intramuscular $pO_2$ in the tibialis anterior muscle (IM) before and after iso- or hypervolemic hemodilution

| Time (h) | Isovolemic IM $pO_2$ (mmHg) | Change (%) from initial value | Hypervolemic IM $pO_2$ (mmHg) | Change (%) from initial value | Difference (%) (iso-hyp) |
|---|---|---|---|---|---|
| Before | 21.6±5.8 | – | 22.2±5.9 | – | −2.8% |
| 1 | 17.0±4.8 | −21.3%* | 23.3±4.5 | +4.9% | −37.1%* |
| 4.5 | 22.0±6.6 | +1.9%** | 24.0±8.1 | +8.1%** | −9.1%* |
| 24 | 24.7±4.6 | +14.4%** | 29.0±5.6 | +30.6%* | −17.4%* |

* $p<0.01$; ** $p<0.05$.

### 4.1.2.9 Blood pH, Plasma Lactate, and Pyruvate Concentration

The pH value of arterial blood decreased significantly only after isovolemic hemodilution (Table 71, Fig. 85). Lactate concentration decreased significantly 1 h after isovolemic hemodilution, after hypervolemic hemodilution only in tendency (similar temporal couse; Table 72, Fig. 85). This was similar with the pyruvate concentration (Table 73, Fig. 85).

The lactate/pyruvate quotient changed 1 h after iso- and hypervolemic hemodilution and decreased significantly ($p<0.05$) to values between 20 and 25 (by about 18%). At the remaining measuring times the lactate/pyruvate quotient remained unchanged with both hemodilutions.

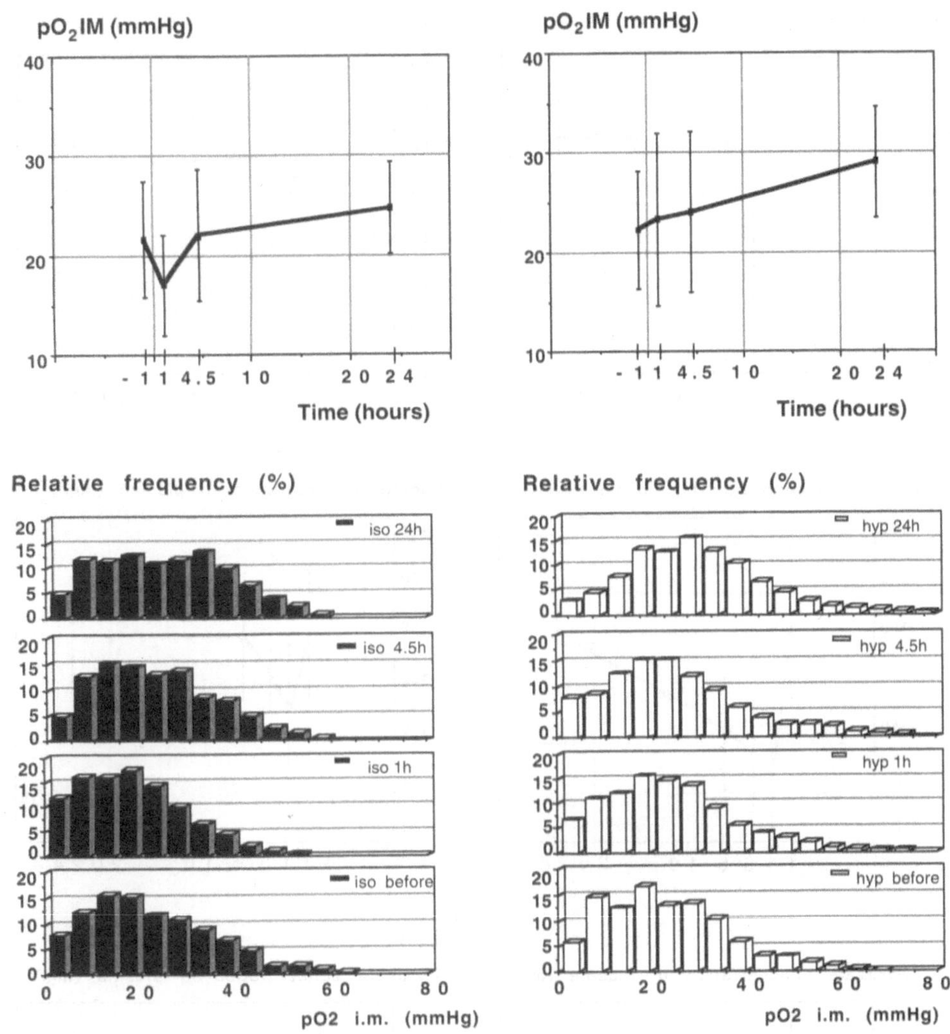


**Fig. 84.** Intramuscular oxygen partial pressure before and 1, 4.5, and 24 h after iso- (*left*) and hypervolemic (*right*) hemodilution. *Above*, means; *below*, histographic distributions (relative frequencies)

### *4.2.10 Summary of the Relative Changes of Parameters*

Figure 86 summarizes the changes in the various parameters after iso- and hypervolemic hemodilution as presented above.

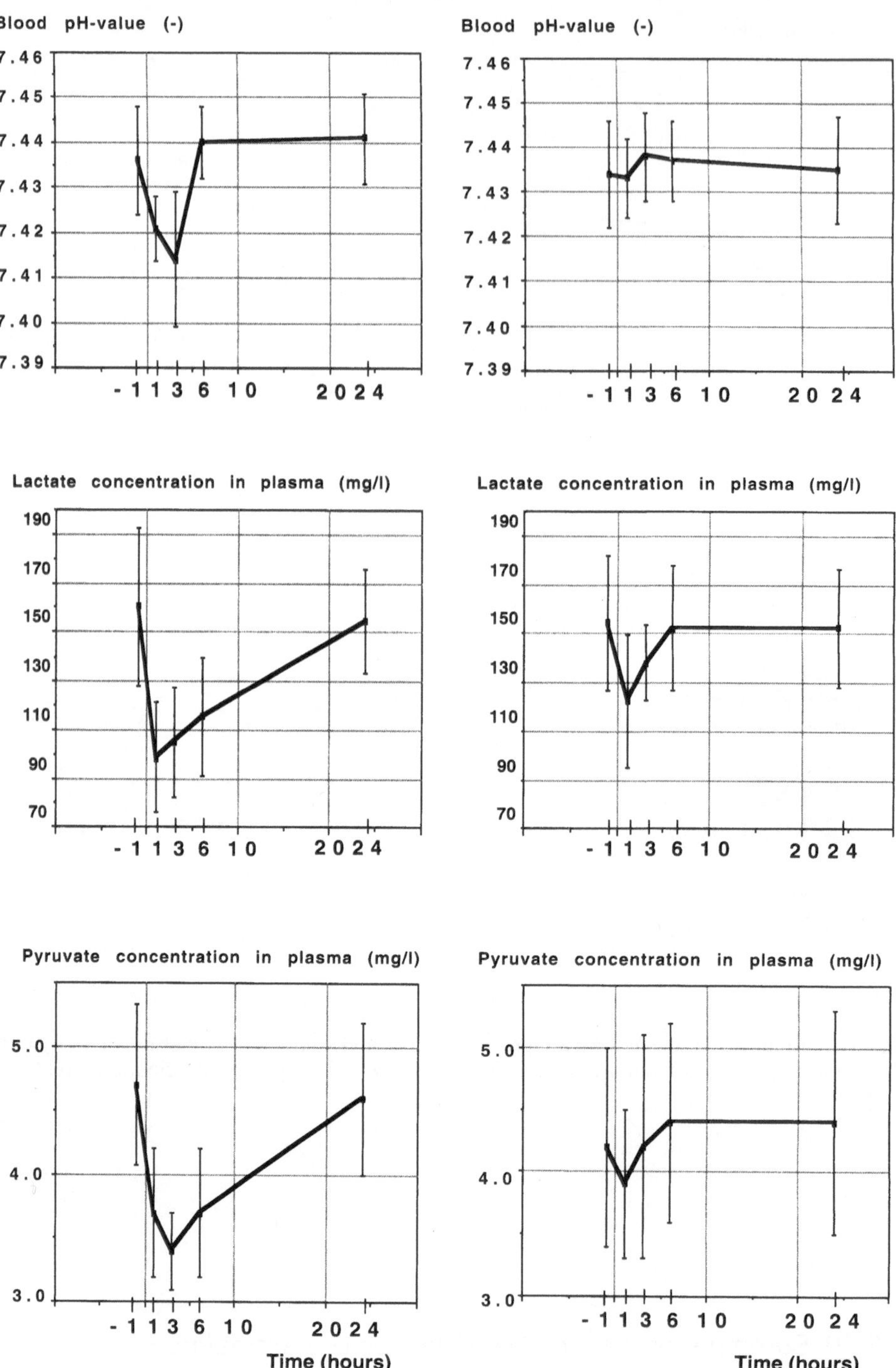


**Fig. 85.** Metabolic parameters (pH value in blood, lactate, pyruvate concentration in plasma) before and 1, 3, 6, and 24 h after iso- (*left*) and hypervolemic hemodilution (*right*)

**Table 71.** pH value in arterialized blood (pH) before and after iso- or hypervolemic hemodilution

| Time (h) | Isovolemic pH[−] | Change (%) from initial value | Hypervolemic pH[−] | Change (%) from initial value |
|---|---|---|---|---|
| Before | 7.436 (7.425/7.448) | – | 7.434 (7.422/7.446) | – |
| 1 | 7.421 (7.410/7.428) | −0.2%* | 7.433 (7.423/7.442) | ±0% |
| 3 | 7.414 (7.400/7.430) | −0.3%* | 7.438 (7.424/7.448) | +0.05% |
| 6 | 7.440 (7.432/7.450) | +0.05% | 7.437 (7.424/7.447) | +0.04% |
| 24 | 7.441 (7.431/7.450) | ±0% | 7.435 (7.421/7.448) | ±0% |

Because there are no significant differences in the group comparison (iso-hyp), the differences are not indicated in this table.
* $p<0.01$.
[a] Median (2.5/97.5 percentiles)

**Table 72.** Plasma lactate concentration (lactate) before and after iso- or hypervolemic hemodilution

| Time (h) | Isovolemic Lactate (mg/l)[a] | Change (%) from initial value | Hypervolemic Lactate (mg/l)[a] | Change (%) from initial value | Difference (%) (iso-hyp) |
|---|---|---|---|---|---|
| Before | 160.7±24.9 | – | 154.5±27.9 | – | + 3.9% |
| 1 | 98.8±22.6 | −38.5%** | 122.5±26.9 | −20.7% | −24.0% |
| 3 | 105.0±22.5 | −34.7% | 138.0±15.5 | −10.7% | −31.4%** |
| 6 | 115.3±24.6 | −23.3% | 152.3±25.8 | −1.4% | −32.1%** |
| 24 | 154.7±22.9 | −3.7% | 152.5±24.3 | −1.3% | +1.4% |

* $p<0.01$; ** $p< 0.05$.

**Table 73.** Plasma pyruvate concentration (pyruvate) before and after iso- or hypervolemic hemodilution

| Time (h) | Isovolemic Pyruvate (mg/l)[a] | Change (%) from initial value | Hypervolemic Pyruvate (mg/l)[a] | Change (%) from initial value | Difference (%) (iso-hyp) |
|---|---|---|---|---|---|
| Before | 4.7±0.6 | – | 4.2 (3.4/5.0) | – | +10.6% |
| 1 | 3.7±0.6 | −21.2%* | 3.9 (3.2/4.4) | −7.1% | −5.4% |
| 3 | 3.4±0.3 | −27.7%* | 4.2 (3.2/5.0) | ±0% | −23.5%* |
| 6 | 3.7±0.8 | −21.2% | 4.4 (3.5/5.1) | +4.5% | −18.9% |
| 24 | 4.6±0.6 | −2.1% | 4.4 (3.3/5.2) | +4.5% | +4.3% |

* $p<0.01$.
[a] Median (2.5/97.5 percentiles)

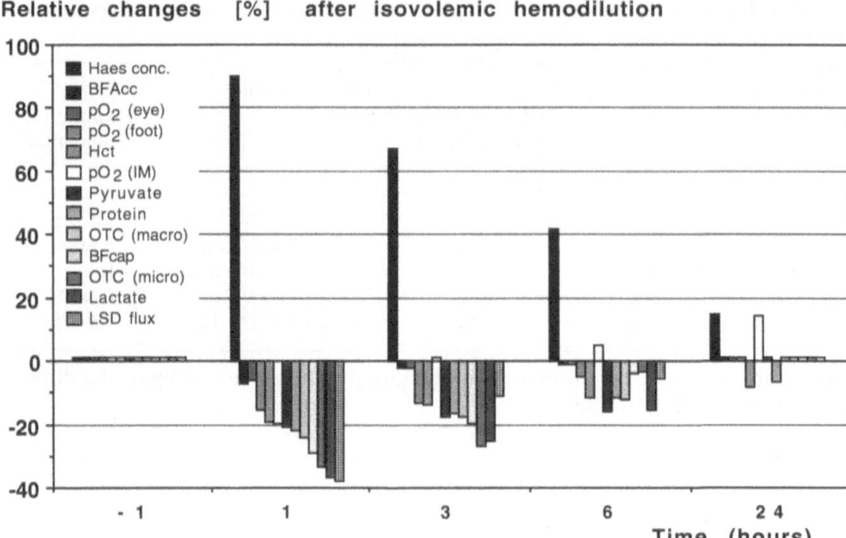


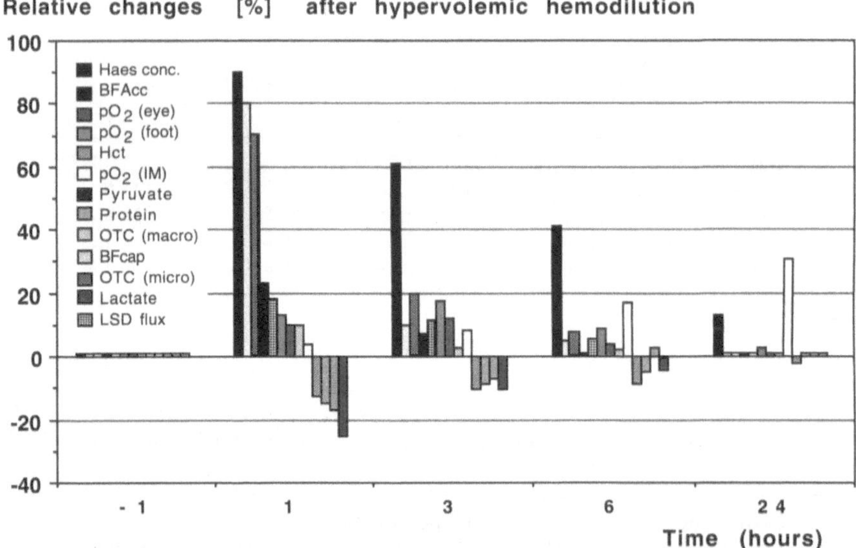


**Fig. 86.** Relative changes (percentages) of parameters (versus the initial values) at 1, 3, 6, and 24 h after iso- (*above*) and hypervolemic hemodilution (*below*)

## 4.2 Multiple Dilution in PAOD II

H. KIESEWETTER, J. BLUME, A. BIRK, and F. JUNG

With hematocrit values between 45% and 48% hyper- or isovolemic hemodilution may be considered. For multimorbid patients especially 6% Haes 200/0.5 is the appropriate colloidal solution. A controlled study [171] tested whether hypervolemic is superior to isovolemic hemodilution in multimorbid elderly patients with PAOD II.

Sixty patients with PAOD II (see Sect. 2.1.1) were included in the study. After the wash-out phase they were allocated at random to three groups of 20 patients each. Groups 1 and 3 received hypervolemic dilution with 500 ml 6% Haes 200/0.5 (Haes-steril 6%; Fresenius; group 1) or Ringer lactate (group 3) three times per week in a double-blind, placebo-controlled design. With isovolemic hemodilution, 500 ml 6% Haes 200/0.5 was infused twice per week, and 250 ml blood was withdrawn after each infusion (group 2). Therefore 1–3 l blood was withdrawn from the patients. At hematocrit below 42% no isovolemic hemodilution was performed. All patients received physical therapy twice per week during the wash-out phase (3 weeks) and during the therapy phase (6 weeks). Figure 87 presents the study design. The groups were homogeneous with regard to the confirmatory and explorative parameters.

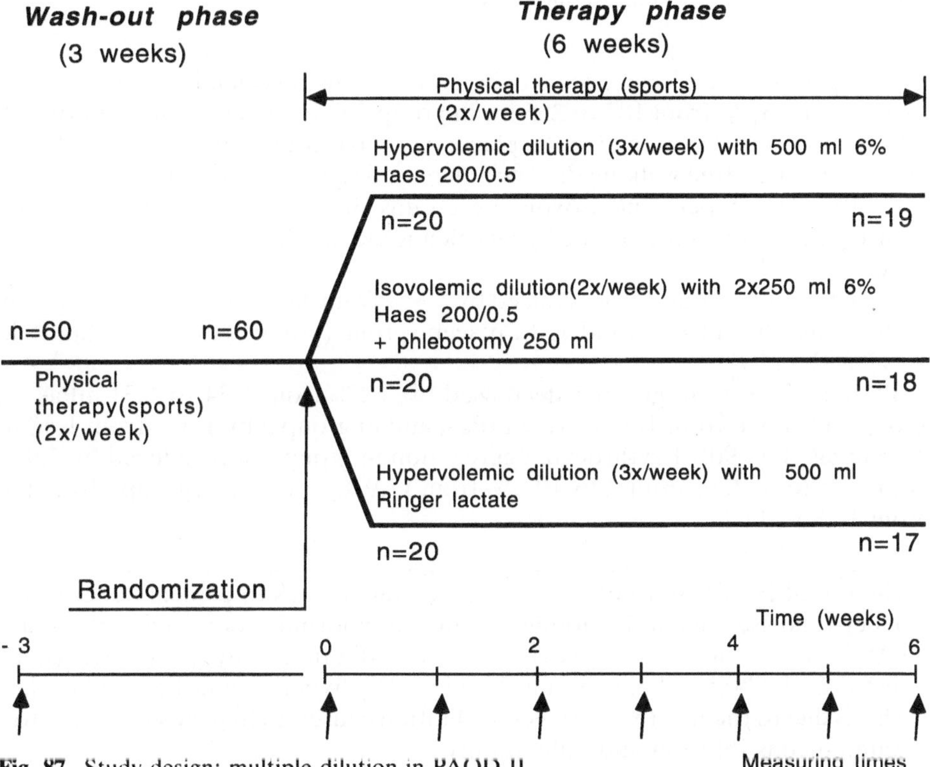


**Fig. 87.** Study design: multiple dilution in PAOD II

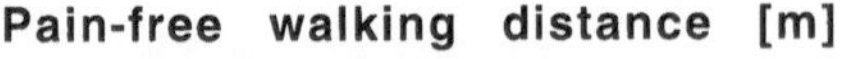


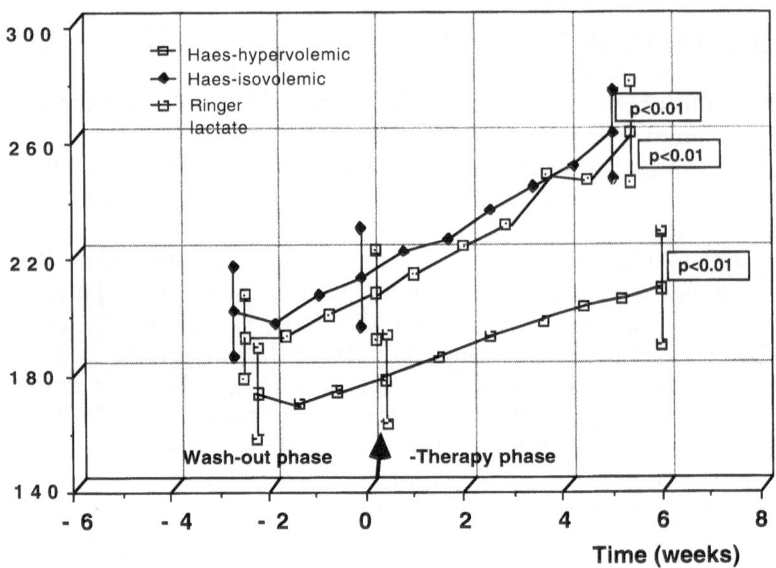


**Fig. 88.** Pain-free walking distance in the three goups for the time of treatment (*p*: significance level in the group comparison – initial value to final value; limits of 1 SD, same symbols as the corresponding standardized measuring points)

The pain-free walking distance in group 1 (hypervolemic hemodilution) increased by 37% from 187 to 255 m, in group 2 (isovolemic hemodilution) by 30% from 194 to 253 m, and in the placebo group (group 3) by 20% from 167 to 201 m. The pain-free walking distance increased significantly in all three groups ($p<0.01$). The hyper- and isovolemic groups differed significantly from the control group ($p<0.05$), but the hypervolemic did not differ from the isovolemic group (Fig. 88).

Hematocrit in group 1 was reduced by 5.8% from 48% to 45%, in group 2 by 16.5% from 48% to 41%, and in the placebo group (group 3) by 2.7% from 48% to 47% (Fig. 89).

Plasma viscosity in group 1 decreased by 2.2% from 1.34 to 1.31 mPas, in group 2 by 4.3% from 1.38 to 1.32 mPas, and in group 3 by 1.5% from 1.37 to 1.35 mPas (Fig. 90). Erythrocyte aggregation in group 1 was reduced by 7.9% from 17.8 to 16.4, in group 2 by 10.6% from 17.9 to 16.0, and in group 3 by 3.4% from 17.8 to 17.2.

> The use of HAES-steril 6% 200/0.5 (Fresenius) leads to clinical benefit for hyper- and isovolemic hemodilution in multimorbid elderly patients with PAOD II. Compared to isovolemic hemodilution only a slightly (not significantly) better clinical result is achieved by hypervolemic hemodilution. This is due to the fact that isovolemic dilution causes no hypervolemia due to simultaneous infusion and phlebotomy.

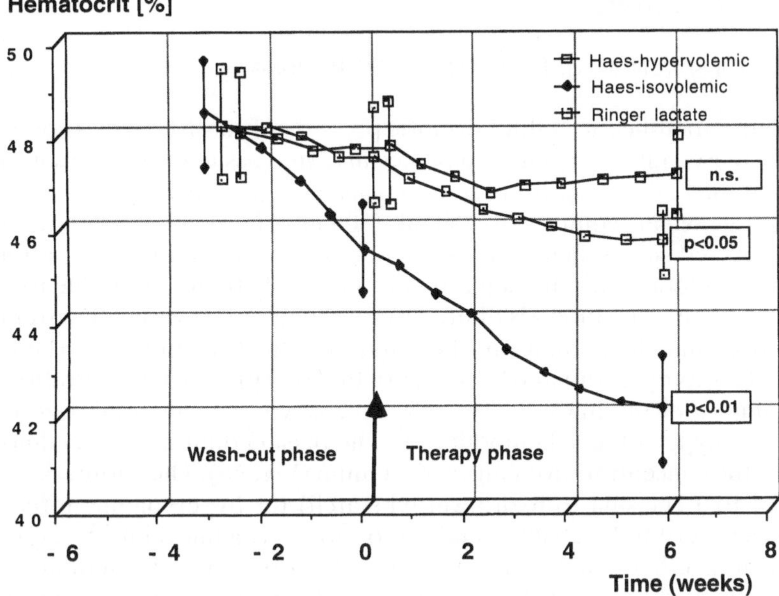


**Fig. 89.** Systemic hematocrit of the three goups for the time of treatment (*p*: significance level in the group comparison – initial value to final value; limits of ±1 SD, same symbols as the corresponding standardized measuring points)

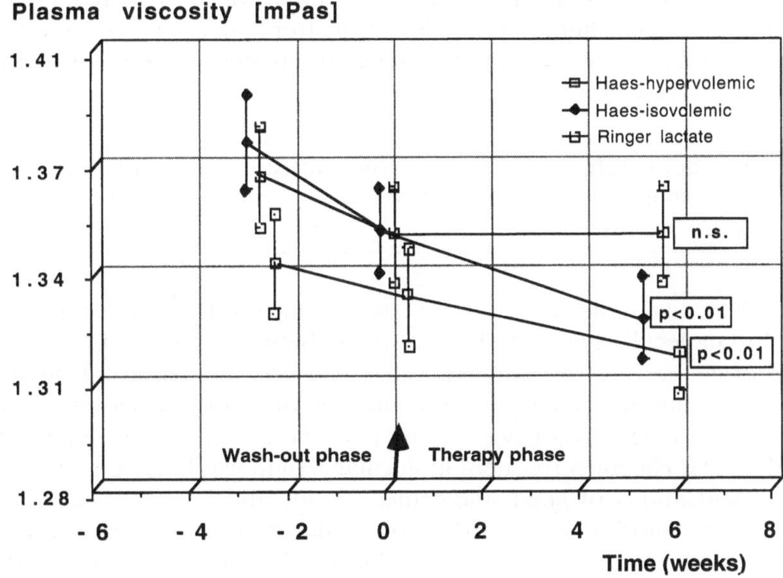


**Fig. 90.** Plasma viscosity of the three goups for the time of treatment (*p*: significance level in the group comparison – initial value to final value; limits of 1 SD same symbols as the corresponding standardized measuring points)

## 4.3 Summary

H. KIESEWETTER, J. KOSCIELNY, and F. JUNG

The hyperoncotic colloid-osmotic pressure of the 10% Haes solution causes an increased intravascular volume because free tissue water flows into the vascular system [206]. With a volume expansion effect of about 50% an increase in intravascular volume of 750 ml (500 ml Haes and 250 ml tissue water) is expected immediately after hypervolemic hemodilution, after isovolemic hemodilution only an increase of 250 ml (only tissue water due to a phlebotomy of 500 ml). The blood is diluted by overloading the vascular system [245]. After isovolemic hemodilution the dilution effect is more marked due to the phlebotomy. Estimated by means of the total protein concentration (Fig. 67) the dilution of plasma was 22% 1 h after isovolemic hemodilution but only 14% after hypervolemic hemodilution. The plasma dilutions were almost confirmed by the concentration changes of albumin (Fig. 68). Therefore, the mixing ratio is 4.1 to 1 (plasma to hydroxyethyl starch) for hypervolemic infusion of 500 ml Haes-steril 10% (200/0.5) and 3.7 to 1 for isovolemic dilution. Consequently, the hydroxyethyl starch concentration after isovolemic hemodilution was significantly higher at all measuring times than after hypervolemic hemodilution (Fig. 61).

If the infusion was performed quickly so that no renal output of the Haes solution could ensue, a mean hydroxyethyl starch concentration of 10.3 g per liter plasma would be expected immediately after isovolemic hemodilution for the above mixing ratio, and one of 9.0 g after hypervolemic hemodilution. The actually measured mean hydroxyethyl starch concentrations were only 9.4 g 1 h after isovolemic hemodilution and 76 g after hypervolemic hemodilution so that apparently 95 or 140 mg has been discharged renally or passed into the extravascular space.

> One hour after the end of the infusion 91% (isovolemic) or 84% (hypervolemic) of the hydroxyethyl starch was in the intravascular system.

The mean molecular weight of pure hydroxyethyl starch solution is 200 kDa. Most molecules have a molecular weight between 7 and 20 kDa (see Fig. 62–65). During the infusion and immediately afterwards the molecular distribution shifted (unsteady condition) but changed only slightly between 1 and 24 h after the end of the infusion. Within this period the mean molecular weight was about 100 kDa. The most frequent molecular weight was between 40 and 60 kDa. The concentrations of small molecules (7–40) and large molecules (>120) were relatively more decreased than the concentration of medium-sized molecules (41–120). In accordance with the results of Förster [11, 69, 70], these concentration shifts can be explained by the renal elimination of the smaller molecules (<40) [17, 18, 52, 53, 69, 70, 342] and by the splitting of high molecular weight molecules (>120) in mean molecular weight hydroxyethyl starch molecules (41–120) during and immediately after the infusion. The velocity of the enzymatic degradation depends on the degree and place of substitution of the hydroxyethyl starch [17, 18, 204, 205, 344, 407]. The precise biochemical mechanisms of the splitting (degradation) are still discussed [11, 70, 245, 286, 342]. A small part of the large hydroxyethyl starch molecules can be stored in the reticuloendothelial system [245, 286, 342]. The renal output led to a steady decrease in total hydroxyethyl starch concentration (Fig. 61) with an elimination half-life of about 4 h [407].

> The mean molecular weight of hydroxyethyl starch 200/0.5 10% decreased to 100 kDa in the plasma 1 h after the end of the infusion. The elimination half-life was about 4 h.

Hyperamylasemia after administration of hydroxyethyl starch as described in the literature was also found in this study (Fig. 66). It is thought that a part of the increased amylase activity in the serum is caused by the formation of an enzyme substrate complex and another part by an enzyme induction in the liver [83, 245]. The induction could be explained by the structural similarity of hydroxyethyl starch to glycogen [299].

> The increase in amylase after Haes infusion is not to be understood as "induced pancreatitis" since the serum lipase remained constant and the α-amylase clearance did not increase but decreased significantly [83, 204].

The intravascular increase in volume of 750 ml may be the cause for the significant increase in blood flow in the common carotid artery 1 h after hypervolemic hemodilution (by about 23%). At the same time after isovolemic hemodilution there was *no* significant change of the blood flow in the macrocirculation despite the expansion effect of 250 ml (Fig. 73). After the phlebotomy of 500 ml during isovolemic hemodilution a hypovolemia occurred, leading to a decrease in the macrocirculatory blood flow. Only after the infusion of 500 ml hydroxyethyl starch was the decrease in flow only slowly compensated (after 3 h the blood flow had returned to the initial level). If infusion and phlebotomy are carried out simultaneously the blood flow increases directly [23, 182, 185, 187, 262, 273, 388]. The laser Doppler flux corresponds to the circulatory conditions in the macrocirculation. A significant increase by 17% (in the macrocirculation by 23%) in blood flow appeared by hypervolemic hemodilution after 1 h. The decrease after isovolemic hemodilution (about 18%) can also be explained (besides the hypovolemia by the initially performed phlebotomy) by a reduced concentration of flowing erythrocytes in the peripheral macrocirculation (Fig. 82).

As a result of the increase in flow after hypervolemic dilution in the macrocirculation there was also an increase in capillary erythrocyte velocity (Fig. 81; Tables 63, 64). The increase in capillary blood flow of the skin was 88% after 3 h. Afterwards the flow decreased again but did not achieve the initial value after 24 h (Fig. 79). As in the macrocirculation, a decrease in capillary blood flow by 29% was also observed after isovolemic hemodilution.

Elimination of the oxygen deficit after a 3-min arterial stasis follows after isovolemic hemodilution by a prolonged reactive hyperemia due to the reduced oxygen transport capacity (Fig. 80). After hypervolemic hemodilution an increased resting flow in the micro- and macrocirculations even increased the oxygen transport capacity so that the reactive hyperemia is *not prolonged* (Fig. 73, 79).

> The blood flow in the macro- and microcirculation increased after hypervolemic and decreased after isovolemic hemodilution. The vasomotor reserve was increased only after isovolemic dilution.

The effects of iso- and hypervolemic hemodilution on the oxygen supply of skin and muscle also differ (Fig. 83, 84). Whereas decreases in transcutaneous and tissue oxygen pressure were observed during the early phase (up to 3 h after the end of isovolemic hemodilution), hypervolemic dilution led immediately to an increase in this parameter. However, significantly increased oxygen pressures in the muscles resulted from both hemodilutions after 24 h. It must be assumed that this increase in oxygen in the muscular tissue was due to the improved fluidity of blood. Landgraf and Ehrly [226, 227] have published comparable findings after hypervolemic hemodilution.

The decrease in transcutaneous and muscular oxygen partial pressures after isovolemic dilution can be explained by reduced microcirculatory blood flow and oxygen content in arterial blood owing to a strong decrease in hemoglobin concentration (Fig. 73).

> The oxygen supply of skin and muscle improved by hypervolemic hemodilution from the beginning up to 24 h; by isovolemic dilution the muscular oxygen pressure increased only after 24 h.

Improved blood fluidity by hemodilution with mean molecular weight hydroxyethyl starch has been described by different authors [108, 226, 227]. The decreases in plasma viscosity and erythrocyte aggregation (Fig. 69) depend on the initial value [93, 226] and on the infusion flow rate [207]. If plasma viscosity is increased initially, a more marked decrease is found after the end of the infusion [93, 226]. The plasma viscosity and erythrocyte aggregation decreased at the latest 1 h after the end of the infusion when the hydroxyethyl starch was intravascularly lowered to a mean molecular weight of 100 kDa.

Spontaneous thrombocyte aggregation is only slightly influenced by either form of hemodilution, as observed in several studies [173, 178, 180, 182, 341]. It seems probable that there is only a slight "coating effect" concerning the thrombocytes after the administration of mean molecular weight hydroxyethyl starch. The influence of hydroxyethyl starch on platelet adhesion and the number of circulating platelet aggregates has been suggested but not yet confirmed [353, 356]. In contrast, a strong "coating effect" is described for dextran [26].

On the one hand, the decrease in systemic hematocrit value (Fig. 69) after isovolemic hemodilution was due to the removal of cells during phlebotomy, and to the dilution resulting from the infusion of 500 ml Haes-steril 10%. After hypervolemic hemodilution this decrease was caused only by the dilution effect. The gradual reincrease (Fig. 69, 70) in systemic hematocrit after both forms of dilution was caused by the release of mature blood cells (erythrocytes, leukocytes, thrombocytes [96, 376, 377]) and by the steadily decreasing hydroxyethyl starch concentration after the infusion (reduced hypervolemia by renal elimination).

Compared to systemic hematocrit, capillary hematocrit was decreased only half as much after either form of hemodilution (Figs. 77, 78). These findings correlate with those of Mirhasemi [262], who demonstrated with an optical procedure in an animal model that systemic hematocrit is considerably and capillary hematocrit only weakly influenced after normovolemic hemodilution.

The distinct decreases in hematocrit and plasma viscosity (Fig. 69) by isovolemic hemodilution caused an elevated cardiac output and therefore a decreased heart rate (Fig. 71).

A hydroxyethyl starch solution (200/0.5 6% or 10%) reduced hematocrit, plasma viscosity, and erythrocyte aggregation. Plasma viscosity was often reduced by 1 h after the end of the infusion if the hydroxyethyl starch in the intravascular system had a molecular weight of 100 kDa. The effect on capillary hematocrit was significantly weaker than on systemic hematocrit. The rheologic effects were more pronounced after iso- than after hypervolemic hemodilution.

Metabolic parameters such as lactate and pyruvate concentration in the blood decreased in the early phase after both forms of hemodilution (Fig. 85). This was due mainly to dilution effects. Since increased oxygen partial pressure was measured in the peripheral muscles (Fig. 84), and the lactate/pyruvate quotient was reduced at this time, a shift in the metabolic condition toward an aerobic one can be assumed.

After isovolemic hemodilution the blood pH value decreased only during the early phase due to an increased supply of acid valences by the Haes solution [245] and the loss of blood buffer capacity by the phlebotomy [245, 408, 409], but it remained within the physiologic range.

The hypervolemic single dilution with Haes-steril 10% (200/0.5) is superior to isovolemic dilution. If a phlebotomy must be performed, it should be done by a *second* access simultaneously with the infusion or by only one access *after* the initially performed infusion.
The hypervolemic multiple dilution with Haes-steril 6% (200/0.5) is only slightly superior to the isovolemic dilution in the treatment of PAOD.

## 4.4 Practical Comments on Hemodilution

J. Koscielny and H. Kiesewetter

*Form of hemodilution*

- Volume tolerant patients: hypervolemic hemodilution. There are good experiences concerning up to 1 l hydroxyethyl starch/day (10% Haes 200/0.5).
- Other patients: isovolemic hemodilution. Phlebotomy with 250–500 ml and the same quantity of hydroxyethyl starch (6% Haes 200/0.5 or 10% Haes 200/05).

*Performance of hemodilution with phlebotomy*

- One venous access: a) 250 ml hydroxyethyl starch;
  b) 250 ml phlebotomy;
  c) 250 ml hydroxyethyl starch;
  d) possibly 250 ml phlebotomy
- Two venous accesses: a) first arm: infusion of 250–500 ml hydroxyethyl starch (start immediately!);
  b) second arm: phlebotomy of 250 ml (500 ml)

*Care:* Avoidance of a negative volume balance!

*Equipment for hemodilution*

1. Tourniquet
2. Sterile sponges
3. Plaster
4. Hydroxyethyl starch solution (Haes-steril 10% or 6%; Fresenius)
5. One or two indwelling cannulas (size: 1.2 mm, 18 G; or 1.6 mm, 16 G), e.g., Vasofix (Braun Melsungen)
6. Infusion set, e.g., Intrafix Air (Braun Melsungen)
7. "Secretion drainage bag" with reflux blockage (Medinorm) or blood bag without stabilizer (Biotest Pharma)
   - On plasmapheresis, instead of 5–7:
     a) CPDA blood donation bag (Biotest) and
     b) transfusion set, e.g., Sangofix ES (Braun Melsungen)

## *4.5 Possible Side Effects of a Haes Infusion and Their Treatment*

H. Kiesewetter, P. Waldhausen, W. Schimetta, H.-J. Wilhelm, and J. Koscielny

Hemodilution using hydroxyethyl starches is performed frequently in the German speaking countries. The wide use allows thorough analysis of the side effects. In order to improve the safety of hydroxyethyl starch all possible side effects, their frequency, prevention and treatment are described below.

### *4.5.1 Heart and Lung*

On hypervolemic hemodilution with hydroxyethyl starch the heart and lung must be monitored since cardiac decompensation with pulmonary congestion or edema may occur. In five patients with peripheral arterial occlusive disease (PAOD) and a condition with considerably restricted ejection fraction after a severe anterior wall infarction Böhme and Bulik [29] detected cardiac decompensation under a mild hypervolemic hemodilution (daily 250 ml 10% Haes 200/0.5 over several days) with an increase in weight by fluid retention. In theory, this corresponds to 5% of the treatments. A recompensation was achieved by the use of loop diuretics after discontinuing the infusions.

In the following we report on a left ventricular decompensation after a single infusion of 500 ml 6% Haes 200/0.62 in a 62-year-old patient with PAOD, coronary heart disease (CHD) after two anterior wall infarctions, arterial hypertension, disturbed fat metabolism, and chronical obstructive bronchitis – within the framework of a study on ten patients with PAOD. Theoretically, this would correspond to a side effect rate of 10% of the treated patients. The basic drug treatment consisted of an α-blocker, fibrate, naftidrofuryl, theophylline, and mononitrate drug. The initial blood pressure was 150/90 mmHg. The Haes solution was infused hypervolemiccally over 60 min. Due to a paravasate formation the infusion was stopped after a volume administration of 450 ml. Immediately afterwards the patient did not indicate a worsened condition but complained of dyspnea and significant angina symptoms 75 min later. The blood pressure, which was 180/100 mmHg at the end of the infusion, was elevated to 230/115 mmHg. Moist rale was auscultated over the basal pulmonary segments on both sides. After the intravenous administration of 40 mg Lasix and 9 Nitrolingual the blood pressure decreased to values of 180/120 mmHg over the following 30 min. Nevertheless, the patient was hospitalized for further diagnosis and therapy. An ejection fraction of 30% was observed with the performed levocardiography. The patient was discharged with a significantly improved general condition 3 days after hospitalization. At discharge the drug treatment consisted of an ACE inhibitor, fibrate, naftidrofuryl, digitalis, mononitrate, and theophylline drug. The previously administered α-blocker had been discontinued.

The described incidents of Böhme [29] and of our own study group demonstrate that decompensation may occur in patients with considerably restricted cardiac output under hemodilution treatment with volume overload. For this purpose, all these patients should be only diluted with a reduced infusion volume and slow infusion rate (increased duration of infusion) "mild" hypervolemically, at best *isovolemically* with simultaneous or occasional phlebotomy, if a hemodilution treatment becomes clinically necessary. During this process the lung should be auscultated and percussed in addition to the infusion. Progressive dyspnea should cause suspicion. Pretibial edemas, edema of the malleolar region, and an increase in body weight indicate fluid retention due to heart insufficiency. Generally, the fluid must be mobilized again with loop diuretics. During this process *plasma viscosity should not exceed 1.4 mPas*; values above 1.5 mPas must be absolutely avoided [49]. The incidence figures of 5% or 10% are naturally only theoretical figures for cardiac decompensation and were determined in very small populations of multimorbid patients. Greater amounts of hydroxyethyl starches with an unfavorable $C_2/C_6$ ratio such as 6% Haes 200/0.62 ($C_2/C_6$ about 10) may increase the risk of cardiac decompensation. If the contraindications are strictly adhered to (Table 2, Sect. 2.1.8.), the incidence is significantly below 1‰, as was demonstrated by our own investigations on more than 2000 patients.

### 4.5.2 Kidney

Renal function must be monitored by the measurement of serum creatinine and body weight parallel to the infusion. Waldhausen and collaborators [383] observed acute renal failure under hemodilution therapy with 10% Haes 200/0.5 in a 74-year-old woman with cerebral ischemia due to arterial hypertension and in a 76-year-old woman with retinal central artery obstruction due to diabetes mellitus.

The first patient with hemiplegia secondary to a left cerebral infarction received an infusion of 850 g Haes (17×500 ml each time) over a period of 9 days, and the second received an infusion of 500 g (10×500 ml each time within 10 days secondary to a vascular-related vision loss. The patients became increasingly dyspneic with the infusion therapy. The elevated retention values already present on admission increased retention values significantly in spite of the simultaneous administration of loop diuretics. The serum creatinine value in the first patient increased from 1.6 to 5.2 mg/dl, the value in the second patient from 2.5 to 7.4 mg/dl. The infusions were stopped due to clinical deterioration by acute renal failure. The increased retention values were accompanied by fluid retention of several liters. Even the high dosage of a loop diuretic (up to 1.5 g Lasix) did not sufficiently increase diuresis. An antihypertensive agent such as dobutamine or dopamine was not administered. Due to the poor clinical condition in cases of considerably disturbed diuresis with high retention values dialysis therapy was started in both patients. The clinical condition improved again significantly after five or ten sessions within 8 or 17 days, and the retention values had returned to the initial constellations. After 38 days the retention values were even decreased by 7% or 34% compared to the initial values, but remained pathologically increased. No cerebral residues remained in the first patient with left cerebral infarction. The vision in the second patient was significantly improved. In the last 7 years more than 2000 patients at the University Hospital Homburg/Saar and cooperating departments received hemodilution with hydroxyethyl starch without corresponding complications, and two further cases occurred which have not been discussed in detail. Consequently, a theoretical incidence of the acute renal failure of less than 2‰ can be estimated. Exclusion of patients with serum creatinine values above 1.5 mg/dl and careful control of patients with moderately increased values may have meant that the described acute renal failures would have been avoided so that the stated incidence of 2‰ would be significantly smaller if the contraindications (Table 2, Sect. 2.1.8.) were observed.

Casuistic analysis clearly shows that especially in elderly patients the renal function must be followed regularly during infusion treatment with starch solutions (determination of serum creatinine twice per week). Especially patients with creatinine values above 1.5 mg/dl are at risk, for example, patients with diabetes mellitus or arterial hypertension. If serum creatinine values exceed 2 mg/dl during an infusion treatment with hydroxyethyl starch, the therapy *must* be stopped immediately, or gelatin solutions must alternatively be given if a hemodilution is clinically essential.

Furthermore, with each hemodilution it must be ensured that diuresis is maintained or improved by a large quantity of fluid (2–3 l) or an additional administration of electrolyte solution. In order to prevent a possible fluid retention during the the accompanying fluid balancing it is imperative that the patient tolerates the volume. Weight and knuckle circumference measurements, liver size determinations, and lung auscultation and percussion should be carried out in high-risk patients in addition to the infusion. Therefore, the following must be noted:

Heart, lung, and kidney must be monitored regularly. The Haes compatibility is tested by:

1. Taking heart rate and blood pressure: not allowed to increase during the infusion.
2. Auscultation of the lung: moist rales (insufficiency of the left heart) require termination of the dilution.
3. Determination of serum creatinine value: not allowed to exceed 2.0 mg/dl at an initial value of $\leq$ 1.5 mg/dl.
4. Determination of the body weight: not allowed to increase by more than 1 kg per week with normocloric nutrition.

### 4.5.3 Increased Risk of Hemorrhage

Some publications comment on an increased risk of hemorrhage during and after the infusion of hydroxyethyl starch solutions, especially of 6% Haes 450/0.7 [43,

290, 292, 296, 353, 355, 356]. In 1987, Damon and collaborators [43] reported on a consumption coagulopathy with the administration of 6% Haes 450/0.7 (Hetastarch) in a 36-year-old woman with syncope during subarachnoidal hemorrhage and an aneurysm of the right middle cerebral artery (diagnosed by computed tomography and angiography).

The authors' view [43] that the administration of hydroxyethyl starch caused the consumption coagulopathy appears rather questionable. The hydroxyethyl starch that was used had a mean molecular weight of 450 kDa, a substitution degree of 0.7, and a concentration of 60 g/l. This hydroxyethyl starch solution leads to an increase in volume of about 90% after rapid infusion [259]. By rapid infusion a plasma dilution is achieved which is partly responsible for the decrease in factor VIII and fibrinogen concentration [290, 296]. Even if the influence on the coagulation (exceeding the dilution effect; reduction in F VIII:C) by 6% Haes 450/0.7 observed by Stump and Strauss [353, 355, 356] is taken into consideration, the administered quantity in the above article of 500 ml daily over 3 days is probably not sufficient to explain the consumption coagulopathy. At best, a weak "thrombocyte coating" could be found [101, 248]. It is more likely that a rupture of the aneurysmatic area occurred by the relatively strong overloading of the vascular system. By this leak of the hematoencephalic barrier higher quantities of thromboplastin could have been released from the necrotic cerebral zone into the intravascular area. The cerebrum has a large capacity for this coagulatory material [361]. Nevertheless, multiple infusion of especially high-substituted hydroxyethyl starch solutions by the intravascular or intracorporal accumulation of substrates is a certain risk factor for hemorrhagic complications, which is also supported by observations of the study groups by Pindur and Haaß [292].

The risk of such a reaction can be reduced if a hydroxyethyl starch with a mean molecular weight of 200 kDa, a substitution degree of 0.5, and a concentration of 60 g/l is used since the half-life is considerably shorter (about 4 h instead of about 12 h), and this substance improves the fluidity of blood significantly [259, 365]. The daily administration of 500 ml 6% Haes 200/0.5 as hypervolemic hemodilution therefore seems less problematic [48, 181]. There is also no or only a slight substrate-specific influence on factor VIII – in contrast to 6% Haes 450/0.7 [354]. Up to now, consumption coagulopathy has not been observed in the Federal Republic of Germany after the use of hydroxyethyl starch in ischemic attacks, subarachnoid hemorrhage, and retinal obstructions [101, 211, 392]. If necessary, careful controls of bleeding time and coagulation status should be made.

### 4.5.4 Anaphylactoid Reactions

Anaphylactoid (nonimmunogen) reactions possibly caused by activation of plasma enzyme systems such as the complement by kallikrein systems are rather seldom [304, 306, 343]. An antigen antibody reaction of specific antibodies against hydroxyethyl starch molecules has not been demonstrated up to now [11, 70, 216, 231, 305]. The available studies determined a relative frequency of

0.005%–2.7% of incompatibility reactions of different severity independently of the physical-chemical composition of the hydroxyethyl starch solutions [232, 304, 305, 306]. These incompatibility reactions (four degrees of severity) range from skin abnormalities such as flush or urticaria (degree I) to hemodynamic reactions which are not life threatening – infusion increase in pulse rate or drop in blood pressure and dyspnea (degree II) – to shock (degree III) or at worst to cardiac or respiratory arrest (degree IV) [232, 304, 305, 306].

In our own series of patients incompatibility reactions of degree I were observed in less than 2% of the cases (far more than 2000 patients were treated). A reaction of degree II was observed once, but degrees III and IV were not observed. After the administration of a one-fourth ampule adrenaline and 300 ml 0.9% saline solution the hemodynamic reaction of the patient with the anaphylactoid reaction (degree II) diminished.

Therefore, attention must be given to the administration of hydroxyethyl starch.

> In the case of minor incompatibility reactions the infusion must be discontinued. Severe incompatibility reactions (degree III/IV) require the immediate administration of adrenaline, volume in the form of crystalloid solutions and cortisone (one ampule Suprarenin, diluted 1:10, infused over several minutes, at least 500 ml 0.9% NaCl, 1–1.5 g cortisone).

### *4.5.5 Pruritus*

A transitory and only slight pruritus was observed in fewer than 6.9% of our own patients with cerebrovascular accidents (80 persons in a prospective study) treated with hydroxyethyl starch (10% Haes 200/0.5). But the administered Haes quantities were below 150 g per week. Nevertheless, in a control group treated with Ringer lactate the incidence of pruritus was 4.8%. Only 9% of the large group of patients with PAOD (1200 analyzed cases) treated with Haes had slight pruritus. In patients with sudden hearing loss who were treated by Wilhelm and collaborators [392] with up to 700 g Haes per week, a pruritus incidence of 60% was observed. After reduction in the Haes dose by 50% the incidence of pruritus decreased below 30%. These frequencies also coincide well (assuming a dose dependence) with the experiences of Albegger and collaborators [3] in patients with acute sudden hearing loss (about 30% pruritus incidence with the administration of approximately 400 g Haes 200/0.5 per patient). To now, pruritus reactions have been observed after the use of all Haes products (6% Haes 200/0.62; 10% or 6% Haes 200/0.5; 6% Haes 40/0.5; 6% Haes 450/0.7), in contrast to drug information of the German Federal Department of Health [8].

In all, the infusion treatment with hydroxyethyl starch was evaluated as "good" to "very good" by the patients with "sudden hearing loss"; the pruritus was seldom disturbing.

The features of pruritus after Haes administration are: dose dependence; long latency; lack of findings on the skin; resistance only to steroid therapy, $H_1$ antihistamines, and antipruritics.

More fluids should be given in the case of pruritus, which may appear especially in patients with sudden hearing loss and with administration of considerable quantities of Haes (more than 150 g per week). Constant Haes plasma levels with values above 10 g/l should be avoided. The alleviation of pruritus can be achieved by local treatment with antihistamine- or corticoid-containing ointments. Oral administration of the antihistamine Zyrtec is also recommended. Oral administration of calcium can also alleviate pruritus. In rare cases of severe pruritus infusions with amantadine (PK-Merz, 200 mg daily; Merz) should be tried. The infusions can be combined with UV radiations of the affected skin areas [192]. Significant improvement of the pruritus symptoms was also described after the administration of hydroxyzine (Atarax, 3×50 mg per day) [133].

Due to possible pruritus considerable quantities of Haes (more than 150 g/week) should be avoided if not clinically essential. In the case of pruritus local skin treatment with antihistamine or cortisone and UV radiation should be tried; calcium can be given systemically. In severe cases of pruritus the administration of hydroxyzine (3×50 mg daily) or a daily infusion of 200 mg amantadine must be attempted.

## 4.6 Hemodilution Schemes

B. ANGELKORT, R. BACH, A. HAASS, L. HEILMANN, H. KIESEWETTER, J. KOSCIELNY, M. REIM, H.-J. WILHELM, and S. WOLF

### 4.6.1 Hypervolemic Hemodilution in Volume Tolerant Patients with PAOD (Target Hematocrit 40%)

**1. Acute scheme for the 1st month (3x/week to Hct≤42 %)**

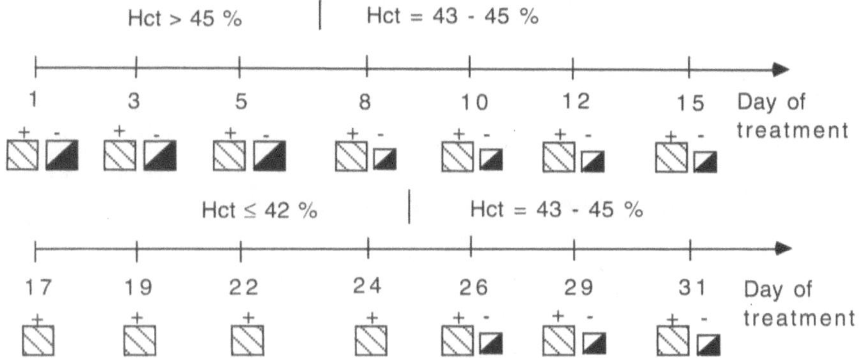


**CAVE: 1. Volume tolerance !**

*Procedure during the Haes infusion:*

1. Measurement of heart rate and blood pressure:
   *are not allowed to increase*
2. Auscultation of the lung:
   *moist rale: breaking off (insufficiency of the left heart)*
3. Creatinine determination twice per week:
   *is not allowed to exceed 2.0 mg/dl with an initial value < 1.5 mg/dl*
4. Body weight (BW) determination:
   *is not allowed to increase more than 1 kg per week with normocaloric nutrition*

**In case of poor volume tolerance adjust the infusion volume to clinical condition !**

**CAVE: 2. Avoidance of hypovolemia and anemia (Hct ≤ 35%) !**

*The infusion is always started before the phlebotomy at the other arm. (2 accesses)*

*The first infusion of 250 ml is given before the phlebotomy of 250 ml, the second after the phlebotomy. (1 access)*

**2. Long-term scheme from the 1st month on (2x/month to Hct≤42 %)**

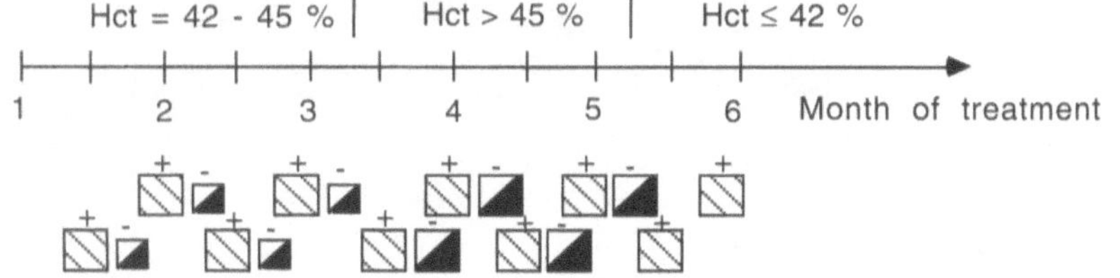


*Legend:*

- 500 ml 6% or 10% Haes 200/0.5 (dependent on volume tolerance)
- 400 ml whole blood
- 250 ml whole blood
- \+ infusion - phlebotomy

## 4.6.2 *Isovolemic Hemodilution in Small Volume Tolerant Patients with PAOD (Target Hematocrit 40%)*

**1. Acute scheme for the 1st month (3x/week to Hct≤42 %)**

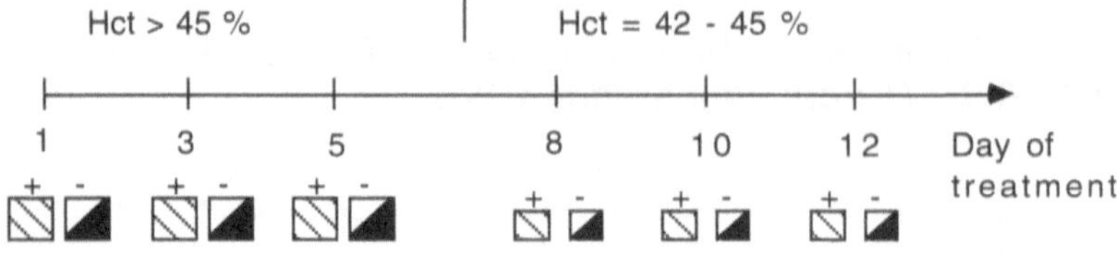


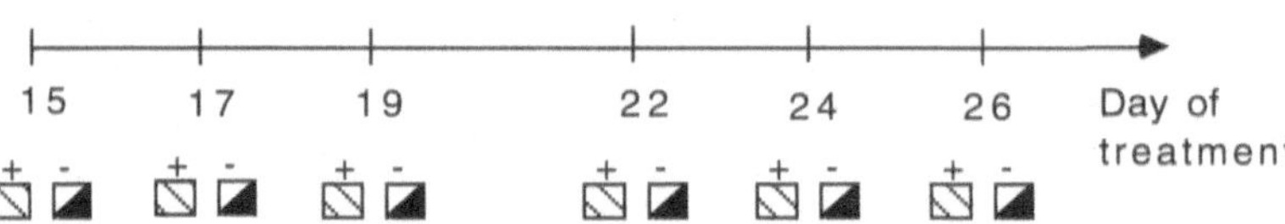


**CAVE: 1. Volume tolerance !**

*Procedure during the Haes infusion:*

1. Measurement of heart rate and blood pressure:
   *are not allowed to increase*
2. Auscultation of the lung:
   *moist rale: breaking off (insufficiency of the left heart)*
3. Creatinine determination twice per week:
   *is not allowed to exceed 2.0 mg/dl with an initial value < 1.5 mg/dl*
4. Body weight (BW) determination:
   *is not allowed to increase more than 1 kg per week with normocaloric nutrition*

***In case of poor volume tolerance adjust the infusion volume to clinical condition !***

**CAVE: 2. Avoidance of hypovolemia and anemia (Hct ≤ 35%) !**

*The infusion is always started before the phlebotomy at the other arm. (2 accesses)*
*The first infusion of 250 ml is given before the phlebotomy of 250 ml, the second after the phlebotomy. (1 access)*

**2. Long-term scheme from the 1st month on (2x/month to Hct≤42 %)**

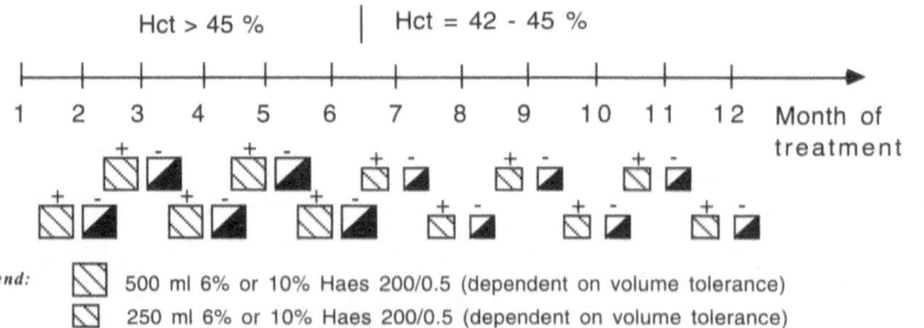


*Legend:*
- 500 ml 6% or 10% Haes 200/0.5 (dependent on volume tolerance)
- 250 ml 6% or 10% Haes 200/0.5 (dependent on volume tolerance)
- 500 ml whole blood
- 250 ml whole blood
- \+ infusion - phlebotomy

### 4.6.3 Bag Plasmapheresis

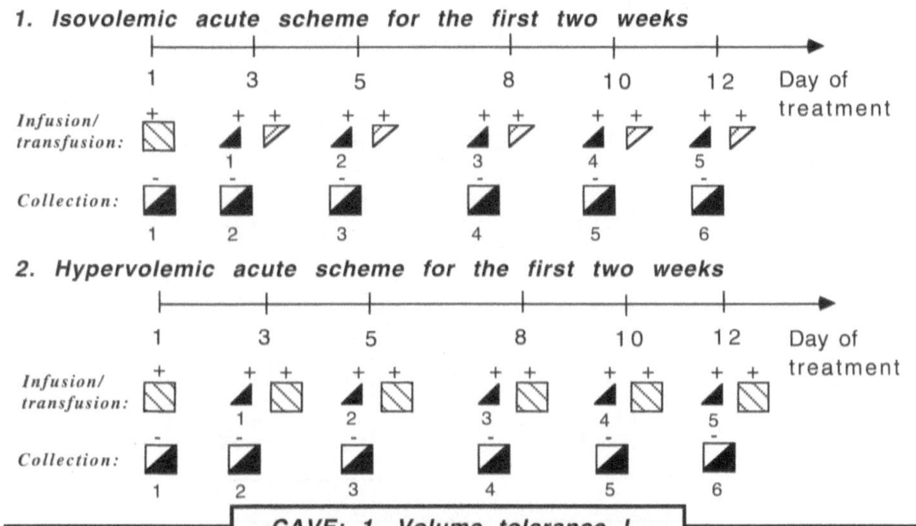


**CAVE: 1. Volume tolerance !**

*Procedure during the Haes infusion:*

1. Measurement of heart rate and blood pressure:
   *are not allowed to increase*
2. Auscultation of the lung:
   *moist rale: breaking off (insufficiency of the left heart)*
3. Creatinine determination twice per week:
   *is not allowed to exceed 2.0 mg/dl with an initial value < 1.5 mg/dl*
4. Body weight (BW) determination:
   *is not allowed to increase more than 1 kg per week with normocaloric nutrition*

**CAVE: 2. Avoidance of hypovolemia and anemia (Hct ≤ 35%) !**

*The infusion is always started before the phlebotomy at the other arm. (2 accesses)*
*The first infusion of 250 ml is given before the phlebotomy of 250 ml, the second after the phlebotomy. (1 access)*

**3. Iso*- and hypervolemic long-term scheme from the 15th day on**

**in isovolemic plasmapheresis the Haes volume has to be halved for the autotransfusion of erythrocytes ! (cf. isovolemic acute scheme)*

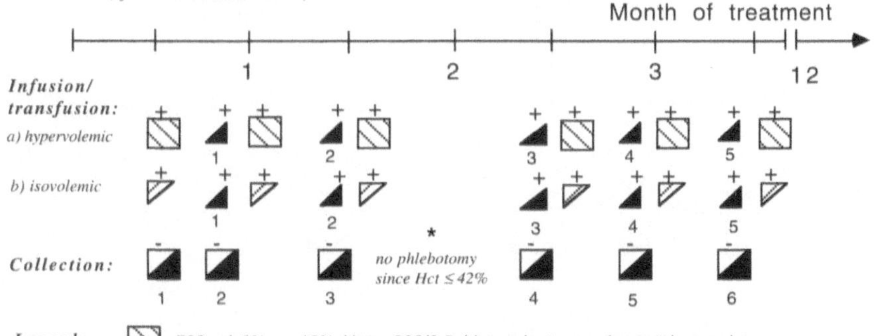


*Legend:*

- 500 ml 6% or 10% Haes 200/0.5 (dependent on volume tolerance)
- 250 ml 6% or 10% Haes 200/0.5 (dependent on volume tolerance)
- 500 ml whole blood
- 250 ml blood cells

### *4.6.4 Mild Hypervolemic Hemodilution in Volume Tolerant Patients with Ischemic Heart Disease*

**1. Acute scheme for the 1st month (2x/week to Hct≤42 %)**

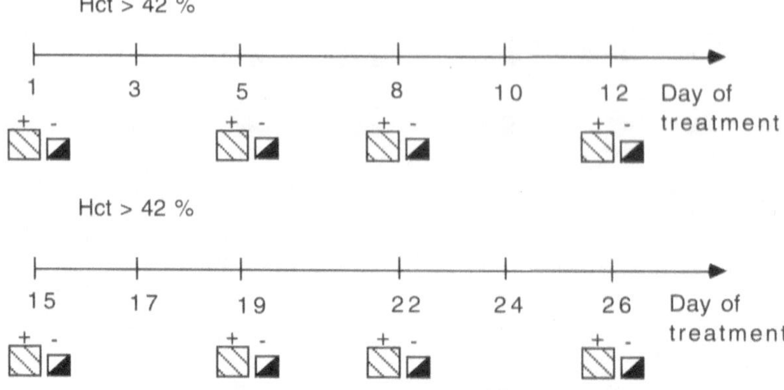


**CAVE: 1. Volume tolerance !**

*Procedure during the Haes infusion:*

1. Measurement of heart rate and blood pressure:
   *are not allowed to increase*
2. Auscultation of the lung:
   *moist rale: breaking off (insufficiency of the left heart)*
3. Creatinine determination twice per week:
   *is not allowed to exceed 2.0 mg/dl with an initial value < 1.5 mg/dl*
4. Body weight (BW) determination:
   *is not allowed to increase more than 1 kg per week with normocaloric nutrition*

**In case of poor volume tolerance adjust the infusion volume to clinical condition !**

**CAVE: 2. Avoidance of hypovolemia and anemia (Hct ≤ 35%) !**

*The infusion is always started before the phlebotomy at the other arm. (2 accesses)*
*The first infusion of 250 ml is given before the phlebotomy of 250 ml, the second after the phlebotomy. (1 access)*

**2. Long-term scheme from the 1st month on (2x/month to Hct≤42 %)**

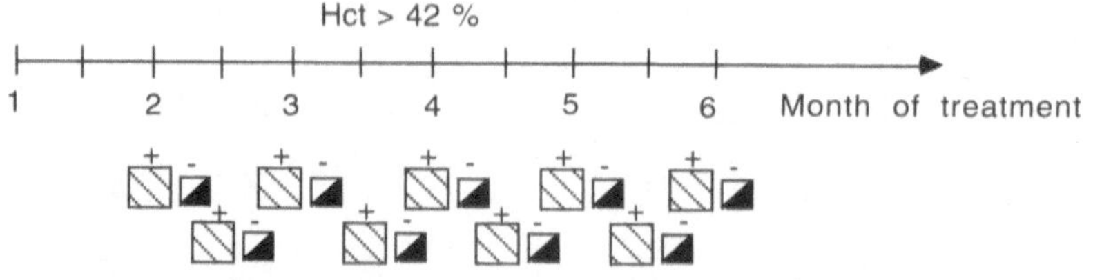


*Legend:*

500 ml 10% Haes 200/0.5

250 ml whole blood

\+ infusion - phlebotomy

## 4.6.5 *Isovolemic Hemodilution in Small Volume Tolerant Patients with Ischemic Heart Disease*

### *1. Acute scheme for the 1st month (2x/week to Hct≤42 %)*

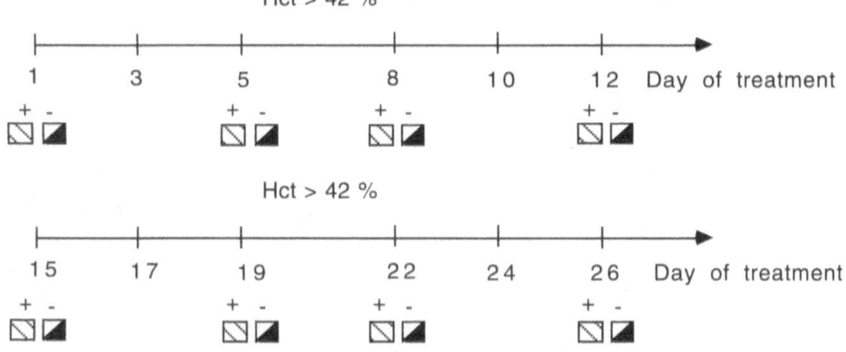


**CAVE: 1. Volume tolerance !**

*Procedure during the Haes infusion:*

1. Measurement of heart rate and blood pressure:
   *are not allowed to increase*
2. Auscultation of the lung:
   *moist rale: breaking off (insufficiency of the left heart)*
3. Creatinine determination twice per week:
   *is not allowed to exceed 2.0 mg/dl with an initial value < 1.5 mg/dl*
4. Body weight (BW) determination:
   *is not allowed to increase more than 1 kg per week with normocaloric nutrition*

***In case of poor volume tolerance adjust the infusion volume to clinical condition !***

**CAVE: 2. Avoidance of hypovolemia and anemia (Hct ≤ 35%) !**

*The infusion is always started before the phlebotomy at the other arm. (2 accesses)*

*The first infusion of 250 ml is given before the phlebotomy of 250 ml, the second after the phlebotomy. (1 access)*

### *2. Long-term scheme from the 1st month on (2x/month to Hct≤42 %)*

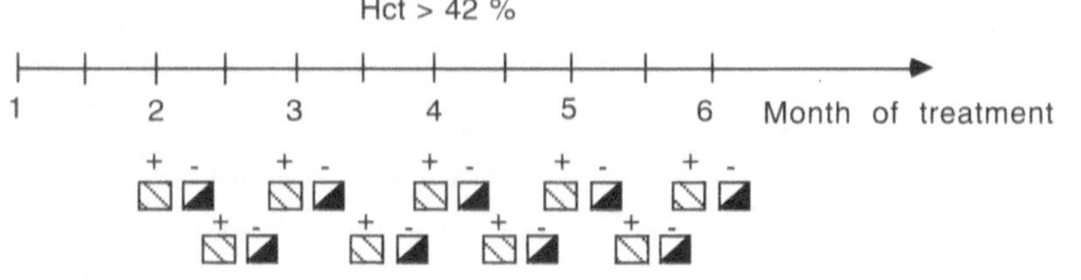


*Legend:*

- ⧅ 250 ml 6% Haes 200/0.5
- ◪ 250 ml whole blood
- \+ infusion - phlebotomy

## 4.6.6. Hemodilution in Acute Ischemic Cerebral Infarction

**1st day :**

A) Acute rapid infusion "loading dose"

500 ml 6% or 10% Haes 200/0.5 (low-sodium) within 45-60 minutes

**contraindication:** acute increase in intracranial pressure
mild intracerebral bleeding is **not a contraindication**

B) Long-term hemodilution treatment

2x 500 ml 6% or 10% Haes 200/0.5 (low-sodium) for 6-12 h each time

- during the infusion of ***10%*** Haes ***always*** add the ***same*** volume of an electrolyte solution (low-sodium)
- ***no*** interruption of the infusion treatment during the night

**2nd day, possibly also 3rd day :**

2x 500 ml 6% or 10% Haes 200/0.5 (low-sodium) for 6-12 h each time

**4th to 10th day :**

1x 500 ml 6% or 10% Haes 200/0.5 (low-sodium) for 6-12 h each time

1.) Begin the therapy as soon as possible, possibly acute treatment by the family or emergency physician
2.) Volume should be according to cardiac load capacity
3.) Decrease the Hct by about 12-15%
4.) If possible increase the CO (cardiac output)
5.) Decrease in Hct is detrimental for CO, therefore acutely no phlebotomy
6.) If Hct after 24h > 45%, then isovolemic hemodilution

**Additional therapy :**

1.) Digitalization according to clinical findings
2.) 3x 5,000 IU heparin s.c. as thrombosis prophylaxis
3.) After exclusion of an intracerebral bleeding:

1st to 3rd day: 1x 500 mg i.v. acetylsalicylic acid
from 4th day on: 1x 500 mg or 2x 250 mg tablets

**CAVE: 1. Cardiac volume load**

*Procedure during the Haes infusion:*

1. Measurement of heart rate and blood pressure:
   *are not allowed to increase*
2. Auscultation of the lung:
   *moist rale: breaking off (insufficiency of the left heart)*
3. Creatinine determination twice per week:
   *is not allowed to exceed 2.0 mg/dl with an initial value < 1.5 mg/dl*

**CAVE: 2. Hypovolemia in isovolemic hemodilution and decrease in CO**

Therefore: - *The infusion is always started before the phlebotomy at the other arm. (2 accesses)*
- *Phlebotomy at the other arm never faster than the infusion. (2 accesses)*

## 4.6.7 *Treatment Scheme for Ischemic Cerebral Infarction in Advanced Age*

Treatment Scheme for Ischemic Cerebral Infarction in Advanced Age

| Beginning/duration of therapy | I. Occurence of infarction ≤ 3 h | II. Occurence of infarction ≤ 3 h | III. Patients with hypertension | IV. Infarction patients with dysphagia |
|---|---|---|---|---|
| | | | | **CAVE: access via CVC** |
| Immediately after discovery (immediately!) | – 500mg ASA i.v.<br>– 40mg dexamethasone i.v.<br>– 2 X 10mg pirenzepin i.v.<br>– 250 X 500ml 6% Haes 0/0.5<br>– 2 × 5,000 I.U. heparin s.c. | – 100mg ASA p.o.<br>– antacid (e.g. aluminum-hydroxide)<br>– 2 × 5,000 I.U. heparin s.c. | – nimodipine in the perfusion according to BW<br>– antacid (e.g. aluminum-hydroxide) | – 500mg ASA i.v. (2× per week)<br>– 2 × 10mg pirenzepin i.v.<br>– infusion therapy according CVP<br>– cephalosporin<br>– 2 × 5,000 I.U. heparin s.c. |
| 1st to 5th day | – 100mg ASA p.o.<br>– gradual reduction of the dexamethasone dose<br>– antacid /e.g. aluminum-hydroxide)<br>– 250–500ml 6% Haes 200/0.5 (provided clinical improvement after the first infusion)<br>– 2 x 5,000 I.U. heparin s.c. | – 100mg ASA p.o.<br>– antacid (e.g. aluminum-droxide)<br>– 2 × 5,000 I.U. heparin s.c. | – nimodipine in the perfusion according to BW<br>– possibly: selective β-blockers and/or ACE inhibitors | – 500mg ASA i.v.<br>– 2 × 10mg pirenzepin i.v.<br>– infusion therapy according CVP<br>– cephalosporin<br>– 2 × 5,000 I.U. heparin s.c. |
| > 5th day | – 100mg ASA p.o.<br>– antacid (e.g. aluminum-hydroxide) | – 100mg ASA p.o.<br>– antacid (e.g. aluminum-hydroxide)<br>– 2 × 5,000 I.U. heparin s.c. | – nimodipine p.o.<br>– 100mg ASA P.O.<br>– antacid (e.g. aluminum-hydroxide) | – 500mg ASA i.v. (2× per week)<br>– 2 × 10mg pirenzepin i.v.<br>– infusion therapy according CVP<br>– cephalosporin<br>– 2 × 5,000 I.U. heparin s.c. |

i.v.: intravenous s.c.:subcutaneous p.o.: per os BW: body weight CVP: central venous pressure CVC: central vein catheter

## 4.6.8 Hemodilution over 5 Days After Cerebral Accident (Acute Scheme)

*(provided there are no indications for a local or systemic lysis or complete heparinization!)*

On discovery of the patient single dose of 500 to* 1,000 ml 6% Haes 200/0.5 over 30 to 60 minutes ("loading dose")

**Also in case of bleeding! In case of bleeding the administration of acetylsalicylic acid is contra-indicated. During the administration of volume the possible emergence of cerebral edema should be observed!*

### 1st to 5th day

| Time | Duration of infusion | Medication |
|---|---|---|
| 7-9 a.m. | 2 h | 400 mg naftidrofuryl in 250 ml saline solution (0.9%)<br>+ 250 mg acetylsalicylic acid per os<br>+ 0.3 ml (7,500 IU) heparin s.c. |
| 9-10 (11) a.m. | 1 (2) h | 500 ml hydroxyethyl starch 200/0,5 |

| | |
|---|---|
| if Hct>45%: with phlebotomy (500 ml) | PV≥1.39mPas: 6% Haes 200/0.5 |
| if Hct>42%: with phlebotomy (250 ml) | PV<1.39mPas: 10% Haes 200/0.5 |
| if Hct≤42%: without phlebotomy | Cave: Avoidance of hypovolemia! |

| Time | Duration of infusion | Medication |
|---|---|---|
| 5-6 (7) p.m. | 1 (2) h | 500 ml hydroxyethyl starch 200/0.5 |
| 7-9 p.m. | 2 h | 400 mg naftidrofuryl in 250 ml saline solution (0.9%)<br>+ 250 mg acetylsalicylic acid per os<br>+ 0.3 ml (7,500 IU) heparin s.c. |
| 9 p.m. -7 a.m. | 10 h | 500 ml saline solution (0.9%) |

### 6th to 8th day

Instead of Haes solutions crystalloid solutions should be infused !

### 9th to 13th day

In case of a progressive improvement 500 ml Haes solution should be infused again daily and instead of the second Haes solution a crystalloid solution should be infused !

**CAVE: 1. Volume tolerance !**

*Procedure during the Haes infusion:*

1. Measurement of heart rate and blood pressure:
   *are not allowed to increase*
2. Auscultation of the lung:
   *moist rale: breaking off (insufficiency of the left heart)*
3. Creatinine determination twice per week:
   *is not allowed to exceed 2.0 mg/dl with an initial value < 1.5 mg/dl*

**In case of poor volume tolerance adjust the infusion volume to clinical condition !**

**CAVE: 2. Avoidance of hypovolemia and anemia (Hct ≤ 35%) !**

*The infusion is always started before the phlebotomy at the other arm. (2 accesses)*
*The first infusion of 250 ml is given before the phlebotomy of 250 ml, the second after the phlebotomy. (1 access)*

### *4.6.9 Hemodilution in Placental Insufficiency, Pregnancy-Related Hypertension and for Thrombosis Prophylaxis During a Cesarian Section*

| Therapy phase over two weeks | | Target hematocrit 30 - 38 % | |
|---|---|---|---|
| **1. Patients with a normal heart and placental insufficiency** | | | |
| From 14th week of pregnancy | | Therapy phase 1st-14th day (possibly longer) | Therapy (daily) |
| Hematocrit (Hct) | Hemoglobin (Hb) | | |
| > 38 % | > 13 g/dl | If Hct exceeds 38 %, again hemodilution therapy (about 1-2 % of the cases) | 500 ml 10% Haes 200/0.5 within 4 hours + 500 ml Ringer solution within 4 hours |

| **2. Patients with pregnancy-related hypertension** | |
|---|---|
| In case of blood pressures of systolic < 165 mmHg and diastolic < 95 mmHg | In case of blood pressures of systolic > 165 mmHg and diastolic > 95 mmHg |
| Treatment according to 1. | Reduction in blood pressure until the day of delivery with hydralazine 3 ml/h + magnesium sulphate 1g/h + 500 ml 10% Haes 200/0.5 within 4h/day (absolutely) to avoid volume deficiency !!! If the heart rate increases over 120/min with this treatment, then administration of 3x 50mg metoprolol |

| **3. For thrombosis prophylaxis during a (cesarian) section** | |
|---|---|
| During the anesthesia induction: | 1st infusion of 500 ml 10% Haes 200/0.5 (completion until the end of the operation) |
| On the evening of the operation day: | 2nd infusion of 500 ml 10% Haes 200/0.5 |
| On the evening of the 1st postoperative day: | 3rd infusion of 500 ml 10% Haes 200/0.5 |
| In case of insufficient mobilization after the 7th postoperative day repetition of the same infusion scheme. | |

| **4. Patients with renal insufficiency** | |
|---|---|
| 1) If serum-creatinine > 2 mg/dl (= 1/2 GFR): | **Absolute contraindication** |
| 2) If serum-creatinine > 1.2 - 1.5 (-2) mg/dl: | **Attention !!!** (GFR: glomerular filtration rate) |
| Guarantee of daily creatinine control after beginning of the therapy, sufficient water supply for all patients before, during and after implementation of the hemodilution therapy (3 liter fluid/day) ! | |

| **5. Patients with severe decompensated cardiac insufficiency** |
|---|
| **Absolute contraindication** |

| **6. Patients with severe disturbances of coagulation** |
|---|
| **Absolute contraindication** |

Comment: dilution limit: Hct ≤ 30% and Hb ≤ 10 g/dl

## 4.6.10 Hemodilution over 10 Days in Acute Venous Circulatory Disturbances of the Retina

**Hemodilution over 10 Days in Acute Venous Circulatory Disturbances of the Retina**

| Patients | **Hemodilution therapy over 10 days** **Target hematocrit 38% – 40%** | |
|---|---|---|
| | Hematocrit (Hct) | 1st – 10th day (daily control of Hct and therapy according to Hct) |
| 1.<br>with a normal heart | Hct > 45%<br>Hct 42% – 45%<br>Hct < 42% | 500ml 10% Haes 200/0.5 – 60 minutes combined with phlebotomy of 500ml<br>250ml 6% Haes 200/0.5 – 60 minutes combined with phlebotomy of 250ml<br>250ml 10% Haes 200/0.5 – 60 minutes |
| 2.<br>with compensated cardiac insuffiency | Hct ≤ 42%<br>Hct < 42% | 250ml 6% Haes 200/0.5 – 60 minutes combined with phlebotomy of 250ml<br>250ml 6% Haes 200/0.5 – 60 minutes |
| with arterial hypertension | Systolic blood pressure < 170mmHg: treatment after therapy scheme 1 or 2<br>Systolic blood pressure ≤ 170mmHg: first reduction of blood pressure, then treatment after therapy scheme 1 or 2<br>**Daily control of blood pressure several times in all patients** | |
| with renal insuffiency | Serum-creatinine > 2mg/dl: **Absolute contraindication**<br>Serum-creatinine > 1.2mg/dl: **Relative contraindication**<br>Guarantee of daily control after beginning of the therrapy, sufficient water supply for all patients! | |
| Patients with severe decompensated cardiac insuffiency<br>or<br>severe disturbances of coagulation | **Absolute contraindication** | |

Additional rheologic therapy: daily 300mg pentoxifylline in 250ml Ringer solution and 1,200mg pentoxifylline per os

### *4.6.11 Hemodilution over 8 Days in Acute Arterial Circulatory Disturbances of the Retina*

After confirmation of the diagnosis single dose of 500 ml 6% Haes 200/0.5 within 30 minutes ("loading dose") and 500 mg acetylsalicylic acid per os as well as the determination of blood fluidity, -picture, -lipids, -glucose, -creatinine, uric acid and state of coagulation !

In case of proven risk factors such as hypertension, diabetes mellitus, hyperuricemia and hyperlipoproteinemia these must be treated !

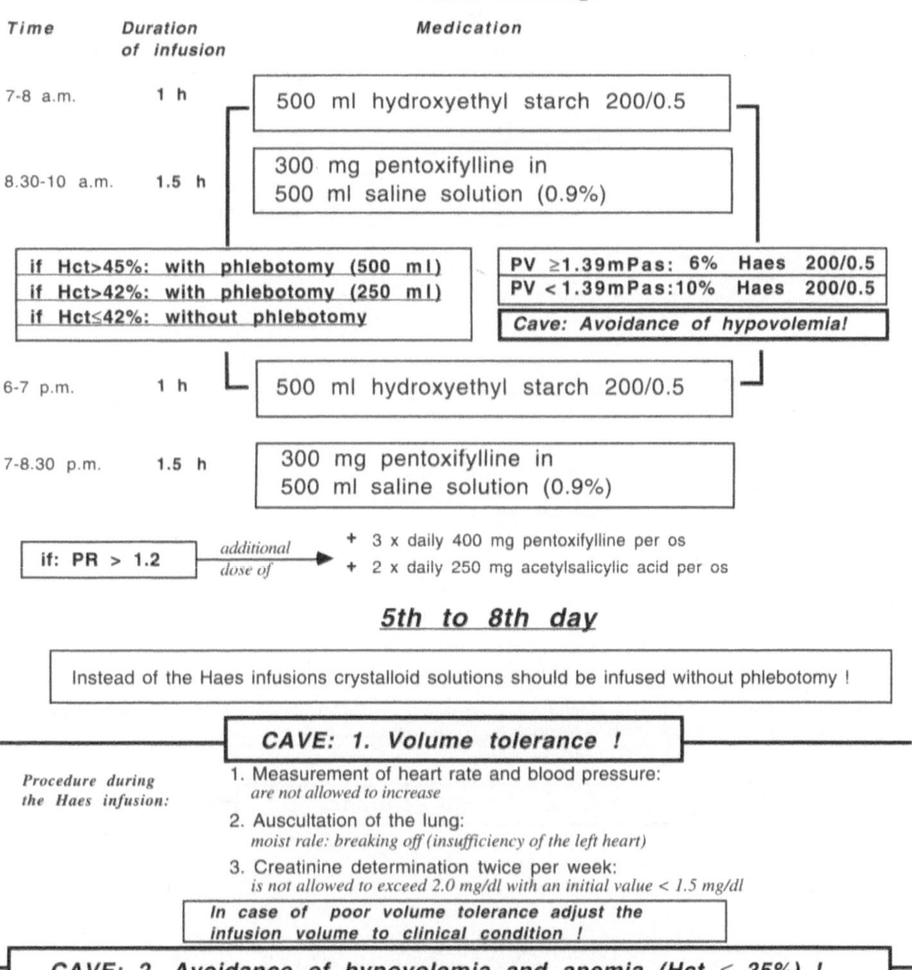

1st to 4th day
Time
Duration of infusion
Medication
7-8 a.m.
1 h
500 ml hydroxyethyl starch 200/0.5
8.30-10 a.m.
1.5 h
300 mg pentoxifylline in 500 ml saline solution (0.9%)
if Hct>45%: with phlebotomy (500 ml)
if Hct>42%: with phlebotomy (250 ml)
if Hct≤42%: without phlebotomy
PV ≥1.39mPas: 6% Haes 200/0.5
PV <1.39mPas:10% Haes 200/0.5
Cave: Avoidance of hypovolemia!
6-7 p.m.
1 h
500 ml hydroxyethyl starch 200/0.5
7-8.30 p.m.
1.5 h
300 mg pentoxifylline in 500 ml saline solution (0.9%)
if: PR > 1.2
additional dose of
+ 3 x daily 400 mg pentoxifylline per os
+ 2 x daily 250 mg acetylsalicylic acid per os
5th to 8th day
Instead of the Haes infusions crystalloid solutions should be infused without phlebotomy !
CAVE: 1. Volume tolerance !
Procedure during the Haes infusion:
1. Measurement of heart rate and blood pressure:
are not allowed to increase
2. Auscultation of the lung:
moist rale: breaking off (insufficiency of the left heart)
3. Creatinine determination twice per week:
is not allowed to exceed 2.0 mg/dl with an initial value < 1.5 mg/dl
In case of poor volume tolerance adjust the infusion volume to clinical condition !
CAVE: 2. Avoidance of hypovolemia and anemia (Hct ≤ 35%) !


*The infusion is always started before the phlebotomy at the other arm. (2 accesses)*
*The first infusion of 250 ml is given before the phlebotomy of 250 ml, the second after the phlebotomy. (1 access)*

## 4.6.12 *Hemodilution over 10 Days after Sudden Hearing Loss or Acute Symptomatic Hearing Loss (Acute Scheme)*

*(1. When venous thrombosis is suspected (condition after established thrombosis, e.g. extremities, known hypercoagulation): complete heparinization with administration of fluid 2. When no rheologic parameter is changed: no hemodilution !)*

| On admission of the patient single dose of 500 to 1000 ml 6% Haes 200/0.5 * ("loading dose") and 250 mg acetylsalicylic acid as effervescent tablet as well as determination of blood fluidity, -picture, -lipids, -glucose and creatinine |
|---|
| In case of proven risk factors such as hypertension, diabetes mellitus and hyperlipoproteinemia these must be treated ! |

* *If 1 liter 6% Haes 200/0.5 is administered, then at least a second liter in crystalloid solution form (e.g. 0.9% saline solution) intravenously or 1 liter drinking volume (water, tea) must be administered !*

**1st to 10th day**

| if: Hct ≤ 42%, PV < 1.34 mPas (fibrinogen < 400 mg/dl) and PR < 1.05 |
|---|
| 2 x daily administration of 500 ml crystalloid solution + possibly 400 mg naftidrofuryl |

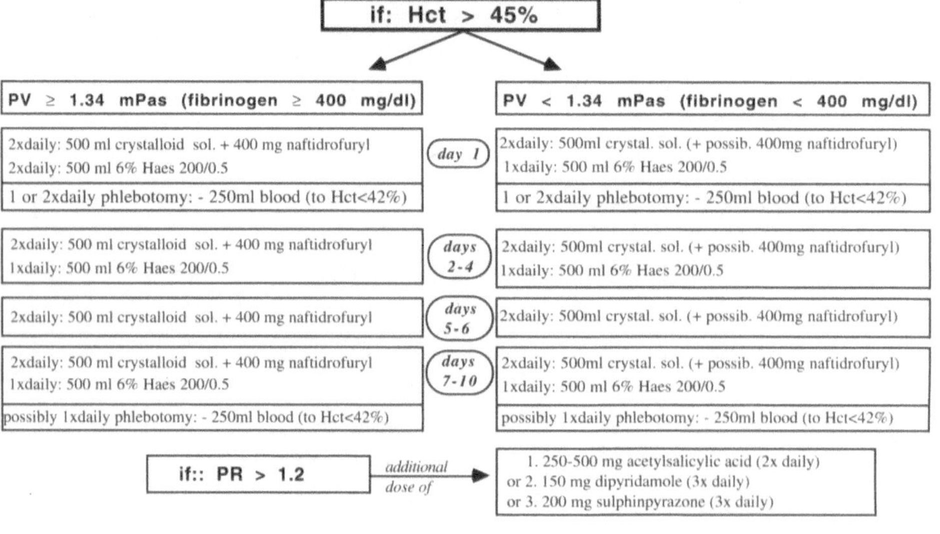


*Target range for the blood flow parameters:*

**1. Hematocrit (Hct): ≤ 42%**
**2. Plasma viscosity (PV): 1.14-1.33mPas; <u>alternatively:</u> fibrinogen concentration: 200-400mg/dl**
**3. Platelet reactivity index (PR) according to Grotemeyer: < 1.05**

**CAVE: 1. Volume tolerance !**

***Procedure during the Haes infusion:***

1. Measurement of heart rate and blood pressure:
   *are not allowed to increase*
2. Auscultation of the lung:
   *moist rale: breaking off (insufficiency of the left heart)*
3. Creatinine determination twice per week:
   *is not allowed to exceed 2.0 mg/dl with an initial value < 1.5 mg/dl*

***In case of poor volume tolerance adjust the infusion volume to clinical condition !***

**CAVE: 2. Avoidance of hypovolemia and anemia (Hct ≤ 35%) !**

*The infusion is always started before the phlebotomy at the other arm. (2 accesses)*

*The first infusion of 250 ml is given before the phlebotomy of 250 ml, the second after the phlebotomy. (1 access)*

## 4.6.13 Long-Term Scheme Subsequent to the Acute Scheme

(for patients with condition after cerebrovascular accident, "sudden hearing loss")

***1. Long-term scheme for volume tolerant patients (2 x hemodilution/month to Hct < 45 %, then 1x/month)***

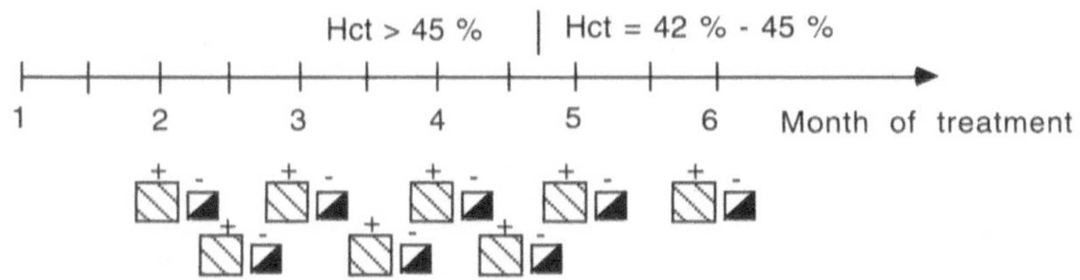


***2. Long-term scheme for small volume tolerant patients (2 x hemodilution/month to Hct < 45 %, then 1x/month)***

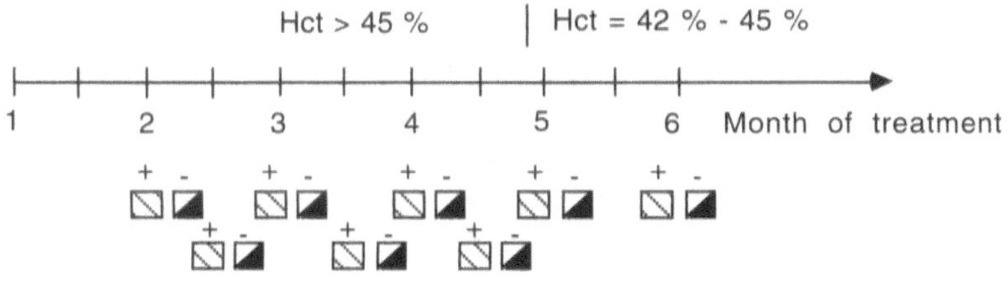


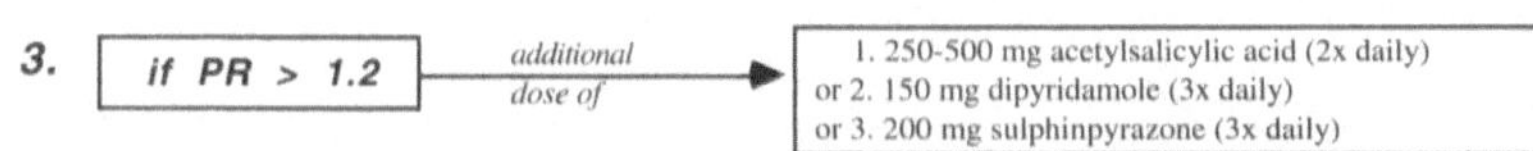


**4.** ***if 1.29 mPas < PV ≤ 1.39 mPas*** → *additional dose of* 1. 200 mg naftidrofuryl (3x daily) or 2. 400 mg pentoxifylline (3x daily)

***CAVE: 1. Volume tolerance !***

*Procedure during the Haes infusion:*

1. Measurement of heart rate and blood pressure:
   *are not allowed to increase*
2. Auscultation of the lung:
   *moist rale: breaking off (insufficiency of the left heart)*
3. Creatinine determination twice per week:
   *is not allowed to exceed 2.0 mg/dl with an initial value < 1.5 mg/dl*
4. Body weight (BW) determination:
   *is not allowed to increase more than 1 kg per week with normocaloric nutrition*

***In case of poor volume tolerance adjust the infusion volume to clinical condition !***

***CAVE: 2. Avoidance of hypovolemia and anemia (Hct ≤ 35%) !***

*The infusion is always started before the phlebotomy at the other arm. (2 accesses)*
*The first infusion of 250 ml is given before the phlebotomy of 250 ml, the second after the phlebotomy. (1 access)*

*Legend:*

- 500 ml 6% or 10% Haes 200/0.5 (dependent on volume tolerance)
- 250 ml 6% or 10% Haes 200/0.5 (dependent on volume tolerance)
- 250 ml whole blood
- \+ infusion  - phlebotomy

## 4.6.14 Long-Term Scheme Subsequent to the Acute Scheme

**For Patients with Condition After Venous Circulatory Disturbances in the Retina**

***1. Long-term scheme (1 x hypervolemic hemodilution/month if Hct < 42%)***

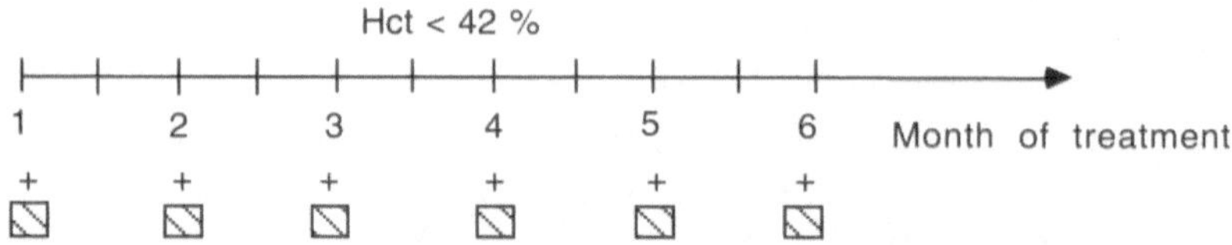


***2. Long-term scheme (1 x isovolemic hemodilution/month if Hct < 42%)***

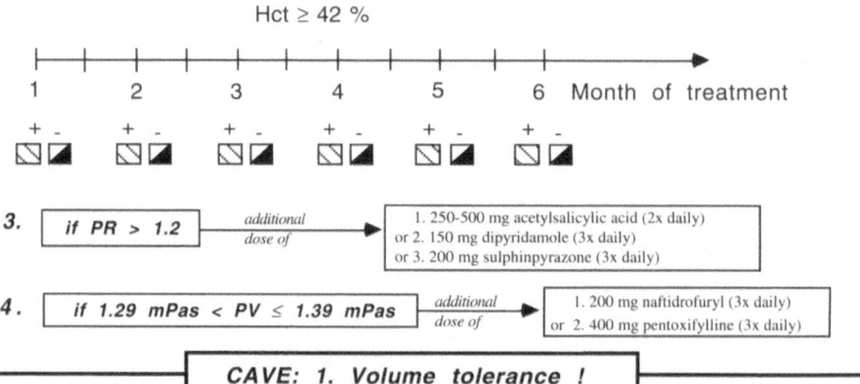


**CAVE: 1. Volume tolerance !**

***Procedure during the Haes infusion:***

1. Measurement of heart rate and blood pressure:
   *are not allowed to increase*
2. Auscultation of the lung:
   *moist rale: breaking off (insufficiency of the left heart)*
3. Creatinine determination twice per week:
   *is not allowed to exceed 2.0 mg/dl with an initial value < 1.5 mg/dl*
4. Body weight (BW) determination:
   *is not allowed to increase more than 1 kg per week with normocaloric nutrition*

***In case of poor volume tolerance adjust the infusion volume to clinical condition !***

**CAVE: 2. Avoidance of hypovolemia and anemia (Hct ≤ 35%) !**

*The infusion is always started before the phlebotomy at the other arm. (2 accesses)*
*The first infusion of 250 ml is given before the phlebotomy of 250 ml, the second after the phlebotomy. (1 access)*

***Legend:***

- ⧅ 500 ml 6% or 10% Haes 200/0.5 (dependent on volume tolerance)
- ◪ 250 ml whole blood
- \+ infusion
- \- phlebotomy

# 5 Methods

F. Jung, H. Kiesewetter, C. Mrowietz, and S. Wolf

## 5.1 Colloidal and Protein Chemistry Parameters

### 5.1.1 Blood Withdrawal Conditions and Obtaining of Samples

Blood samples for determining colloidal and protein chemistry parameters are obtained in standardized manner without tourniquet [164] from the antecubital vein, with the subject remaining seated [219] and using 10 ml sterilized disposable syringes with large-lumen needles [4]. Then blood samples are immediately converted into serum [19] according to general guidelines and the serum samples are stored at −30°C in sealed polystyrene tubes [19] for later analysis. The blood samples obtained for the molecular weight distribution are decanted after centrifugation (15 min at 110 *g*) and the supernatant dissolved with acetone and frozen afterwards at −80°C [51].

### 5.1.2 Methods of Measurement

*Hydroxyethyl Starch Concentration.* The methods of detection developed by Förster et al. [71] allow precise determination of the hydroxyethyl starch concentration in serum without interference with other polysaccharides and glucose.

In the first step 1 ml serum is mixed with 0.5 ml concentrated potash solution and boiled over 45 min. By this procedure not only proteins but especially glucose and polysaccharides which can disturb the measurement are destroyed. Then, 12 ml pure alcohol (about 100%) is added, well mixed, and stored over 24 h at 4°C; due to the polysaccharide sedimentation about 95%–96% of the hydroxyethyl starch can now be determined. Afterwards, centrifugation for 60 min is performed and the supernatant is decanted. In the second step the sediment is absorbed with 5 ml twice-normal hydrochloric acid and incubated for a period of 60 min to split the starch chains. After cooling the hydrolysate is filled in 10 ml volumetric flasks. The centrifuge tubes are cleaned with 4 ml twice-normal sodium hydroxide (NaOH) and the volumetric flasks filled up to the mark. Now, "free glucose" can be determined in hydrolysate by hexokinase glucose-6-phosphate dehydrogenase (hexokinase) [325] and further with *o*-toluidine [144].

The relatively tight hydroxyethyl groups are obviously not influenced by this preparation. Consequently, hydroxethyl-substituted glucose molecules and nonsubstituted glucose molecules result from the hydrolysis of hydroxyethyl starch. The hydroxyethyl-substituted glucose molecules are not recorded by the enzymatic prodecure with hexokinase whereas the reaction of the carbonyl group with *o*-toluidine is not influenced by substitution. But it is not necessary to identify all fission products of hydrolysis. It is sufficient for the enzymatic detection always to determine the same quantity of the hydroxyethyl starch used. It is required that a calibration value of the hydroxyethyl starch used be carried along since hydroxyethyl starch groups cannot be split off in the organism. Therefore, the identification of hydroxyethyl starch with *o*-toluidine serves as control for the enzymatic detection. Values higher by several percent are found on detection with *o*-toluidine depending on the contamination of test solution or other (still unknown) disturbing factors.

By this procedure, except for the low molecular weight (i.e., non-alcohol-precipitable) hydroxyethyl starch shares, about 95%–96% of the hydroxyethyl starch molecules are determined, with a recovery rate of 92.3% for enzymatic and of 93.8% for *o*-toluidine detection [71].

*Molecular Weight Distribution.* The molecular weight distribution is performed with a low-angle laser-light scattering (LALLS) combined with a concentration detector and a data processing system [50, 51]. For this purpose a differential refractometer, an RI-detector (Refracto Monitor III, LDC/Milton Roy, USA) is used [50]. The LALLS detector is equipped with a special flow cell (cell volume 10 μl) and an "inline filter" (cellulose acetate membrane filter of 0.2-μm pore) so that the scatter intensity (I) can be measured at a very small scattering angle (<6°) and greatest possible protection against contamination. In the case of such a small scattering angle the scatter intensity equals the extrapolated light scatter intensity at an angle of 0° in classic-dependent light scatter experiments; the concentration dependence can also be neglected at first approximation due to very small concentrations on chromatographic measurements in the detector cell (within the range of μg/ml). For this reason, this system can be used as absolute detector for exclusion chromatography. The direct proportional connection between scatter intensity (I) and the product of the mean molecular weight (MMw) and concentration (c) applies: $I \approx MMw \times c$. During measurement the substance is separated according to the different retention volumes of different molecular weights. The LALLS detector generates the scatter intensity profile of the sample; the scatter intensity (I) at a definite retention volume (V) is proportional to the product of mean molecular weight (MMw) and concentration (c). In order to calculate the mean molecular weight the corresponding concentration obtained by the RI detector is needed. The volume in the system capillaries is also taken into consideration for the determination of measuring volumes. The corrected chromatograms are subdivided in narrow, equidistant intervals, and a molecular weight is calculated for each interval.

Such a calculated mean molecular weight represents a monodisperse sector of the total molecular weight distribution, i.e., within such an interval the calculated mean molecular number corresponds to the mean molecular weight (MMn = MMw).

The following signal recording is done by a picture system equipped with an analogue/digital transformer which generates the desired sum or semilogarithmic curves of the ascertained data. The coefficient of variation, dependent mainly on disturbing aggregates in the sample, is smaller than 1% for this system [51, 62].

*α-Amylase Activity.* The α-amylase activity is determined by means of the test system Testomar Amylase (Behringwerke). This test is based on a method of the kinetic dye-test developed by Wallenfells [385]. The principle is based on the fact that α-amylase 4-nitrophenyl oligosaccharides such as, in this case, split *p*-nitrophenylmaltoheptaosid into p-nitrophenylmaltosid and glucose. Through further α-glucosidase catalyzed splitting yellow 4-nitrophenol is set free from *p*-nitrothenylmaltosid and is determined photometrically at 405 nm at a measuring temperature of 25°C. The precision in series during activities at the standard limit in serum samples by manual and mechanized measurement shows a coefficient of variation between 1% and 3.5% [267]. The precision from day to day at same enzyme activities is, with a coefficient of variation between 2% and 5%, only insignificantly worse [267]. The area of measurement for this method is up to 300 U/I [266]. Quality control is carried out according to the instructions by the manufacturer (Behringwerke). Hyperamylasemia is observed after the administration of hydroxyethyl starch [83].

*Total Protein Concentration.* Determination of the total protein concentration uses the biuret method developed by Weichselbaum [386] and modified for clinical purposes by Doumas et al. [47]. The principle of the biuret method is based on the accumulation of copper ions in the alkaline pH value area to the peptide bonds of proteins and peptides. The intensity of the resulting violet dyeing is linear to the amount of peptide bond and therefore to the protein concentration in a wide area. A requirement for the reaction is the presence of at least two peptide bonds (tripeptide). This is met by all blood protein fractions. The biuret reagent contains copper sulfate, sodium potassium tartrate, potassium iodide, and sodium hydroxide. To obtain a reaction as complete as possible bivalent copper is kept in solution in the alkaline environment as tartrate complex while potassium iodide prevents the autoreduction of bivalent copper. Then the concentration of the analysis sample is determined at 546 nm by a photometrical method after 30 min of incubation at room temperature. Bovine serum albumin of a particular concentration is used as standard for the photometrical measurement. The coefficient of variation according to the modified method by Doumas et al. [47] is given between 3% and 4% in series and from day to day. The reference range for clinically healthy adults aged between 20 and 60 years is 6.6–8.7 g/dl in serum [300]. An interference, which can be observed with other infusion solutions, does not exist between hydroxyethyl starch and biuret reagent [200].

*Albumin Concentration.* The albumin concentration is also determined by means of a microzone electrophoresis on a membrane film [364]. The electrophoretical separation of serum proteins is carried out on a prepared cellulose acetate microfilm, both ends of which are in contact with the electrode buffer. After applying the sample a fractionation of proteins is performed at constant stress (200–250 V) with direct current at a flow time of about 20 min in a buffer solution with a pH value of 8.6. The serum proteins move toward the anodes while breating down in desmoid form into singular fractions. The coloring of proteins on the film is performed with special protein dyes (such as Ponceau S, Amidoblack 10 B). Dye which is nonspecifically adsorbed to the film is washed out in decoloration baths. Quantitative estimation of the electropherogram is performed photometrically with a special evaluation device after having made the film transparent. This provides, besides an extinction place curve (giving the optical densities) and the percentage of the singular fractions, the corresponding protein concentrations (e.g., albumin concentration) in g/dl [364]. Since the serum protein electrophoresis is not standardized, each laboratory must indicate its own reference ranges [364]. In this case, the biochemical laboratory of the University of Frankfurt conducted by Förster has given a reference range of 3.5–5.5 g/dl for the albumin concentration in serum. The coefficients of variation in series and from day to day are below 3.5% for all individual protein concentrations [364]. Quality control is done according to the guidelines of the manufacturer (Behringwerke) [364]. The parameters used, methods of measurement, and reference ranges (measuring ranges) are indicated in Table 74.

**Table 74.** Parameters, methods of measurements, and reference ranges for laboratory chemistry parameters

| Parameter of measurement | Symbol | Method of measurement | Reference range |
|---|---|---|---|
| Haes concentration | Haes | Hexokinase enzym test | None, mg/dl |
| Haes concentration | Haes | o-Toluidine test | None, mg/dl |
| Mean molecular weight | Mw | LALLS detector | None, Da |
| Molecular weight distribution | MMw | LALLS detector | None, %/Da |
| α-amylase activity | α-amyl. | Dye test | (to 300 U/l) |
| Total protein concentration | Protein | Biuret reaction | 6.0–8.7 g/dl |
| Albumin concentration | Albumin | Electrophoresis | 3.5–5.5 g/dl |

## 5.2 Hemorheologic and Blood Picture Parameters

### 5.2.1 Blood Withdrawal Conditions and Obtaining of Samples

Blood samples for the determination of hemorheologic parameters were obtained in standardized manner without tourniquet [164] from the antecubital vein, with the subject remaining seated [219] and using sterilized disposable syringes with large-lumen needles [4]. During the storage period the blood samples were kept at room temperature in sealed polystyrene tubes. Rheological parameters were measured within 2 h after obtaining the blood samples [157]. To determine spontaneous thrombocyte aggregation a blood sample is anticoagulated with sodium citrate; the platelet-rich plasma is produced according to guidelines for standardized measurements by Breddin and collaborators [34]. Furthermore, for the measurement of blood picture parameters a blood sample is anticoagulated with dipotassium EDTA (concentration 2 mg/ml blood) [394].

### 5.2.2 Methods of Measurement

*Plasma Viscosity.* Plasma viscosity describing the internal friction or viscosity of blood plasma is a proportional constant. It is determined after centrifugation of venous blood at 1500 revolutions over 5 min [145, 146] by a capillary viscosimeter [157] and calculated from the quotient of shear stress and shear degree. The shear stress is determined by the driving pressure and capillary geometry; the shear degree is four times the plasma velocity with regard to the vascular diameter [153]. Quality control uses deep frozen (storage −30°C) plasma from citrate anticoagulated whole blood, measurement by a capillary viscosimeter. Method of measurement and quality control are described in [153]. The reference range in healthy adults is 1.14–1.34 mPas [157]. The coefficient of variation is 1.14% in series and 1.8% from day to day [153].

*Hematocrit.* Hematocrit is measured with the impedance device determining the Ohm's fraction of an alternating current resistance. The alternating-current voltage falling proportionally to the resistance of the blood column between the elctrodes of the measuring chamber is recorded, and the hematocrit is indicated [194]. Quality control uses a standard electrolyte solution, the conductivity of which corresponds to that of a blood sample with hematocrit of 45%. The method of measurement is described in [194] and the quality control in [153]. The reference range is 39%–52% by volume for adult men (adult women 35%–50%). The coefficient of variation is 0.4% in series and 2.4% from day to day [153].

*Erythrocyte Aggregation.* Erythrocyte aggregation is the reversible process of red blood cells sticking together in the form of so-called rolls of coins, which occurs under normal physiological conditions; under pathologic conditions erythrocytes form clumps [196]. Since erythrocytes have a negative surface tension, they push each other off due to Coulomb forces. This means that they can approach only up to a distance of about 30 mn [40]. Thus, erythrocytes in normal saline solution are unable to aggregate. To enable the membranes to accumulate connecting links between the erythrocyte membranes must be formed, for example, high molecular weight proteins with a diameter greater than 30 nm (fibrinogen, alpha-2-macroglobulin, immunglobulin M). The erythrocyte aggregation index is determined photometrically with the mini-erythrocyte aggregometer [196]; quality control is described in [193]. As erythrocyte aggregation depends on hematocrit [196], this value must be adjusted to a prefixed value before determining the aggregation index. For practical and theoretical reasons a value of 45% is chosen. The reference range is 8–21. The coefficient of variation is 5.2% in series and 7.1% from day to day [193].

*Erythrocyte Rigidity.* Since an erythrocyte can easily change its shape, it can pass vessels with a diameter smaller than its own during rest. Erythrocyte deformability is founded on the fact that the blood cells are particles with a very large surface and liquid contents. Thus, erythrocytes are comparable to an incompletely filled water pillow which can adapt its outer form to the influence of the surrounding forces. The passage time of individual erythrocytes through a monoporous membrane, which is measured by a "selecting erythrocyte rigidometer" [310], is the measure of the deformability of erythrocytes. This monoporous membrane is a plastic tissue which has a single measuring pore (pore length 27 μm; pore diameter 4.5 μm), and which is smaller than the diameter of an erythrocyte during rest. Thus, the passing blood cells change their shape while passing the hole; the passage time is the longer the more rigid a blood cell is. The passage time of 250 singular passages is measured; the mean value is calculated and shown. The design of quality control is described in [193]. The reference range is 0.83–1.19. The coefficient of variation is 7.5% in series and 6.1% from day to day, at an interindividual variation range of 8.3% [193].

*Spontaneous Thrombocyte Aggregation.* Thrombocyte aggregation, like erythrocyte aggregation, is a nonspecific connection of cells mainly by fibrinogen molecules. During the second phase, irreversible aggregates are formed, and thrombocytes are destroyed mechanically. Thrombocyte aggregation is also quantified as a matter of routine [34]. Spontaneous thrombocyte aggregation is determined according to the method by Breddin [34]. For the description of the aggregation curve the angle of ascent $\alpha_2$ was chosen. For determination of the reference range a study on 124 healthy subjects was carried out by Breddin [34]. This revealed an age dependence for the $\alpha_2$ parameter of spontaneous thrombocyte aggregation. A significantly increased spontaneous thrombocyte aggregation (angle $\alpha_2$>40°) was detected in about 15% of those aged 10–29 years, 11% aged 30–39 years, 28% aged 40–49, and 28% aged 50–59 years.

*Platelet Reactivity Index.* For examination of the platelet function the thrombocyte function system described by Wu and Hoak [404] was modified by Grotemeyer [91]. This system is chosen due to the mechanical test investigation and because in vitro manipulations of the platelets are no longer necessary. The test procedure is based on the dissolution of platelet aggregates (occurring in vivo or resulting from blood sampling) in but with immediate fixation in EDTA. After the withdrawal of blood by applying the two-syringe technique, 0.3 ml blood is added to 1 ml EDTA (11.7 mmol sodium EDTA in 1/15 mmol/l sodium potassium hydrogen phosphate, pH 7.4) or 1 ml EDTA formalin (11.7 mmol sodium-EDTA and 1% formaldehyde in 1/15 mmol/l sodium potassium hydrogen phophate, pH 7.4) and well mixed immediately. Both samples are filled in 2-ml centrifuge tubes (Grainer) and centrifuged at 820 rpm for a period of 20 min. The platelet number was determined from the supernatant fluid by means of a thrombocyte counter (Sysmex Hematology System TOA PL-100; Digitana, Hamburg). Deviations in platelets counts were known to be less than 5% in platelets of healthy subjects. With the EDTA formalin test, the platelet count in supernatant whole blood is reduced by the number of platelet aggregates. Results of measurements in the two samples are expressed in a quotient, with the EDTA formalin platelet count in the denominator. The quotient is larger in the presence of more platelet aggregates. The index for measuring platelet reactivity (PR) is:

$$\frac{\text{Erythrocytes (EDTA formalin)} \times \text{platelets (EDTA)}}{\text{Erythrocytes (EDTA)} \times \text{platelets (EDTA) formalin}} = \text{PR}$$

A PR value greater than 1.05 raises is suspicious; values over 1.2 are highly pathological [91].

*Hemoglobin Concentration.* The hemoglobin concentration in the capillary blood of the finger pad or in the EDTA blood is determined by the cyanogen methemoglobin method [394]. Hemoglobin (FE II) is oxidized by sodium ferricyanide over methemoglobin (FE III) in cyangen methemoglobin which shows a typical absorption spectrum at 546 nm. For this preparation a defined volume of a transformation solution is mixed with 0.02 ml blood and measured photometrically as extinction with the transformation solution. The difference between extinction of the preparation solution and transformation solution (neutral value) multiplied with a constant factor which depends on the used transformation solution results in the hemoglobin concentration in g/dl. The hemoglobin value is subject to a very slight daily variation and is smaller than the coefficient of variation of the method of measurement (about 2%) [394]. The reference range of this method is 13–18 g/dl for the hemoglobin content in adult men [332].

*Mean Corpuscular Volume and Thrombocyte Count.* The mean corpuscular volume of erythrocytes (MCV) and the frequency distribution of erythrocytes and thrombocytes is determined by the Coulter counter procedure [35]. The counter unit of the apparatus with an automatic registration device includes a measuring capillary with a diameter of 100 μm and a length of 50 mm and two direct current electrodes. The counting process is carried out with the highest possible electric amplification of the measuring signal and is finished within 20 s. The lowest threshold value at which erythrocytes or thrombocytes can still be counted is previously determined with regard to the respective electric adjustment. Volume calibration is performed with latex particles of known volume distribution and with the known value of the MCV of a blood sample [35]. Further technical details of the coincidence correction with other corpuscular blood particles, the influence of electric current, and the failure range of the apparatus (coefficient of variation 3%) are described by Adam et al. [1]. Variations during 1 day which are significant below the coefficient of variation and interindividual differences of the erythrocyte volume distribution are described in [24]. The reference range of this method for MCV is 80–94 $\mu m^3$

for healthy adults [332] and 140 000–440 000 per $mm^3$ for the thrombocyte count [394].

*Mean Corpuscular Hemoglobin Concentration.* The mean corpuscular hemoglobin concentration (MCHC) is also calculated by the Coulter counter procedure as described above [35]. After determination of the erythrocyte count, and simultaneous Hb and MCV determination, the MCHC is determined as a derived parameter with an integrated electronic system in the same precise way as for the method of measurement. The reference range of this method for the MCHC is 32–36 g/l for adults [332]. During the period of examination a quality control for rheologic parameters [193] and blood picture parameters [1] ensures the laboratory analyses. The parameters used methods of measurement, and reference ranges are given in Table 75.

**Table 75.** Parameters, method of measurement, reference ranges for hemorheologic and blood picture parameters

| Parameter of measurement | Symbol | Method of measurement | Reference range |
|---|---|---|---|
| Plasma viscosity | PV | Capillary tube plasma viscosimeter | 1.14 – 1.34, mPas |
| Hematocrit | Hct | Impedance method | M: 39 – 52, %<br>W: 34 – 50, % |
| E aggregation | SEA | E aggregometer | 8 – 21, none |
| E rigidity | SER | E rigidometer | 0.83 – 1.19, none |
| T aggregation | sTA | T aggregometer | (See text), degree |
| T reactivity | PR | Coulter counter procedure | (See text), none |
| Hemoglobin concentration | Hb | Cyanogen methemoglobin method | 11 – 18, g/dl |
| Mean e volume | MCV | Coulter counter procedure | 80 – 94, $mm^3$ |
| Mean Hb content | MCHC | Electronic counting procedure | 32 – 36, g/dl |
| T count | Tc | Coulter counter procedure | 140 – 440, count/nl |

E, Erythrocyte; T, thrombocyte.

## 5.3 Metabolic Parameters

### 5.3.1 Blood Withdrawal Conditions and Obtaining of Samples

For blood gas analysis and measurement of hemoglobin arterialized capillary blood is used which appears spontaneously without bruising after skin puncture at the hyperemized lobe of the ear [268] or at the finger pad [112]. With regard to its composition this arterialized capillary blood corresponds to arterial blood since it comes mainly from the arterioles [239], and it does not differ at all in blood gas analysis if the withdrawal conditions are precisely observed [239]. Local hyperemia is caused chemically with a preparation containing nicotinic acid ester such as Finalgon ointment. After 5 min the drug is removed with dry cellulose, and the place of the skin concerned is disinfected with an alcohol solution. As soon as the place is dry, the lower rim of the lobe of the ear or the finger pad is scratched about 5 mm deep with an one-way lancet. After absorption of the first blood drop the spontaneously extravasating blood is filled without air bubbles in heparinized glassy capillaries. The capillary is sealed on both sides with cement and mixed magnetically by means of a steel pin. Immediately (within a period of 15 min) after withdrawal the blood gas analysis is performed.

For determination of pyruvate or lactate concentration in blood venous blood is obtained without tourniquet from the antecubital vein [164] with the subject remaining seated [219], with a sterilized monovette (5 ml) containing lithium heparinate (concentration of 10 IU/ml blood) for anticoagulation. The anticoagulated blood content of one monovette is immediately deproteinized with ice-cold 0.6 *M* perchloric acid (ratio 1:1), well mixed and centrifugated at 110 *g* for 10 min. The supernatant fluid remains available for the total enzymatic pyruvate determination according to the method of Czok and Lambrecht [42] at room temperature for 3 days [229]. From the blood of the other monovette plasma is obtained by centrifugation under standardized conditions, which is afterwards deproteinized with ice-cold 0.6 *M* perchloric acid (ratio 1:1). After another centrifugation (at 110 *g* for 10 min) the supernatant fluid is available for the total enzymatic lactate determination according to the method of Noll [279] at room temperature for 3 days [331].

## 5.3.2 Methods of Measurement

*Plasma Pyruvate Concentration.* The pyruvate determination is performed with deproteinized supernatant blood as described in Sect. 5.3.1, completely enzymatically and with following photometrical measurement. First, the supernatant fluid is brought to reaction with the following solutions: (a) lactate dehydrogenase dissolved in aqua destilata, (b) 2.2 *M* dipotassium hydrogen phosphate, and (c) 0.012 *M* reduced nicotinamide, adenine dinucleotide (NADH). Oxydation of NADH to $NAD^+$ occurs which is proportional to the substrate quantity measured photometrically at 340 (334, 366) nm. In accordance with the extinction change the pyruvate concentration is calculated stoichiometrically [42]. The coefficient of variation of this method is 4%; the reference range for the pyruvate concentration 3.6–5.9 mg/l for adults with a healthy metabolism at rest [229]. The quality control of this enzyme test is performed according to the guidelines of the manufacturer (Boehringer Mannheim) [27].

*Plasma Lactate Concentration.* The determination of lactate is carried out with deproteinized supernatant plasma obtained in accordance to the guidelines described in Sect. 5.3.1, completely enzymatically and following photometrical measurement. First, the supernatant is brought to reaction with the following reagents: (a) 0.027 *M* nicotinamide adenine dinucleotide ($NAD^+$), (b) 2 mg lactate dehydrogenase per ml supernatant, (c) 0.5 *M* glycin buffer with pH 9.0, and (d) 0.4 *M* hydrazine. This leads to reduction of $NAD^+$ to NADH, the increase in which measured at the extinction change at 340 (334, 360) nm is directly proportional to the lactate concentration [279]. The coefficient of variation for this enzyme test is 2.3% [279]. A good precision in series and a variation from day to day which is below the coefficient of variation of the method of measurement is described by Schwab et al. [331]. The reference range of the lactate concentration in plasma is 57–220 mg/l in adults with a healthy metabolism at rest [225]. The quality control of this enzyme test is performed according to the guidelines of the manufacturer (Boehringer Mannheim) [27].

*pH Value in Blood.* The pH value in blood is determined according to the principle of Astrup and Schröder [14] with a glass electrode chain and modified by Bates [20] and Johansson et al. [151]. Construction and function are explained below. The glass electrode in its simplest form is a thin-walled round-bottom glass flask containing an electrolyte solution (e.g., calomel solution $Hg_2Cl_2$) with known pH (inner reference solution). A lead electrode is immersed in the electrolyte solution. The prepared round-bottom flask is inserted as glass electrode into the outer measuring solution (blood) of unknown pH value. For the afflux of a potential difference a glass reference electrode is needed which is in conducting contact (electrolyte bridge) with the measuring solution through an electrolyte solution (e.g., potassium chloride). Measuring solution (blood) and electrolyte bridge are separated by a diaphragm. Due to the protode effect of glass potential differences appear at the outer and inner glass layers which in wide limits are linearly dependent on the pH values of the inner and outer solutions. Since the pH value on the inner side of the glass layer (inner reference solution) is left constant, the measurable potential difference is dependent exclusively on the pH value of the solution of the outer opposite side (measuring solution, blood) and can be read immediately. For blood gas analysis a modified capillary glass electrode according to Astrup [14] with an open connection between blood and potassium chloride solution is used which also serves as supply to the $pO_2/pCO_2$ measuring chamber. Measurements of the pH value and other blood parameters are performed constantly at 37°C ± 0.1°C to avoid changes of the potential of the inner reference solution due to its temperature dependence (Nernst's equation) and to obtain standardized measuring conditions for blood. This is achieved by internal heating with temperature regulation. The coefficient of variation measured in series is less than 0.1% [268]. The reference range of this method for arterial and arterialized capillary blood is 7.370–7.450 in healthy adults [338]. In the case of correct withdrawal technique the pH value of peripheral venous blood is not more than 0.030 U lower than for arterialized capillary blood [75]. The quality control of blood gas parameters is performed in accordance with the guidelines for buffer gas solution by Maas et al. [247], which are also established by the German Medical Society. Table 76 shows the parameters, methods of measurement, and corresponding reference ranges for metabolic parameters.

**Table 76.** Parameters, methods of measurement, and reference ranges for metabolic parameters

| Parameter of measurement | Symbol | Method of measurement | Reference range |
|---|---|---|---|
| Lactate concentration in plasma | Lactate | LDH/GPT enzyme test | 57–220 mg/l |
| Pyruvate concentration in plasma | Pyruvate | NADH/LDH enzyme test | 3.6–5.9 mg/l |
| pH value in blood | pH | Glass electrode chain | 7.370–7.450, none |

## 5.4 Measurement of Oxygen Partial Pressure and $O_2$ Saturation

*Conjunctival $pO_2$.* The conjunctival oxygen partial pressure is measured polarographically according to Clark's principle [141]. The anode consists of silver-silver chloride and the cathode of platinum. The electrodes are installed in an electrolyte solution behind a membrane permeable to gas and water-repellent. The strength of the electric current measured between the electrodes is determined by the quantity of oxygen diffusing through the membrane. The quantity of the diffusion current is predetermined by the concentration of oxygen in the measuring solution so that a direct correlation exists between oxygen partial pressure of the lacrimal fluid and measured strength of the electric current, which is given by a calibration curve as conjunctival oxygen partial pressure [61]. The reference range of this method for oxygen partial pressure is 35–65 mmHg in healthy adults [61].

*Transcutaneous $pO_2$.* The measurement of transcutaneous oxygen partial pressure is carried out polarographically with a silver-platinum electrode with integrated heating device according to Clark's principle [141]. Measurements are performed at heating temperatures of 43°C at the forearm and back of the foot. The reference range of this method for oxygen partial pressure is 65–97 mmHg in healthy adults [155].

*Intramuscular $pO_2$.* Intramuscular oxygen histograms are measured according to the method developed by Fleckenstein et al. [66] with the macroelectrode type $pO_2$ histograph KIMOC (Eppendorf Geraetebau; Hamburg). Since the measurement has not been standardized, it is described below. Prior to the examination the patients are adapted to room temperature; the waiting period before measurement is about 1 h in a pleasantly warm room. The temperature of the skin surface is controlled prior to the measurement, which is only started up on exceeding a temperature of 27°C. The $pO_2$ measurements are performed in the tibialis anterior muscle. After preparation of the measuring site and subcutaneous local anesthesia a disposable puncture cloth is put around the needle insertion site. The puncture site is situated lateral to the tibial edge at the level of the greatest muscle cross-section. Then an access for the $pO_2$ probe is laid by means of an Abbokath vascular catheter at an angle of about 30° to the longitudinal axis of the muscle fiber in cranial direction. The measurement of $pO_2$ values is not started prior to a 15 min period of rest. The measuring probe is positioned under control of the $pO_2$ measuring values to ensure that the measurement is started in the muscular tissue. The automatically operating (microprocessor controlled) advance of the probe is with the so-called *Pilgerschrittverfahren* (pilgrim's pace procedure). A length of stride of 1.0 mm with a retrograde step of 0.3 mm is chosen so that an effective length of stride of 0.7 mm – at a measuring interval of 1.4 s – results. Then 21 successive measurements are carried out, resulting in a puncture channel of 1.47 cm. A measuring cyle consists of 21 measurements, afterwards the probe returns to its initial position. After each measuring cycle the probe is turned by 120°. By the first grind of the measuring probe another tissue area is measured with each new advance since the puncture channel is palpated into another preferential direction. To be able to evaluate a muscular area as great as possible puncture angle and direction are slightly changed after the second turn. Therefore, a new puncture channel is determined with each measurement. On the whole, 200 individual values are recorded and used for the drawing up of an oxygen partial pressure histogram. The intramuscular reference range for the $O_2$ puncture electrode at an oxygen partial pressure is 16.4–58.3 mmHg; the coefficient of variation in series is 20% [154].

*Blood $pO_2$ Ex Vivo.* The determination of the $pO_2$ in blood (arterial, capillary, and venous) is performed polarographically with a platinum electrode coated with an oxygen-permeable membrane [14], as modified by Gleichmann et al. [82]. The collection of samples is explained in Sect. 5.2.1. Construction and function are explained below. The platinum cathode melted in a glass stick is surrounded by a tubular capsule, the open end of which is sealed with an oxygen-permeable membrane. The space of this capsular is filled with an electrolye solution (e.g., potassium chloride and a buffer system) of defined concentration so far that the point of the platinum cathode is in conducting contact with a silver/silver chloride reference electrode. A sufficient reduction stress of 600–800 mV is imposed on the platinum electrode to reduce the molecular oxygen passing the membrane and reaching the surface of the electrode. By means of the electrodes, which are set free at the reference electrode, four hydroxyl ions ($OH^-$) per molecule oxygen ($O_2$) are produced at the platinum electrode. Now the hydroxyl ions react with protons, which originate from the electrolyte solution, to water; for this reason a buffer system in the electrolyte solution is necessary. The strength of the current produced in this system by the constant stress of 600–800 mV is proportional to the number of oxygen molecules per time unit reduced at the platinum cathode. The strength of the current obtained by the given stress with the oxygen-free electrolyte solution serves for the zero adjustment. A stress of 600–800 mV is chosen for the following reasons: (a) In this range of stress the strength of the current is mainly independent of the imposed stress since electrons are available in surplus for the complete reduction of oxygen. (b) The electrolyte solution is composed in such a way that it does not contain other particles which could be reduced in this range of stress. Furthermore, the measuring conditions consider the oxygen autoexpenditure of the platinum electrode so that the measurement remains uninfluenced. The $pO_2$ electrode is combined with a pH and $pCO_2$ electrodes and has the same temperature (37°C ± 0.1°C) as the electrodes or measuring chamber. By this device the $pO_2$ of the blood sample, i.e., the concentration of the physically saturated oxygen, is inferred from the reduction current produced by oxygen molecules arriving at the platinum cathode per time unit under constant diffusion conditions between measuring solution (blood) and measuring system. The $pO_2$ can be determined within the range of 80–150 mmHg with a coefficient of variation of 2%–4% and within a range from 30–60 mmHg with a coefficient of variation of 5%–8% [268]. On correct collection of blood samples (as described in Sect. 5.2.1) a common range between 70 and 100 mmHg [268] is given for arterialized capillary blood or arterial blood, and for venous blood from the cubital vein without tourniquet a range between 20 and 40 mmHg [412] in healthy adults. A confidence range of 99% ± 10 mmHg is assumed. The quality control of blood gas parameters is performed in accordance to the guidelines with the buffer gas solutions of Maas et al. [247], established by the German Medical Society. However, at normal values the considerable age dependence of arterial or capillary pO should also be taken into consideration. This is considered in the following formula [241]:

$$\mathbf{pO_2\ (mmHg) = 102\text{–}0.33 \times years\ of\ life}$$

*Total Oxygen Saturation.* The oxygen saturation ($SO_2$) is determined nomographically by the conductor nomogram (Radiometer, Copenhagen) based on the oxygen standard dissociation curve an the proof factors for temperature, $pH_2$ value, and pO determined by experiments [13]. By this indirect procedure a sufficient approach (below 1% deviation) toward the actual oxygen saturation is achieved if no $pO_2$ values smaller than 50 mmHg are used for the nomographic clearing [268]. The reference range for the nomographically established oxygen saturation is between 0.94–0.98 [22] (Table 77).

**Table 77.** Parameters and methods of measurement and reference ranges of oxygen parameters

| Parameter | Symbol | Method | Reference range |
|---|---|---|---|
| *$O_2$ partial pressures:* | | | |
| Transcutaneuos (arm, foot) | $pO_2$-tc | Clark's sensor | 65–97 mmHg |
| Transconjunctival (eye) | $pO_2$-tCb | Clark's sensor | 35–65 mmHg |
| Intramuscular (tib. ant. m.) | $pO_2$-IM | Clark's sensor | 16.4–58.3 mmHg |
| Arterial (blood) | $pO_2$-art | Astrup | 70–100 mmHg |
| Capillary (blood) | $pO_2$-cap | Astrup | 70–100 mmHg |
| Venous (blood) | $pO_2$-ven | Astrup | 20–40 mmHg |
| $O_2$-saturation (art./cap.) | $SO_2$ | Nomogram | 0.94–0.98, none |

## 5.5 Measurement of Blood Flow and Pressure

*Blood Flow in the Common Carotid Artery.* The volume flow in the common carotid artery is measured by means of the *M*obile *A*rtery and *V*ein *I*maging *S*ystem (MAVIS). This is a 30-channel pulsed ultrasound Doppler system by means of which an ECG is recorded before each measurement and angle between vascular axis and Doppler probe is automatically determined so that velocity and blood volume can be measured. The probe diameter is 1.0 cm, the time frequency 25 ms. The variation range of the method is below 7% [64]. The reference range of the method is between 210 and 380 ml/min for adults with a healthy vascular system [320].

*Resting Flow in Nail Fold Capillaries.* The capillary blood flow in the main capillaries can be estimated by measuring erythrocyte velocity and capillary geometry. Since the results depend considerably on the way in which these measurements are performed, video capillaroscopy is described in detail below [163]. The capillaroscopy is performed by means of a direct light microscope with an objective, optovar 1.0–2.0, cold light source with green light filter (in the wavelength range of hemoglobin absorption), video camera, video timer (to insert date and time), video recorder, monitor, and picture-analyzing system. According to the adjustment of the optovar the magnification of 275–550 times is possible. The pictures are recorded by means of the ¾″ video recorder and evaluated with a picture-analyzing system. Erythrocyte velocity (v) is calculated as the quotient of the distance (s) traveled by the erythrocytes in the capillaries in a given time ($\delta t$). The mean erythrocyte velocity for young and healthy subjects is $0.60 \pm 0.21$ mm/s in the arterial capillary loop [163]. Before the performance of the microscopy the surface temperature at the nail fold is controlled; only at a constant temperature above 27°C is the recording started [163]. The erythrocyte velocities indicated in Sect. 4.1.2 are temporal (repeated measurements in one capillary) and spacial (measurements in different capillaries) mean values (Fig. 91). The mean capillary blood flow (BFcap) is calculated according to the continuity theorem as a product of mean erythrocyte velocity (v) and capillary cross-section area. The capillary area is calculated from the erythrocyte column diameter measured on the assumption of a circular cross section [163]:

$$\mathbf{BFcap} = \pi / 4 \times d^2 \times v$$

where BFcap = mean capillary blood flow ($10^{-9}$ ml/s), v = mean erythrocyte velocity (mm/s), and d = erythrocyte column diameter (μm). The calculation of a relative error results in a value of 6%.

*Reactive Hyperemia in Nail Fold Capillaries.* Additionally, a function test with regard to the regulation of the microcirculation is performed. For this purpose, the velocity is measured after a 3-min ischemia produced with a tourniquet at the upper arm by a stasis at 300 mmHg. After release of the stasis a reactive hyperemia is physiologically to be expected; the course is recorded by repeated velocity measurements after stasis (10, 30, 60, 120, 180, and 240 s). The

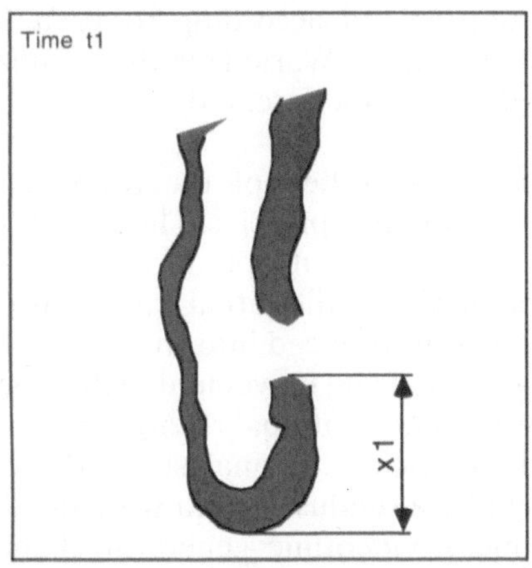


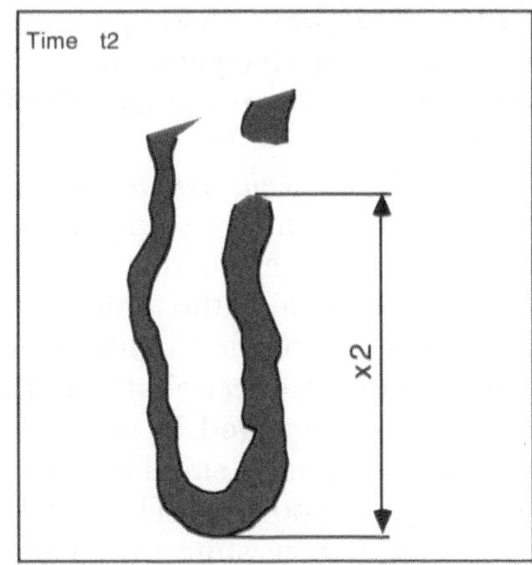


1)Recording of an identical capillary area at different times (each time about 5 min.)

2) Recording of time t1 and t2 (video timer)

3) Measurement of distances x1 and x2

4) Calculation of mean velocity: $v = \frac{(x2 - x1)}{(t2 - t1)}$

5) Spacial meaning: Measurement of all visible capillaries

6)Temporal meaning: Repeated measurement of capillaries for a period of 5 min. } $v_{mean}$

**Fig. 91.** Scheme determining mean erythrocyte velocity

period of time between release of the stasis and adjustment of the erythrocyte velocity under resting conditions is described as duration of the reactive hyperemia, in which the height of the amplitude between resting velocity and maximum velocity after stasis is also recorded as a further parameter. About 80% of healthy subjects show a duration of hyperemia of more than 180s [163]. Figure 92 shows a typical course of reactive hyperemia.

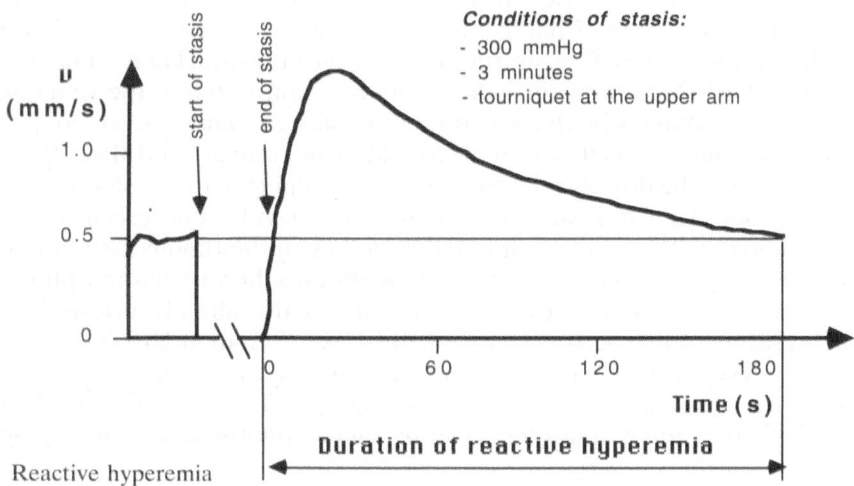


**Fig. 92.** Reactive hyperemia

*Blood Pressure.* Blood pressure is determined according to Riva Rocci, corresponding to the performance guidelines of the World Health Organization [403]. Measurements are carried out with the subject seated.

*Video Fluorescein Angiography.* The vascular bed of the retina is most suitable for the in vivo study of arterioles and precapillaries. The vessels of the retina are arranged at one level and visible without operation. Due to the methods available at the moment the capillaries of the retina can be visualized only under pathologic conditions. The dye is introduced into the circulation by injection into an antecubital vein. Its distribution and movement in the vessels of the retina are observed. To measure flow velocity continual recording by a video system is especially suitable since a direct electronic analysis of the optical signals became possible. The system includes a fundus camera with an adapted video system consisting of a video camera, videotime generator (Panasonic WJ-810), video recorder (Sony VO-5800PS), two video monitors (Panasonic WV-5470), and a picture-analyzing system (Microvideomat 3, Zeiss). The operating system of the video analyzer is changed to allow tracking of the eye movements. The automatic control circuit of the amplifier of the low-light camera (Bosch Type TCY 9A with SIT tube) is disconnected to establish a linear relationship between the light intensity and video signal. The video camera is connected with the fundus camera by means of a special adapter (f = 107 mm) without use of a beam splitter. Therefore the whole available light is used for observation, and the numeric aperture of the system is doubled. The magnification of retina: videotarget is 1:2.5 under an observation angle of 21°. The adapter permits an optic resolution of 8 μm. For the recording of fluorescein angiograms, a filter combination with a relatively wide spectrum of pseudofluorescein (barrier GG 520, exciter 485; Zeiss) is chosen. This is necessary for analysis of the video fluorescein angiograms since the pupil must the visible as a bright center of the picture and the vessels at the fundus before the influx of fluorescence. At the beginning of the video fluorescein angiography, the patient receives an intravenous catheter (Abbokath catheter G20). Pulse and blood pressure are measured. Then the retinal image is recorded by using red-free light. Prior to the injection of the dye the exciter filter is inserted in the lighting ray path and the barrier filter in the observation ray path. Then 5 ml/70 kg body weight of a 10% fluorescein sodium solution is infused into the vein quickly as bolus. Simultaneously the videotimer is started, and the video picture is recorded. Fluorescein flow into the retinal vessels is registered after 10–15 s, and the picture of the flow is recorded until the beginning of the wash-out phase. This takes about 30 s. Afterwards, the recording of the video fluorescein angiogram is interrupted. Only after 2–3 min, the recording of the fundus is resumed. These late images provide particularly good insight into the vascular morphology. The patient does not notice the injection due to the already inserted catheter. Indisposition rarely occurs. Occasionally – less often than 1/10 000 – circulatory collapse occurs. For emergency cases a bed and an emergency bag for shock treatment are beside the camera for angiography. The discomfort to the patient by the light is many times less than by fundus photos and photoangiograms.

The video fluorescein angiograms are analyzed densitometrically by the picture-analyzing system Microvideomat 3. The change in light intensity brought about by the influx of a fluorescent indicator into the retinal vessels is registered at several points. Data are obtained for each video frame. Intensity curves, so-called dilution curves, are obtained by plotting these data against the time axis (Fig. 93).

Typically, one measuring area is positioned on a retinal arteriole at the margin of pupil, a second on the same vessel distant from the pupil, and a third on the corresponding venule. During recording, the measuring areas must keep their normal position in relation to the retina. The fast involuntary eye movements of the patients are highly problematic in the drawing up of indicator-dilution curves by means of the videoanalyzer. The influx of fluorescein not only leads to the appearance of fluorescence inside the retinal vessels but is also associated with a change in the background light by filling the choroid layer. Therefore, an alteration in the position of the measuring areas in relation to the retina leads to false data. To avoid this pitfall a reference area with constant size and shape is defined on the electronic image of the retina. The reference area is composed of all picture points which appear brighter than any other adjustable gray value. Due to the used combination of exciter and barrier filter the optic disk with its physiologic excavation is mostly the brightest point of the fundus picture. During the influx of fluorescein there is no change in brightness of this excavation, and the fluorescence of the retinal vessels is usually weaker than the reflected light on the pupil. For this reason, the excavation of the pupil is generally chosen as reference area. The origin of the coordinate system is put into its center of gravity, to which all further measurings of fluorescence refer. The position of the measuring areas is kept constant in this coordinate system. If the reference area moves on the video picture, the measuring areas are carried along.

The appearance of fluorescein in a vessel is characterized by a rise in the dilution curve (Fig. 93). Following an indistinct maximum, the intensity slowly decreases. The initial value is not reached even after a longer period of time. This

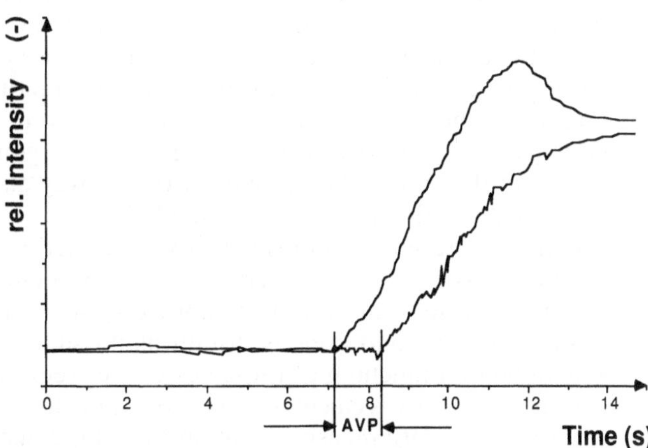


**Fig. 93.** Dye intensity curve after administration of sodium fluorescein

is due to the recirculation of dye and the deposition of sodium fluorescein in the vessel walls. By the extravasation of small amounts of dye through the vessels of the choroidea the contrast between fluorescence of the retinal vessels and the fundus is additionally diminished.

The dilution curves show various characteristics that can be used for evaluation: the rise, the maximum, and the more or less well pronounced decrease in dye registered over the measuring area. The course of the dilution curve depends on several factors such as the duration of the injection, individual vascular condition of the patient, arterial and venous blood pressure, cardiac output, and resistance in the pulmonary system. Therefore, the slope of the dilution curve is somewhat variable and not characteristic of retinal circulation. The same applies to the points of inflection, which were assessed by Körber and collaborators [208] in their first video-fluorescence angiograms. They also show a range of variation that is too great. Since the maxima of the dilution curves cannot be defined exactly, the can not be used for the assessment of retinal circulation times. Therefore, the most appropriate parameter is the initial rise in the dilution curve, i.e., the instant at which fluorescein is detected in the vessels for the first time. These parameters are reliably reproducible. With these experiences minimal transit times are assessed. They are defined as the period of time between the appearance of dye at two points separated by a defined distance.

According to the position of the measuring points, the following parameters are estimated.

1. The *arm-retina time* is the period between the injection of dye into the antecubital vein and its first appearance in the retinal arteries. It allows a rough estimation of the macrocirculation. A measuring area is positioned on a retinal artery next to the rim of the optic disk. The first measurable rise in intensity in this measuring area defines the time of influx of the indicator into the retinal vessel [399].
2. The *arteriovenous passage time* is defined as the interval between the first influx of fluorescein into a retinal artery and its appearance in the corresponding retinal vein. It is the shortest circulation time of the indicator through a corresponding area of retinal microcirculation. The measurement is made by focusing one measuring area on an artery and a second one on the corresponding vein. The time difference between the first intensity rise in the artery and the first rise in the corresponding vein represents the arteriovenous passage time. Both measuring areas are generally positioned on the vessels at the rim of the optic disk. In this way also retinal vessels in other areas of the retina can be examined [399].
3. The mean arterial dye-bolus velocity is defined as the mean velocity of the dye bolus inside a retinal artery. The measurement is performed by focusing on an artery near the rim of the optic disk with one measuring area and by positioning a second area as distant as possible on the same artery. There should be no branching of these vessels between the two measuring points. The mean velocity is calculated from the time difference ($\delta t$) between the rise in intensity at both measurement areas and the distance (s) between the two points. A velocity profile according to a newtonian fluid is assumed. The

arterial mean dye bolus velocity is thus calculated as: MDV = v = s/2 × δt) [399].

The distance between the two measuring points is determined on the monitor and multiplied by a magnification factor calculated for the emmetropic eye. The curve of the fundus is neglected. According to Littmann [240], an error of about 5% results; this error is in a justifiable order of magnitude. Parameters and measurement methods are presented in Table 78.

**Table 78.** Parameters and methods of measurement for blood flow parameters

| Parameter | Symbol | Method | Reference range |
|---|---|---|---|
| E velocity (art.) | v | Videomicroscopy | 0.39–0.81 mm/s |
| Reactive hyperemia | DrH | Videomicroscopy | > 180 s |
| Blood flow (com. carot. a.) | Bfcca | MAVIS | 210–280 ml/min |
| Arm-retina time | ART | Video fluorescence ang. | 4.6–17.8 s |
| AV passage time | AVP | Video fluorescence ang. | 0.7–2.2 s |
| Mean dye velocity | MDV | Video fluorescence ang. | 3–9.8 mm/s |

## 5.6 Laser Doppler Flux

In the following the laser Doppler technique is described used for the skin blood flow determination in four areas of the back of the foot. The Periflux system [363] (Perimed) is used as measuring system. A 2 mW helium-neon laser (wavelength 632.8 nm) with an optical light guide and a probe holder to establish a firm distance between light guide and skin surface is used as light source. The light intensity on the skin surface is about 1 mW/mm$^2$ so that measurements for long periods are possible without spoiling the patient [368].

As soon as the beam leaves the light guide it diverges. Therefore the intensity decreases rapidly with increasing distance so that the measurement can also be performed without danger at the human eye. A part of the reflected light strikes the surface of two photodetectors (UDT 450, United Detector Technology) or the light feed pipe lying in front of it. The area of these light guides is 1 mm$^2$. The received light signal consists of two parts; one Doppler-shifted – by reflection at moved particles – and one non-frequency-shifted originating from reflection at resting layers. On the whole the signal is composed of a direct stress part, a component of a basic frequency and a component with an overlying frequency. The direct stress part is proportional to the light intensity striking the photodetector. The homodyne term contains only components with Doppler-shifted frequencies whereas the heterodyne component consists of a mixture of Doppler-shifted and non-Doppler-shifted signals. The homodyne part of the signal is now neglected with regard to the heterodyne part. This is permissible as long as the hematocrit or particle count in the measuring area is not too great.

**Table 79.** Parameter and method of measurement for laser Doppler flux

| Parameter | Symbol | Method | Reference range | |
|---|---|---|---|---|
| Laser Doppler flux | LDF | Laser Doppler | 20–46 | PU |

The manufacturer therefore indicates that no measurement can be performed in dilated vessels or at the lip.

The initial signal of photodetectors consists of a small alternating current signal (RMS 2–5 mV) overlaid by direct stress (2–5 V). The signals are filtrated by a tape pass (75–15 000 Hz) and normalized to compensate variations of the light intensity of the transmitter, the optical conduction of the light guides, and the qualities of the photodetectors. The signal of the differential amplifier is conducted through a filter network with an overlying function H(f) and a Butterworth deep-pass with a borderline frequency of f=15 kHz. To maintain a continuous initial signal the measuring signal is squared and meaned, and the disturbing signal is suppressed. After passing the deep-pass the signal is led to an indicator instrument on a recording instrument. This writer signal corresponds to the mean flow of the red cells multiplied by the accompanying cell count. The measurements are performed as follows:

15 min before the measurement the apparatus is switched on to obtain a sufficient stability of the measurement. The temperable laser holder is fixed to the skin area concerned by means of double-sided adhesive tape; according to Ranft et al. [298] it is measured at a heating temperature of 44°C. Due to its geometry distance between skin and laser probe head is guaranteed by this laser holder after inserting the laser probe head. After a 3-min period of rest – to exclude possible effects by manual manipulation or microcirculatory caused by temperature – the measurement is performed, or the initial signal registered by the recording instrument is indicated as usable measuring signal. The method of measurement is automated so that immediately after finishing the measurement the results are available as a curve. Ranft et al. [298] indicate for the flow figure a range of 20–46 PU (10 PU = 1 V) as reference for adults.

## 5.7 Oxygen Transport Capacity

### 5.7.1 Macrocirculation

The oxygen transport capacity (OTC) in the sytem of the great vessels is determined as the product of blood flow (BF) and oxygen content ($CaO_2$:

$$OTC = BF \times CaO_2 \text{ ml } (O_2/s) \tag{1}$$

where: $CaO_2 = CaO_2\text{chem} + CaO_2\text{ phys}$

$$CaO_2 = SO_2 \times Hb \times 1.34 + (\alpha \times 100/760) \times pO_2 \text{ (ml } O_2\text{/100 ml blood)} \tag{2}$$

$SO_2$: oxygen saturation (guide nomogram)
Hb: cyanogen methemoglobin method (finger pad; EDTA blood; g/dl)
1.34: Hüfner's figure for $O_2$-binding capacity (ml $O_2$/g Hb)
$\alpha$: Bunsen's solubility coefficient (0.02356 for $O_2$)
$pO_2$: arterial oxygen partial pressure (lobe of the ear mmHg)
BF: arterial blood flow (ml blood/s)

The arterial oxygen content consists of the chemically bound and the physically saturated share of oxygen. By Eq. 2 one also determines the hemoglobin concentration of blood (withdrawal of blood from the finger pad under defined conditions [112] yields a value almost identical with the arterial hemoglobin concentration), the oxygen saturation (determined by means of the guide nomogram: from the pH concentration, the arterial oxygen partial pressure, and temperature [268]) and the arterial oxygen partial pressure. The arterial pH and $pO_2$ values are determined by means of the Astrup method [14] from blood samples withdrawn from the hyperemized lobe of the ear [268]. The oxygen binding capacity of hemoglobin is taken as 1.34 ml $O_2$ per gram hemoglobin, according to Hüfner [143], and not as the stoichiometrically calculated figure of 1.39 ml $O_2$ per gram hemoglobin. The oxygen content calculated in this way differs by about 0.3% by volume from that measured for Hb values from 10–18 g/dl and is within the range of error of the methods [378]. Therefore, a very small relative error, which must also be within the range of error of the methods, can be assumed with regard to the oxygen transport capacity, which is calculated by the measured blood flows and the oxygen content determined as described above. Analysis of variance on this calculated parameter revealed a relative error of about 5%.

### 5.7.2 Microcirculation (Nutritive Main Capillaries)

The oxygen transport capacity in the area of the microcirculation ist not easy to determine. The problem lies in the quantification of the oxygen content of the capillary blood, which is calculated by the same equations as for the macrocirculation However, by Eq. 2 the hemoglobin value in the capillaries must be determined first. For this purpose, capillary hematocrit is estimated and used for the calculation of the capillary hemoglobin concentration. Capillary hematocrit is determined using light microscope and computer; the procedure is described in the following section. Analysis of variance on this calculated parameter revealed a relative error of about 7%.

## 5.8 Capillary Hematocrit

An absolute determination of capillary is not possible by optical procedures [57]. However, it is possible to quantify the influence of hemodilution on capillary hematocrit as change with regard to the initial value. This procedure is based on measurement of the optical density of capillaries on the video and the quantification of the erythrocyte column diameter and lengths or frequency of plasma gaps [159].

Since the lighting of capillaries is done with a wavelength in the range of the hemoglobin absorption, the capillaries filled with cells appear dark on the video monitor. The more densely the capillaries are filled with blood cells, the more darker (compared to the surrounding tissue in which no absorption ensues) the capillaries appear. Therefore it is possible to deduce from a change in the optical density to a change in the hematocrit in the capillaries.

Furthermore, the capillary hematocrit is determined mainly by the diameter of the erythrocyte column and then by length and frequency of plasma gaps. This can be also determined by means of the computer [159].

*Optical Measurement of Density.* To eliminate the influence of fluctuations of the reflected light (e.g., by slightest movements of the finger, changes in lighting, changes in focusing the capillaries on the optical density of capillaries, the optical density of the tissue directly situated beside the capillary is also quantified and the difference between these two values estimated as optical differential density. The procedure is illustrated in Fig. 94. By the differential density it can be estimated whether the packing density of the cell column in a

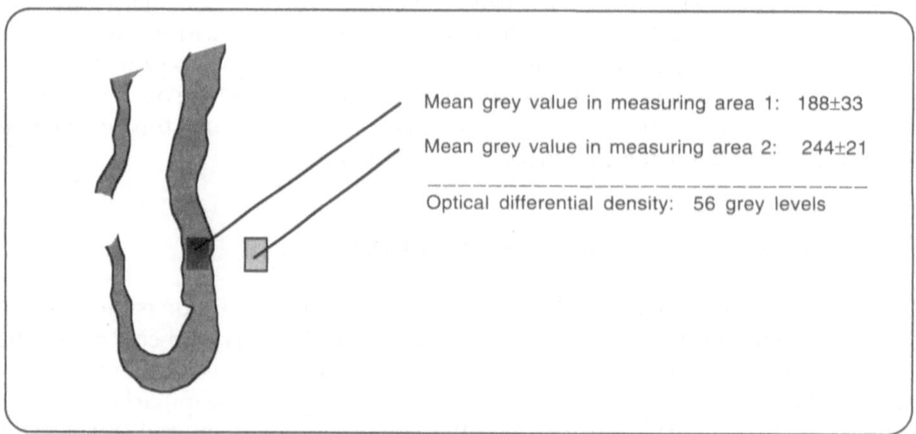


**Fig. 94.** Scheme for determining the optical differential density

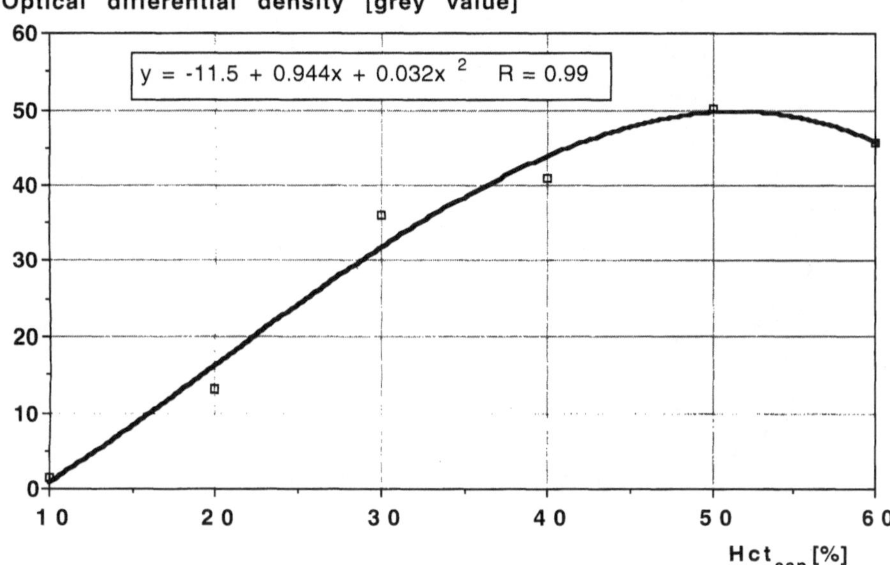


**Fig. 95.** Dependence of optical differential density on capillary hematocrit

capillary has changed by hemodilution. Figure 95 shows the dependence of the optical differential density on the capillary hematocrit. In wide ranges (10<Hct<40) there is a linear proportional dependence of the optical differential density on the predetermined cell density; after a maximum at 50% it decreases again.

*Erythrocyte Column Diameter.* To quantify the erythrocyte column diameter well focused, vertically running capillaries in the middle of the picture are chosen. Determinations of the diameter are performed 50 μm distal to the parietal capillary, if possible, over a length of 100 μm. The measurement is carried out interactively to ensure that the measurement is performed only in a well focused vascular area (without plasma gaps), and that distortions (e.g., by drops of perspiration or contortions of the capillaries from the depth of focus) are excluded. Figure 96 shows the area of measurement. To determine the diameter a line histogram over a picture line is first made. This graph is smoothed with a median filter (over three pixels). Then the course of the curve is differentiated, and the local coordinates of maximum and minimum are determined in the curve of gradients. The distance between maximum and minimum is indicated as erythrocyte column diameter in micrometers over the known magnification. Since the erythrocyte column is not strictly cylindrical but marginated by chance, this procedure is repeated in at least 50 picture lines, and a mean value for the erythrocyte column diameter is determined from the 50 measurements. Before the analysis one checks whether an image depth of at least 30 gray levels exists; only in this case is an analysis carried out. Otherwise, another image with a greater contrast is chosen.

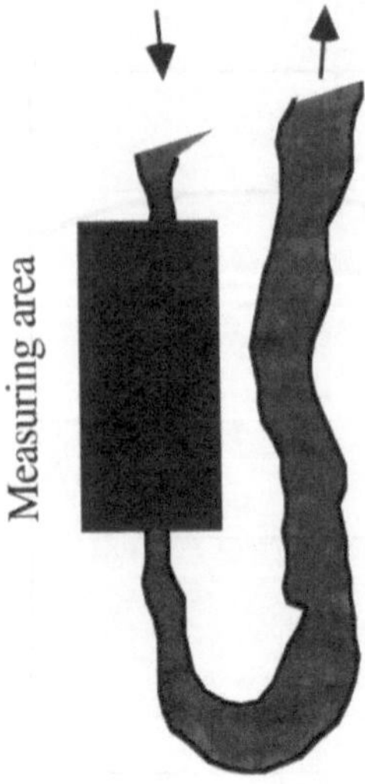


**Fig. 96.** Area of diameter determination

*Plasma Gap Quantification.* On the digitalized picture a central line is laid through the capillary, and the distribution of gray values is recorded over the picture points along the central line (Fig. 97). A gray value of 0 corresponds to the color black and a gray value of 255 to the color white. Therefore the plasma gaps in the gray value distribution appear as high values; the width of this peak corresponds with the length of the plasma gap. While the optical differential density and the plasma gaps can be quantified quite precisely, the measurement of the erythrocyte column diameters – if a U-Matic video recorder an objective with numerical aperture of 0.20 is used – is indicated by a clear inaccuracy. Under these conditions the resolution is 2.52 μm on measurement in horizontal direction, the error (on measurements of lengths about 10 μm) is 6% with a coefficient of variation of 6.1% [162]. With better resolution (which is technically possible today by the use of digital mass recorders instead of a video recorder) differences in erythrocyte column diameters may be determined which now become lost within the range of the error. Since the erythrocyte column

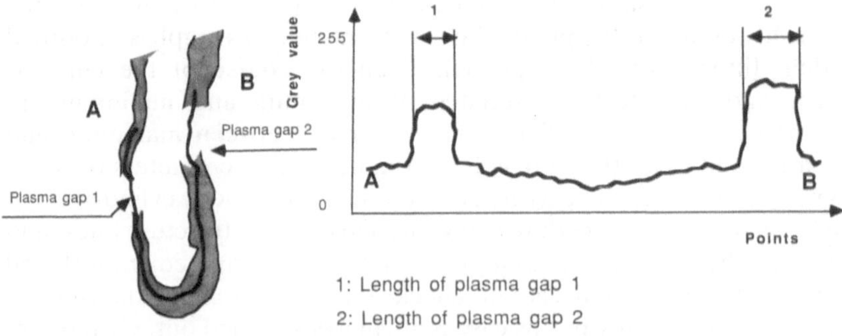


**Fig. 97.** Quantification of plasma gaps

diameter is of considerable importance for the determination of capillary hematocrit, this must be taken into consideration with respect to the results presented here.

*Calculation.* To analyze capillary hematocrits in each subject 60 sharply focused video images per measuring time are recorded by the computer (IBAS I–II; Zeiss), digitalized, and stored. These pictures are chosen every time after the same time pattern. In Chap. 3 these times are: before (–1 h), 1, 3, 6, and 24 h after hemodilution. After analyzing the 60 video images a mean plasma gap length is calculated [159]. Knowing the optical differential density of the cell column and the mean plasma gap length, the hematocrit value after hemodilution can be determined. Capillary hematocrit at the beginning of hemodilution is estimated to Liposky [238]. (After this estimation the capillary hematocrit is 33% of the systemic hematocrit value.) By means of this estimated value capillary hematocrit after hemodilution is calculated according to Klitzman and Duling [202]. This calculation is possible since the packing density of the red blood cells in the capillaries is not changed by hemodilution (see Figs. 74, 75). This procedure is presented step-by-step in the following.

1. Estimation of the initial value from the systemic hematocrit before hemodilution (–h) according to Lipowsky [238].
2. On this value a mean cell count/capillary can be calculated according to Klitzman and Duling [202]:

   $$n_{before} = Hct_{cap} \times \pi \times r^2 \times l \,/\, V_E$$

   $n_{before}$: erythrocyte count before hemodilution (–)
   $Hct_{cap}$: capillary hematocrit (%)
   r: erythrocyte column radius (μm)
   l : erythrocyte column length (μm)
   $V_E$: erythrocyte volume (corresponds to the MCV; $mm^3$)

   The standardization on the capillary length yields a mean erythrocyte count per micrometer capillary (Cm).
3. After hemodilution (1, 3, 6, and 24 h after infusion; Sect. 4.1) the count of the missing erythrocyte ($n_{Pl}$) is calculated by the plasma gap difference: mean length of the plasma gap before hemodilution ($Pl_b$ minus mean length after hemodilution ($Pl_a$):

   $$n_{Pl} = (Pl_a - Pl_b) \times C_m$$
4. The count of red blood cells in the capillary after hemodilution ($n_{after}$) and the capillary hematocrit after hemodilution are now determined by:

   $$n_{after} = n_{before} - n_{Pl}$$
   $$Hct_{cap} = n_{after} \times V_E \,/\, (\pi \times r^2\, l)$$
5. The corresponding capillary hemoglobin value is calculated from capillary hematocrit and the simultaneously measured mean corpuscular hemoglobin concentration (MCHC):

   $$Hb_{cap} = Hct_{cap} \times MCHC$$

All other parameters for the determination of the capillary oxygen transport capacity of the microcirculation are available so that it can be calculated by Eqs. 1 and (see Sect. 5.7).

# References


1. Adam W, Schulz J, Kratt E, Nitsche HJ, Kubanek B: Elektronische Zählung von Thrombozyten aus dem Vollblut. Blut 32: 347–352 (1976)
2. Admani AK: New approach to treatment of recent stroke. Br Med J 2: 1678–1679 (1978)
3. Albegger K, Schneeberger R, Franke V, Oberascher G, Miller K: Juckreiz nach Therapie mit Hydroxyäthylstärke (HES) bei otoneurologischen Erkrankungen. Therapiewoche, in press (1991)
4. Alström T, Gräsbeck R, Hjelm M, Skandsen S: Recommendations concerning the collection of reference values in clinical chemistry and activity report. Scand J Clin Lab Invest 35: 1–43 (1975)
5. Angelkort B, Kiesewetter H: Influence of risk factors and coagulation phenomena on the fluidity of blood in chronic arterial occlusive disease. Scand J Clin Lab Invest 41, Suppl 156: 185–188 (1981)
6. Angelkort B, Pirnay D, Kiesewetter H, Maurin N: Hemodilution and pentoxifyllin effects on muscle blood flow and blood fluidity in chronic arterial occlusive disease. Vascular Med 1/3: 150–158 (1983)
7. Arruda AL, Kurtzman NA: Relationship of renal sodium and water transport to hydrogen ion secretion. Ann Rev Physiol 40: 43–66 (1978)
8. Arzneimittel-Schnellinformationen des BGA: Juckreiz nach Infusion von Hydroxyäthylstärke (HES), Pharm Ind 52, Nr. 6 (1990)
9. Asplund K: Randomized trial of hemodilution in acute ischemic stroke. Acta Neurol Scand Suppl 127: 22–30 (1989)
10. Asplund K: Eriksson S, Hägg E: Multicenter trial of hemodilution in acute ischemic stroke. Acta Neurol Scand 73: 530–538 (1986)
11. Asskali F: Einfluß von Substitution und Molekulargewicht auf die Pharmakokinetik von Hydroxyäthylstärke. In: Peter K, Schimetta W, Bergmann H, Gerlach E, Meßmer K, Steinbereithner K, (eds). Hydroxyäthylstärke (HES), aktuelle Theorie und Praxis. Beiträge zur Anaesthesiologie und Intensivmedizin 26, Verlag Wilhelm Maudrich, Vienna, pp: 43–53 (1988)
12. Van Assche FA, Robertson WB, Renaer M: Fetal Growth retardation. Churchill Livingstone, Edinburgh (1981)
13. Astrup P, Engel K, Severinghaus J, Munsen E: The influence of temperature and pH on the dissociation curve of oxyhemoglobin of human blood. Scand J Clin Lab Invest 17: 515–525 (1965)
14. Astrup P, Schröder S: Apparatus for anaerobic determination of the pH of blood at 38 degree centigrade. Scand J Lab Invest 8: 30–36 (1956)
15. Astrup P, Siesjö BK, Symon L: Thresholds in cerebral ischemia – the ischemic penumbra. Stroke 12: 723–725 (1981)
16. Back T, Von Kummer R: Blutverdünnung bei zerebraler Ischämie. Dtsch Med Wschr 114: 350–356 (1989)
17. Banks W, Greenwood CT, Muir DD: Studies on hydroxyethyl starch. Stärke 24: 181–188 (1972)
18. Banks W, Greenwood CT, Muir DD: The structure of hydroxyethyl starch. Br J Pharmacol 47: 172–177 (1973)
19. Barman TE: Enzyme handbook. Springer, Berlin Heidelberg New York (1974)

20. Bates RG: Determiniation of pH. Theory and practice. Wiley, New York, pp: 61–75 (1973)
21. Bauer J (1870): Geschichte der Aderlässe. Munich 1870. (Fritsch Verlag, Munich 1966)
22. Bela U: Untersuchungen zur Bestimmung der Sauerstoffsättigung und der Sauerstoffaffinität des Hämoglobins. Dissertationsschrift, Universität Hamburg (1975)
23. Becsi C, Wehofer D, Weidinger P.: Hämodilution bei peripherer AVK. VASA Supplement 26: 113–115 (1988)
24. Bessmann JD, Johnson RK: Erythrocyte volume distribution in normal and abnormal subjects. Blood 46: 369–375 (1975)
25. BGA; Arzneimittel-Schnellinformationen: Juckreiz nach Infusion von Hydroxyäthylstärke (HES), Pharm Ind 52: Nr 6 (1990)
26. Bloom WL, Harmer DS, Bryant MF, Brewer SS: Coating of vascular surface and cells – a new concept on the prevention of intravsacular thrombosis. Proc Soc Exp Biol (N.Y.) 115: 384–389 (1964)
27. Boehringer Mannheim GmbH: Test-Fibel, Grundlagen und Praxis. Boehringer Mannheim (1976)
28. Böhme H: Hämodilution und Defibrinogenierung zur Behandlung der peripheren arteriellen Verschlußkrankheit. In: Neuere klinische Aspekte zur Hämodilution. L Heilmann, M Beez (eds) Schattauer, Stuttgart, pp: 137–142 (1987)
29. Böhme H, Bulik I: Zur Indikation der Hämodilution bei peripherer arterieller Verschlußkrankheit mit gleichzeitigem Vorliegen einer koronaren Herzkrankheit. Natur und Ganzheitsmedizin 4: 8–13 (1990)
30. Böttiger L, Carlson L: Risk factors for death for males and females. Acta Med Scand 211: 437–442 (1982)
31. Bogousslavski J, Regli F: Unilateral watershed cerebral infarcts. Neurology 36: 373–377 (1986)
32. Bollinger A, Simon HJ, Köhler R, Lüthy E: Wirkung von niedermolekularem Dextran auf Blutviskosität und Extremitätendurchblutung. Z Kreisl-Forsch 57: 456–464 (1968)
33. Bousser MG: "Aicla" Controlled trial of aspirin and dipyridamole in the secondery prevention of athero-thrombotic cerebral ischemia. Stroke 14: 5–14 (1983)
34. Breddin K, Grun H, Krzywanek HJ, Schremmer MM: On the measurement of spontaneous platelet aggregation. The platelet aggregation. Art III. Methods and first clinical results. Thromb Haemost 48: 261–272 (1975)
35. Bull BS, Brecher G, Schneidermann M: Platelet counts with the Coulter counter. Am J Clin Path 44: 678–688 (1965)
36. Canadian Cooperative Study Group: A randomized trial of aspirin and sulfinpyrazone in threatened stroke. N Engl J Med 299: 53–59 (1978)
37. Caplan LR: Are terms such as completed stroke or Rind of continued usefulness? Stroke 14: 431–433 (1983)
38. Carter C; Mcgee D; Reed D; Yano K, Stemmermann G: Hematocrit and the risk of coronary heart disease: the Honolulu heart program. Am Heart J 105: 674–679 (1983)
39. Cerebral Embolism Task Force: Cardiogenic Brain Embolism. Arch Neurol 43: 71–84 (1986)
40. Chien S, Jan KM: Ultrastructural basis of the mechanism of rouleaux formation. Microvasc Res 55: 155–166 (1973)
41. Crowell JW: Determinant of the optimal hematocrit. J Appl Physiol 22: 501–504 (1967)
42. Czok R, Lamprecht W: In: Bergmeyer HU (ed). Methoden der enzymatischen Analyse. Verlag Chemie, Weinheim, pp: 1491–1496 (1974)
43. Damon L, Adams M, Stricker RB, Ries C: Intracranial bleeding during treatment with hydroxyethyl starch. New Engl J Med 317 (15): 965–966 (1987)
44. Diehm C: Bei Störungen der peripheren Durchblutung: häufige Fehldiagnosen. Dt. Ärztebl 87 28/29: 1578–1582 (1990)

45. Dienes HP, Gerharz CD, Wagner R, Weber M, John HD: Accumulation of hydroxyethyl starch (HES) in the liver of patients with renal failure and portal hypertension. J Hepatol 3: 223–228 (1986)
46. Ditzel J; Bang HC; Thorsen N: The effect of dextran 40 on hemorheological factors during the course of acute myocardial infarction. Bibl Anat 10: 132 (1969)
47. Doumas BT, Bayse DD, Carter RJ, Peters JR, T, Schaffer R: A candidate reference method for determination of total protein in serum. I. Development and validation. II. Test for transferability. Clin Chem 27: 1642–1651 (1981)
48. Ehrly AM: Allgemeiner Überblick zur Hämodilution. In: L Heilmann, M Beez (eds). Neuere klinische Aspekte zur Hämodilution. Schattauer, Stuttgart, pp: 3–13 (1987)
49. Ehrly AM, Mann E, Saeger-Lorenz K, Wodniok M: Einfluß einer Saluretika-Kombination (Bemetizid-Triamteren) in verschiedener Dosierung auf die Fließeigenschaften des Blutes bei Patienten mit arterieller Hypertonie. Herz-Kreislauf 22: 22–27 (1990)
50. Eigner W-D: Low Angle Light Scattering. In: Satelle D, Lee W, Ware R (eds). Biomedical applications of laser light scattering. Elsevier, Amsterdam (1982)
51. Eigner W-D: Hydroxyäthylstärke. Krankenhauspharmazie 9: 20–22 (1988)
52. Eisele R, Birnbaum D, Büscher D, Kötter D, Nasseri M: Die unterschiedliche Kreislaufwirkung bei schneller Infusion von Hydroxyäthylstärke (HÄS), Dextran 60 und Blut beim postoperativen Patienten. Infusionstherapie 6: 43–49 (1979)
53. Elliger J: Experimentelle Untersuchung zur Elimination und Gewebespeicherung von mittel- und niedermolekularer Hydroxyäthylstärke ("Haes-steril" und "Expafusion"). Dissertationsschrift, Universität Frankfurt (1984)
54. Ernst E, Marshall M: Acetyl salicylic acid is rheologically inactive and hence an ideal reference medication for clinical trials in hemorheology. Clin Hemorrheol 4: 563–566 (1984)
55. Ernst E, Matrai A, Kollar L: Hämodilution bei der peripheren arteriellen Verschlußkrankheit: eine plazebokontrollierte Doppelblindstudie. Lancet 8548: 1449–1451 (1987)
56. Esps-Study Group: Europäische Studie zur Prävention des Schlaganfalls. Lancet (deutsche Ausgabe) II: 221–225 (1988)
57. Fagrell B, Intaglietta M, Östergren J: Relative hematocrit in human skin capillaries and its relation to capillary blood flow velocity. Microvasc Res 20: 327–335 (1980)
58. Fahraeus R: Die Strömungsverhältnisse und die Verteilung der Blutzellen im Gefäßsystem. Klin Wochenschr 7: 100–105 (1928)
59. Fahraeus R, Lindquist T: The viscosity of the blood in narrow capillary tubes. Am J Physiol 96: 562–567 (1931)
60. Fan F-J, Chen RYZ, Schuessler GB, Chien S: Effects of hematocrit variations on regional hemodynamics and oxygen transport in the dog. Am J Physiol 238: H 545–H 552 (1980)
61. Fatt I, Deutsch TA: The relation of conjunctival $pO_2$ to capillary bed $pO_2$. Critical Care Med 111 (1983)
62. Ferber H, Nitsch E, Förster H: Studies on hydroxyethyl-starch. Arzneim-Forsch / Drug Res 35 (Nr. 3): 615–622 (1985)
63. Fields G: Controlled trial of aspirin in cerebral ischemia. Stroke 8: 301–315 (1977)
64. Fish PJ, Wilson IM, Holt B: In: White P, Lyons EA. (eds.). Ultrasound in medicine. Plenum Press, London: 359–362 (1978)
65. Fisher CM: Lacunes, small deep cerebral infarcts. Neurology 15: 774–784 (1965)
66. Fleckenstein W, Heinrich R, Kersting T, Schomerus H, Weiss C: A new method for the bed-side recording of tissue $pO_2$-histograms. Verh Dtsch Ges Inn Med 90: 439–445 (1984)
67. Forst H, Fujita Y, Racenberg J, Brückner U, Weiss T, Sunder-Plassmann L, Messmer K: Skelettmuskeldurchblutung bei arterieller Verschlußkrankheit: Wirkung verschiedener Therapieverfahren. In: Meßmer, Hammersen: Die Mikrozirkulation des Skelettmuskels. Karger, Basel, pp: 119–135 (1983)
68. Förster H: In: Heilmann L, Ehrly AM. (eds.). Hämorheologie und operative Medizin. Münchner Wissenschaftliche Publikationen, Munich, pp: 118–134 (1987)

69. Förster H: Pharmakologie der Stärke: Verweildauer, Kinetik und mögliche klinische Folgerungen. Vortrag auf dem Workshop: Hydroxyäthylstärke (HÄS) – eine aktuelle Übersicht. St. Paul de Vence (1988)
70. Förster H: Biochemische Grundlagen zur Verwendung von polymeren Kohlenhydraten als Plasmaersatzmittel. In: Peter K, Schmimetta W, Bergmann H, Gerlach E, Meßmer K, Steinbereithner K. (eds.). Hydroxyäthylstärke (HES), Aktuelle Theorie und Praxis. Beiträge zur Anaesthesiologie und Intensivmedizin 26, Verlag Wilhelm Maudrich, Vienna, pp: 27–42 (1988)
71. Förster H, Wicarkzyk C, Dudziak R: Bestimmung der Plasmaelimination von Hydroxyäthylstärke und von Dextran mittels verbesserter analytischer Methode. Infusionstherapie 2: 88–94 (1981)
72. Gaehtgens P: Regulation of capillary haematocrit. Int J Microcirc: Clin Exp 3: 147–160 (1984)
73. Gallery EDM, Delprado AZ, Györy AZ: Antihypertensive effect of plasma volume expansion in pregnancy-associated hypertension. Austr N Zeal J Med 11: 20–24 (1981)
74. Gallery EDM, Hunyor SM, Györy AZ: Plasma volume contraction: a significant factor in both pregnancy associated hypertension (pre-eclampsie) and chronic hypertension in pregnancy. Q J Med 48: 593–602 (1979)
75. Gambino SR: Normal values for adult human venous plasma content. Am J Clin Pathol 32: 294–299 (1959)
76. Gard R: Dopplersonographie multilokulärer Verschlußprozesse der extra- und intracraniellen Arterien. Waderner Druck, Wadern/Saar (1990)
77. Garn SM, Ridella SA, Petzhold AS, Falkner F: Maternal hematologic levels and pregnancy outcomes. Sem Perinat 5: 155–162 (1981)
78. Gelmers HJ, Gorter K, De Weerdt CJ, Wiezer HJA: A controlled trial of nimodipine in acute ischemic stroke. New Engl J Med 4: 203–207 (1988)
79. Gelmers HJ, Krämer G, Hacke W, Hennerici M: Zerebrale Ischämien. Springer, Berlin Heidelberg New York: (1989)
80. Gelmers HJ: A controlled trial of nimodipine in acute ischemic stroke. N Engl J Med 318: 203–207 (1988)
81. Gilroy J, Barnhart MJ, Meyer JS: Treatment of acute stroke with dextran 40. J Am Med Assoc 210: 293 (1969)
82. Gleichmann U, Lübbers DW: Die Messung des Sauerstoffdruckes in Gasen und Flüssigkeiten mit der Platinelektrode unter besonderer Berücksichtigung der Messung im Blut. Pflügers Arch Ges Physiol 271: 431–444 (1960)
83. Gofferje H, Kozlik V: Zur Hyperamylasämie nach Infusion von Hydroxyäthylstärke unterschiedlicher Molekulargewichtsverteilungen. Infusionstherapie 4: 141–144 (1977)
84. Goller B, Schwab J, Schwab KO, Schramm A: Kreislaufstörungen beim alten Menschen. Z Geriatrie Rehab 2: 148–149 (1989)
85. Goslinga H: Viscosity reduction and rehydration by hemodilution with albumin and crystalloids may improve clinical outcome in stroke patients (The Amsterdam Stroke Study). In: Haaß A. (ed). Hemodilution in stroke. Springer, Berlin Heidelberg New York, in press (1991)
86. Goslinga H, Eijzenbach E, Schoute E, Weber JW, Vos J: Effects of normovolemic hemodilution using 20% albumin on rheological hemodynamic parameters and clinical outcome after acute ischemic stroke. Abstracts of the 6th European Conference Clinical Hemorheology 9: 471–472 (1989)
87. Gottstein U: Hemodilution therapy in acute ischemic stroke. In: Kriegelstein J (ed). Pharmacology of cerebral ischemia. Elsevier, Amsterdam, pp: 221–229(1986)
88. Gottstein U, Sedlmeyer J, Heuss A: Behandlung der akuten zerebralen Mangeldurchblutung mit niedermolekularem Dextran Dtsch Med Wschr 7: 223–227 (1976)
89. Gottstein U, Sedlmeyer J, Schöttler M, Gülk V: Der Effekt von niedermolekularem Dextran auf die Unterschenkeldurchblutung von gesunden und von Kranken mit peripheren arteriellen Zirkulationsstörungen. Dtsch Med Wschr 39: 1955 (1970)
90. Gross R: Wie hoch dosiert man Aspirin (ASS) ? Dt Ärztebl 87/24: 1409–1412 (1990)

91. Grotemeyer K-H; Viand R; Beykirch K: Thrombozytenfunktion bei vasomotorischen Kopfschmerzen und Migränekopfschmerzen. Dtsch Med Wschr 108: 775–778 (1983)
92. Grotemeyer K-H, Thrombozytenfunktion und zerebrale Ischämie. In: Grotemeyer K-H, Brune GG. (eds.) Hirninfarkt – Pathophysiologie, Diagnostik, Therapie und Prophylaxe. Arcis Verlag, pp: 21–25 (1988)
93. Groth C, Thorsen G: The effect of rheomacrodex and macrodex on factors governing the flow properties of the human blood. Acta Chir Scand 130: 507–512 (1965)
94. Grotta JC: Hypervolämic hemodilution treatment of acute stroke. Results of a Randomized Multicenter Trial Using Pentastarch. Stroke 20: 317–323 (1989)
95. Grotta JC, Lemak N, Gary H, Field WS, Vital D: Does platelet antiaggregant therapy lessen the severity of stroke? Neurology 35: 632–636 (1985)
96. Grundmann E: Spezielle Pathologie. Urban and Schwarzenberg, München (1986)
97. Haaß A: Hämodilutionsbehandlung bei zerebralen Durchblutungsstörungen. In: Kiesewetter H, Jung Fileds Konservative Behandlung peripherer und zentraler arterieller Durchblutungsstörungen. Ermer-Verlag, Homburg (Saar), pp: 85–94 (1987)
98. Haaß A: Hämorheologische Therapie. Stand und Perspektiven. Nervenarzt 60: 528–539 (1989)
99. Haaß A: Hämodilutionstherapie beim ischämischen Hirninfarkt: sinnvoll. Akt Neurol 16: 213–219 (1989)
100. Haaß A: Therapie des akuten ischämischen Insultes. Nervenheilkunde 8: 35–45 (1989)
101. Haaß A: Hämodilution mit mittelmolekularer Stärke zur Therapie des ischämischen Insultes, der Subarachnoidalblutung und intrazerebralen Blutung. Hämorheologische und gerinnungsphysiologische Probleme. In: Lawin P, Zander J, Weidler B, (eds). Hydroyäthylstärke: Eine aktuelle Übersicht - INA, vol 74. Thieme, Stuttgart, pp: 137–148 (1989)
102. Haaß A: Aggregationshemmung oder Antikoagulation bei zerebraler Ischämie. In: Weber MA (ed). Aggregationshemmung oder Antikoagulation. MMW 137–148 (1991)
103. Haaß A, Decker I, Hamann G, Stoll M, Schimrigk K, Kässer U: Hämodilutionsstudie bei akutem ischämischen Hirninfarkt. In: Ehrly AM (ed) Abstractband der 9. Jahrestagung der Deutschen Gesellschaft für klinische Mikrozirkulation und Hämorheologie, Würzburg 50 (1990)
104. Haaß A, Decker I, Hamann G, Stoll M, Schimrigk K, Kässer U: Hemodilution Therapy of Acute Stroke. A randomized double blind two center trial using hydroxyethyl starch (10% Hes 200/0,5). In: Haaß A. (ed.). Hemodilution in stroke. Springer, Berlin Heidelberg New York, in press (1991)
105. Haaß A, Jost C, Hamann G: Indikationen zur Hämodilution bei Subarachnoidalblutung und intrazerebraler Blutung. Klin Wochenschr 65: 989–1021 (1987)
106. Haaß A, Jung F: Haemodilution and oxygen transport capacity. Neurol 237: 126 (1990)
107. Haaß A, Kloss R, Brenner M, Hamann G, Schimrigk K: ICP-gesteuerte Hirnödembehandlung mit Glyzerin und Sorbit bei intrazerebralen Blutungen. Nervenarzt 58: 22–29 (1987)
108. Haaß A, Kroemer H, Jäger H, Müller K, Decker I, Wagner EM, Schimrigk K: Dextran 40 oder Haes 200/0,5 ? Dtsch Med Wschr 111: 1681–1686 (1986)
109. Haaß A, Kroemer H, Jäger H, Oest A, Schimrigk K: In: Hartmann A, Kuschinsky W. (eds.). Cerebral Ischemia and Hemorheology. Springer, Berlin Heidelberg New York pp: 488–495 (1987)
110. Haaß A, Treib J, Pindur G, Krack P, Wenzel E, Schimrigk K: Influence of hydroxyethylstarch substitution on rheology and coagulation. Abstractband der 30. Frühjahrstagung der Deutschen Gesellschaft für Pharmakologie und Toxikologie. Mainz R117 (1989)
111. Haaß A, Treib J, Stoll M: Hemorheological parameters of hydroxyethylstarch 200/0,62 as a basis for hemodilution. Br J Haematology, in press (1991)
112. Hallmann L: Klinische Chemie und Mikroskopie. Thieme, Stuttgart, pp: 2–6 (1980)

113. Hamann G, Haaß A, Pindur G, Wenzel E, Schimrigk K: Pro-urokinase therapy in stroke. In: Hacke W, Del Zoppo G. (eds.). Thrombolytic therapie in stroke. Springer, Berlin Heidelberg New York in press (1991)
114. Harrison MJG: Influence of haematocrit in the cerebral circulation. Cerebrovasc Brain Metabl Rev 1: 55–67 (1989)
115. Harrison MJG: Influence of haematocrit in the cerebral circulation. In: A. Haaß (ed) Hemodilution in stroke. Springer, Berlin Heidelberg New York (1991)
116. Harrison MJG, Pollock S, Kendall BE, Marshall J: Effect of haematocrit on carotid stenosis and cerebral infarction. Lancet 2: 114–115 (1981)
117. Harrison MJG, Pollock S, Thomas D, Marshall J: Haematocrit, hypertension and smoking in patients with transient ischaemic attacks and in age and sex matched controls. J Neurol Neurosurg Psychiat 45: 550–551 (1982)
118. Hartmann A, Tsuda Y: A controlled study on the effect of pentoxifylline and an ergot alkaloid derivate on regional cerebral blood flow in patients with chronic cerebrovascular disease. Angiology 39: 449–457 (1988)
119. Hayashi S, Nehls DG, Kieck CF, Vielma J, De Girolami U, Crowell RM: Beneficial effects of induced hypertension on experimental stroke in awake monkeys. J Neurosurg 60: 151–157 (1984)
120. Heidrich H, Boccalon H: Prinzipien kontrollierter klinischer Therapiestudien bei peripherer arterieller Verschlußkrankheit. Angio Archiv: 13 (1986)
121. Heilmann L, Hirsche H: Hämorheologische Untersuchungen zur Wirkung des Naftidrofuryls. Ergebnisse einer klinischen Doppelblindstudie. Med Welt 41: 273–276 (1990)
122. Heilmann L, Hojnacki B: Die Hämodilution als Therapieprinzip bei Risikoschwangerschaften. Gyne 11 (1990)
123. Heilmann L, Müntefering H: Hämodilution mit Hydroxyäthylstärke in der Schwangerschaft. Perinat Med vol XIII, Thieme, Stuttgart, in press (1990)
124. Heilmann L: Die Hämodilution – ein hämorheologisches Therapiekonzept in der Geburtshilfe. In: Dudenhausen JW, Saling E. (eds) Perinatale Medizin, XI. Thieme, Stuttgart, pp: 112–113 (1986)
125. Heilmann L: Blood rheology and pregnancy. Bailliere's Clin Haematol 1: 777–779 (1987)
126. Heilmann L: Hämodilution in der Schwangerschaft: Vergleich des niedermolekularen Dextran 10%ig und mittelmolekularer Hydroxyäthylstärke 10%ig. Perfusion 5: 1982–1986 (1989)
127. Heilmann L: Klinische Ergebnisse der Hämodilution mit Hydroxyäthylstärke in der Schwangerschaft. Z Geburtsh Perinat 193: 219–225 (1989)
128. Heilmann L: Thromboseprophylaxe beim Kaiserschnitt mit Hydroxyäthylstärke in der Schwangerschaft. Med Welt 40: 648–651 (1989)
129. Heilmann L: Hämodilutionstherapie in der Schwangerschaft. Gyn. Praxis 14: 465–470 (1990)
130. Heiss WD: Pharmakotherapie der zerebralen Mangeldurchblutung. Therapiewoche 27: 34–42 (1981)
131. Heiss WD: Ansatzpunkte zur Therapie zerebraler Durchblutungsstörungen. Dtsch Med Wschr 111: 186–191 (1985)
132. Heiss WD: Der ischämische Insult. Dt Ärztebl 86: B30–32 (1989)
133. Hermann J, Gall H: Diagnose und Therapie des persistierenden Pruritus nach Infusion von Hydroxyäthylstärke (HÄS). Akt Dermatol 16: 166–167 (1990)
134. Heros RC, Korosue K: Hemodilution for cerebral ischemia. Stroke 20: 423–427 (1989)
135. Herrschaft H: Die Wirksamkeit von Piracetam bei der akuten cerebralen Ischämie des Menschen. Med Klinik 83: 667–677 (1988)
136. Hoffmann U, Bollinger A: In: Kriessmann A. (ed.). Aktuelle Diagnostik und Therapie in der Angiologie. Thieme, Stuttgart, pp: 56–60 (1988)
137. Hollmann W, Hettinger T: Sportmedizin-Arbeits- und Trainingsgrundlagen. Schattauer, Stuttgart (1976)

138. Holthoff VA, Heiss WD, Pawlik G, Neveling M: Positron emission tomography in nimodipine treated patients with acute ischemic stroke. Second International Symposium on Nimodipine. Acute Indications, Miami Beach, Florida: 34 (1990)
139. Holtz J, Giesler M, Bassenge E: Two dilatatory mechanisms of anti-anginal-drugs on epicardial arteries in vivo: indirect flow-dependent endothelium-mediated dilatation and direct smooth muscle relaxation. Z Kardiol 72, Suppl 3: 98–106 (1983)
140. Hossmann KA, Schuier FJ: Experimental brain infarcts in cats. Stroke 11: 583–592 (1980)
141. Huch R, Huch A, Lübbers DW: Transcutaneous $pO_2$. Thieme-Stratton, New York (1981)
142. Hudak ML, Koehler RC, Rosenberg AA, Traystman RJ, Jones JR, MD: Effect of hematocrit on cerebral blood flow. Am J Physiol 251: H63–H70 (1986)
143. Hüfner G: Neue Versuche zur Bestimmung der Sauerstoffcapazität des Blutfarbstoffs. Arch Anat Physiol Jahresband 1894: 130–176 (1894)
144. Hultman E: Rapid specific method for determination of aldo-saccarides in blood. Nature 183: 108–112 (1959)
145. International commendations for standardization in hematology: Recommendations for a selected method for the measurement of plasma viscosity. J Clin Path 37: 1147–1152 (1984)
146. International committee for standardization in haematology: Guidelines for measurements of blood viscosity and erythrocyte deformability. Clin Hemorheology 6: 439–453 (1986)
147. Italian acute stroke study group: Haemodilution in aute stroke. Results of the Italian haemodilution trial. Lancet I: 318 (1988)
148. James TN: Pathology of small coronary arteries. Am J Cardiol, Vol. 20: 679–691 (1962)
149. Jesch F, Hübner G, Zumtobel V, Zimmermann M, Messmer K: Hydroxyäthylstärke (Häs 450/0,7) in Plasma und Leber. Konzentrationsverlauf und histologische Veränderungen beim Menschen. Infusionstherapie 6: 112–118 (1979)
150. Jesdinsky H, Trampisch H: Statistik und Biometrie. in Dölle, Müller-Derlinghausen, Schwabe. Grundlagen der Arzneimitteltherapie. Bibl Institut, Mannheim: 146–165 (1985)
151. Johansson G, Karlberg B, Wikby A: The hydrogen-ion selective glass electrode. Talanta 22: 953–966 (1975)
152. Jouppila P, Jouppila R, Koivula A: Albumin infusion does not alter the intervillous blood flow in severe preeclampsia. Acta Obstet Gynec Scand 62: 345–348 (1983)
153. Jung F: Neue Meßgeräte zur rheologischen Diagnostik und Therapie für Gefäß- und Kreislauferkrankungen. Dissertation an der RWTH Aachen (1985)
154. Jung F, Bock M, Heinrich R, Kiesewetter H, Krawzak B, Wenzel E: Intramuscular oxygen partial pressure in the tibialis anterior muscle of apparently healthy subjects. International $po_2$-Symposium, Frankfurt (1988)
155. Jung F, Kiesewetter H, Mrowietz C, Leipnitz G, Braun B, Wappler M, Scheffler P, Wenzel E: Hemorrheological, microand macrocirculatory effects of naftidrofuryl in an acute study: a randomized, placebo-controlled, double-blind individual comparison. Int J Pharmacol Ther Toxicol 25: 507–514 (1987)
156. Jung F, Kiesewetter H, Körber N, Wolf S, Reim M, Müller G: Quantification of characteristic blood-flow parameters in the vessels of the retina with a picture analysis system for video-fluorescence angiograms: initial findings. Graefes Arch Clin Exp Ophthalmol 211: 133–136 (1983)
157. Jung F, Kiesewetter H, Roggenkamp H, Nüttgens HP, Ringelstein B, Gerhards M, Kotitschke G, Wenzel E, Zeller H: Bestimmung der Referenzbereiche rheologischer Parameter: Studie an 653 zufällig ausgewählten Probanden im Kreis Aachen. Klin Wochenschr 64: 375–381 (1986)
158. Jung F, Koscielny J, Kolepke W, Kiesewetter H, Wenzel E: Einfluß einer iso- bzw. hypervolämischen Hämodilution auf die Fließfähigkeit des Blutes, die Sauerstofftransportkapazität in Makro- und Mikrostrombahn sowie die Gewebesauerstoffversorgung von Haut- und Skelettmuskulatur. In: Lawin P, Zander J, Weidler B, (eds) Hydroxyä-

thylstärke: Eine aktuelle Übersicht – INA, vol 74. Thieme, Stuttgart, pp: 91–115 (1989)

159. Jung F, Koscielny J, Mrowietz C, Wolf, Kiesewetter H, Wenzel E: Einfluß der Hämodilution auf den systemischen und den Kapillarhämatokrit. Infusionstherapie 17: 268–275 (1990)
160. Jung F, Roggenkamp HG, Mrowietz C, Seegert A, Kiesewetter H: In: Kiesewetter H, Ehrly AM, Jung F. (eds.). Hämorheologische Meßmethoden. Münch Wiss Publikationen, Munich: 113–116 (1985)
161. Jung F, Roggenkamp HG, Ringelstein E, Schmidt J, Kiesewetter H: Das Kapillarschlauch-Plasma-Viskosimeter: Methodik, Qualitätskontrolle und Referenzbereich. Biomed Tech 30: 152–158 (1985)
162. Jung F, Toonen H, Mrowietz C, Wolf S, Kiesewetter H, Wenzel E, Gersonde K, Müller G: Fehleranalyse, biologische Einflußfaktoren und Varianz der periungualen Videokapillarmikrospie. Biomed Technik 35, Heft 9: 195–204 (1990)
163. Jung F, Wappler M, Nüttgens HP, Kiesewetter H, Wolf S, Müller G: Zur Methodik der Videokapillaroskopie: Bestimmung geometrischer und dynamischer Größen. Biomed Tech 32: 204–213 (1987)
164. Junge B, Hoffmeister H, Fedderson HM, Röcker L: Standardisierung der Blutentnahme. Dtsch Med Wschr 103: 121–129 (1987)
165. Kannel WB, Castelli MD, Gordon T, Mcnamara PM: Serum cholesterol, lipoproteins and the risk of coronary heart disease. The Framingham study. Anal Intern Med 74: 1–12 (1971)
166. Kannel W, Gordon T, Wolf A, Mc Namara P: Hemoglobin and the risk of cerebral infarction: the Framingham Study. Stroke 3: 409–420 (1972)
167. Kannel W, Wolf A, Castelli WP, D'agostino RB: Fibrinogen and risk of cardiovascular disease. Jama 258: 1183–1186 (1987)
168. Kaste M, Folgenholm R, Waltimo O: Combined dexamethasone and low-molecular-weight dextran in acute brain infarction: double blind study. Br Med J 11: 1409–1410 (1976)
169. Katz PM, Ackermann RH, Alpert NM, Correia JA, Babikian VL, Burbank KM: The effects of hemodilution on cerebral blood flow and oxygen metabolism in ischemic stroke disease. Journal of Cerebral Blood Flow and Metabolism 7: 40 (1987)
170. Keller TS, Mc Gillicuddy JE, La Bond VA, Kindt GW: Modification of cerebral ischemia by cardiac output augmentation. J Surg Res 39: 420–432 (1985)
171. Kiesewetter H, Blume J, Birk A, Jung F: Hyper- oder isovolämische Hämodilution bei Patienten mit p-AVK II. Angio Archiv, in press (1991)
172. Kiesewetter H, Blume J, Jung F, Gerhards M, Leipnitz G: Gehtraining und medikamentöse Therapie bei der peripheren arteriellen Verschlußkrankheit. Dtsch Med Wschr 112: 873–878 (1987)
173. Kiesewetter H, Blume J, Jung F, Gerhards M, Spitzer S, Leipnitz G, Wenzel E: Beutelplasmapherese bei Patienten mit peripherer arterieller Verschlußkrankheit im Stadium IIb. Klin Wochenschr 66: 284–291 (1988)
174. Kiesewetter H, Blume J, Jung F, Radtke H, Bulling B, Gerhards M, Prünte C, Reim M: Hämorheologische Aspekte peripherer arterieller Verschlußkrankheit. Med Welt 35: 896–901 (1984)
175. Kiesewetter H, Blume J, Jung F, Spitzer S, Bach R, Birk A, Schieffer H, Wenzel E: Hämodilution bei multimorbiden Patienten mit peripherer arterieller Verschlußkrankheit. Schweiz Med Wsch 119: 1862–1867 (1990)
176. Kiesewetter H, Blume J, Jung F, Spitzer S, Gerhards M, Waldhausen P, Wenzel E: Iso- und hypervolämische Hämodilution mit Hydroxyäthylstärke (Hes 200/0,5 10%) an Patienten mit p-AVK IIb. WMW 17: 396–401 (1989)
177. Kiesewetter H, Blume J, Jung F, Spitzer, Wenzel E: Haemodilution with medium molecular weight hydroxyethyl starch in patients with peripheral arterial occlusive disease stage II b. J Intern Med 227: 107–114 (1990)
178. Kiesewetter H, Erlenwein S, Jung F, Wenzel E, Vogel W, Dyckmans J, Bach R, Hahmann H, Schieffer H, Bette L: Isovolämische Hämodilution bei Patienten mit koronarer Herzkrankheit. Klin Wochenschr 66: 8–14 (1988)

179. Kiesewetter H, Jung F: Kombination von physikalischer Therapie, Hämodilution und/oder eines Rheologikums bei Patienten mit peripherer arterieller Verschlußkrankheit. In: Heilmann L, Becz M Cechs. Neuere klinische Aspekte zur Hämodilution. Schattauer, Stuttgart, pp: 151–166 (1985)

180. Kiesewetter H, Jung F: Rheologische Therapie der peripheren arteriellen Verschlußkrankheit im Stadium IIb. Angio. 8/1: 21–31 (1986)

181. Kiesewetter H, Jung F: Durchblutungsstörungen. Hämatocrit als Risikofaktor, Hämodilution als mögliche Therapie. Arzneimitteltherapie 5: 151–162 (1987)

182. Kiesewetter H, Jung F: Hämodilution bei der peripheren arteriellen Verschlußkrankheit im Stadium II, Ergebnisse aus vier klinischen Studien. In: Heilmann L, Ehrly AM. (eds) Hämorheologie und operative Medizin. MWP: 143–152 (1988)

183. Kiesewetter H, Jung F: Rheologische Therapie bei der peripheren arteriellen Verschlußkrankheit. Angio 10/3: 109–115 (1988)

184. Kiesewetter H, Jung F: Hämodilution bei der peripheren arteriellen Verschlußkrankheit im Stadium II b nach Fontaine. CorVas 3: 78–84 (1989)

185. Kiesewetter H, Jung F, Blume J, Bulling B, Franke RP: Vergleichende Untersuchung von niedermolekularer Dextran- oder Hydroxyäthylstärkelösungen als Volumenersatzmittel bei Hämodilutionstherapie. Klin Wochenschr 64: 29–37 (1986)

186. Kiesewetter H, Jung F, Blume J, Gerhards M: Isovolämische Hämodilution bei peripherer arterieller Verschlußkrankheit im Stadium IIb. Deutsch Med Wschr 35: 1307–1312 (1986)

187. Kiesewetter H, Junge F, Blume J, Gerhards M: Hämodilution bei Patienten mit peripherer arterieller Verschlußkrankheit im Stadium II b: Prospektive randomisierter Doppelblind-Vergleich von mittelmolekularer Hydroxyäthylstärke und kleinmolekularer Dextranlösung. Klin Wochenschr 65: 324–330 (1987)

188. Kiesewetter H, Junge F, Ladwig, KH, Waterloh E, Roebruck P, Schneider R, Kotitschke, Bach R: Prädiktorfunktion hämorheologischer Parameter im Hinblick auf die Inzidenz manifester Durchblutungsstörungen: Konzept der Aachen-Studie. Klin Wochenschr 64: 653–662 (1986)

189. Kiesewetter H, Junge F, Lazar H, Roggenkamp HG, Leipnitz G, Kiehl R: Hematocrit as a risk factor for vascular disease. Klin Wochenschr 64: 974–978 (1986)

190. Kiesewetter H, Jung F, Roggenkamp HG: Einfluß der Fließfähigkeit des Blutes auf die Versorgung des Gewebes. In: Heilmann I, Kiesewetter H, Ernst E. (eds.) Klinische Rheologie und Beta-1-Blockade. Zuckschwerdt, Munich (1984)

191. Kiesewetter H, Jung F, Spitzer S, Wenzel E: Die Fließeigenschaften des Blutes und ihre klinische Bedeutung beim arteriellen Gefäßpatienten. Internist 30/7: 420–428 (1989)

192. Kiesewetter H, Jung F, Spitzer S, Wenzel E: Therapeutische Plasmapherese zur Steigerung der Fließfähigkeit des Blutes. Ztschr für Natur und Ganzheitsmedizin 32/3: 14–17 (1990)

193. Kiesewetter H, Jung F, Wenzel E: Hämorheologie. Münchn. Med Wschr 127: 113–114 (1985)

194. Kiesewetter H, Lazar H, Radkte H, Thielen W: Hämatocritbestimmung durch Impedanzmessung. Biomed Tech 27: 171–175 (1982)

195. Kiesewetter H, Radtke H, Jung F: Determination of yield point: methods and review. Biorheology 19: 363–374 (1982)

196. Kiesewetter H, Radtke H, Schneider R, Mussler K, Scheffler A, Schmid-Schönbein H: Das Mini-Erythrozyten-Aggregometer: Ein neues Gerät zur schnellen Quantifizierung des Ausmaßes der Erythrozytenaggregation. Biomed Techn 27: 209–213 (1982)

197. Kiesewetter H, Spitzer S, Jung F, Birk A, Waldhausen P, Bach R, Schieffer H, Wenzel E: Die Plasmaviksosität als neuer Risikofaktor in der Angiologie. Epidemiologische Daten der Aachen-Studie und das Ergebnis einer Studie zur Beutelplasmapherese bei erhöhter Plasmaviskosität. Natur Ganzheitsmedizin 30/4: 124–130 (1989)

198. Kiyohara Y, Fujishima M, Ishitsuka T, Tamaki K, Sadoshima S, Omae T: Effects of hematocrit on brain metabolism in experimentally induced cerebral ischemia in spontenously hypertensive rats (SHR). Stroke 16: 835–840 (1985)

199. Kiyohara Y, Ueda K, Hasuo Y, Fujii I, Yanai T, Wada J, Kawano H, Shikata T, Omae T, Fujishima M: Hematocrit as a ris factor of cerebral infarction: long-term prospective population survey in a Japanese rural community. Stroke 17: 687–692 (1986)
200. Kleine OT: Interferenz von Infusionslösungen mit der Biuretreaktion in einem vollmechanisierten und manuellen System. Med Welt 30: 102–107 (1979)
201. Kleinhauer E: Hämatologie. Springer, Berlin Heidelberg New York (1985)
202. Klitzman B, Duling BR: Microvascular hematocrit and red cell flow in resting and contracting striated muscle. Am J Physiol: 237 (1979)
203. Köhler H: Zur Pharmakokinetik von Häs. Habilitationsschrift, Universität Mainz (1977)
204. Köhler H, Kirch W, Horstmann HJ: Die Bildung hochmolekularer Komplexe aus Serumamylase und kolloidalen Plasmaersatzmitteln. Anaesthesist 26: 623–625 (1977)
205. Köhler H, Kirch W, Roloff B, Weihrauch TR, Prellwitz W, Höffler D: Beeinflussung der Serumamylase durch kolloidale Volumenersatzmittel. 82. Tagung der Deutschen Gesellschaft für Innere Medizin, Wiesbaden (1976)
206. Köhler H, Zschiedrich R, Clasen A, Linfante A, Gramm H: Blutvolumen, kolloidosmotischer Druck und Nierenfunktion von Probanden nach Infusion mittelmolekularer 10% Hydroxyäthylstärke 200/0,5 und 10% Dextran 40. Anaesthesist 31: 61–67 (1982)
207. Költringer P, Eber O: Hämorheologische Parameter und Mikrozirkulation. In: Hydroxyäthylstärke: therapeutische Hämodilution und Volumenersatz. Suppl 2. Wiener Schockgespräche (1988)
208. Körber N, Gesch M, Kiesewetter H, Reim M, Schmidschönbein, H.: Fernsehfluoreszenzangiographie der Retina. Neue technische Aspekte. Albrecht v. Graefes Arch Klin Exp Ophthal 213: 65–70 (1980)
209. Körber N, Gesch M, Kiesewetter H, Angelkort B: Effect of hemodilution on retinal blood flow – television fluorescein angiographic measurements. Clin Hemorheology (1981)
210. Körber N, Kiesewetter H, Jung F, Blume M, Gerhards M: Hydroxyäthylstärke-Lösung bei Patienten mit Fundus aterioskleroticus und Zerebralsklerose. Fort Med 103: 775–777 (1985)
211. Körber N, Nüsser D, Paulmann H, Wolf S: Erfahrungen mit einer hämorheologisch konzipierten Therapie bei arteriellen und venösen Gefäßprozessen der Retina. Med Welt 37: 1543–1546 (1987)
212. Koide T, Wieloch J, Siesjo BK: Chronic dexamethasone pretreatment aggravates ischemic brain damage by inducing hyperglycemia. J Cereb Blood Flow Metab 5 (Supplement 1): 251–252 (1985)
213. Koller M, Haenny P, Hess K, Weniger D, Zangger P: Adjusted hypervolamic hemodilution in acute ischemic stroke. Stroke 21: 1429–1434 (1990)
214. Korbmacher G, Ringelstein EB: Risk and benefit of anticoagulation in patients with acute hemispheric infarctions: preliminary results of a prospective study. In: Poeck K, Ringelstein EB, Hacke W. (eds) New trends in diagnosis and management of stroke. Springer, Berlin Heidelberg New York 1987
215. Korosue, Ishida K, Matsuoka H, Nagao T, Tamaki N, Matsumoto S: Clinical, hemodynamic and hemorheological effects of isovolemic hemodilution in acute cerebral infarction. Neurosurgery 23: 148–153 (1988)
216. Kraft D, Laubenthal H, Schimetta W, Scheiner O: Immunologische Aspekte der Hydroxyäthylstärke (HES) – Nebenwirkungen. In: Peter K, Schimetta W, Bergmann H, Gerlach E, Meßmer K, Steinbereithner K. (eds). Hydroxyäthylstärke (HES). Aktuelle Theorie und Praxis. Beiträge zur Anaesthesiologie und Intensivmedizin 26, Verlag Wilhelm Maudrich, Vienna: 57–62 (1988)
217. Kramer HJ: Bluthochdruck bei älteren Menschen. In: Grotemeyer KH Brune GG. (eds) Hirninfarkt. Pathophysiologie, Diagnostik, Therapie und Prophylaxe. Arcis Verlag: 26–30 (1988)
218. Krause D: Physikalische Therapie peripherer arterieller Durchblutungsstörungen im Stadium II nach Fontaine. Ther Ggw 11: 117 (1978)
219. Kreutz FH: In: Roka L (ed) Optimierung der Diagnostik. Springer, Berlin Heidelberg New York, pp: 149–163 (1972)

220. Kreyszig E: Statistische Methoden und ihre Anwendung. Vandenhoeck & Ruprecht Verlag, Göttingen (1979)
221. Kroemer H, Haaß A, Müller K, Jäger H, Wagner EM, Heimburg P, Klotz U: Haemodilution therapy in ischaemic stroke: plasma concentrations and plasma viscosity during long-term infusion of dextran 40 or hydroxyethyl starch 200/0,5. Eur J Clin Pharmacol. 31: 705–710 (1987)
222. Krogh A: Studies on the physiology of capillaries. II. The reactions of local stimuli of the blood-vessels in the skin and web of the frog. J Physiol 55: 412–422 (1921)
223. Von Kummer R: Hämodilution bei zerebraler Ischämie: Therapieversuch ohne gesichertes pathophysiologisches Konzept. Nervenarzt 60: 523–527 (1989)
224. Von Kummer R, Scharf J, Back T, Reich H, Machens G, Wildemann B: Autoregulatory capacity and the effect of isovolemic hemodilution on local cerebral blood flow. Stroke 19: 594–597 (1988)
225. Kühnle HF, Von Dahl K, Schmidt FH: Die Bestimmung von Lactat und ß-Hydroxybutyrat in kleinen Plasmamengen. J Clin Chem Clin Biochem. 15: 171 (1977)
226. Landgraf H, Ehrly AM: In: Heilmann L, Beez M. (eds.). Neuere klinische Aspekte zur Hämodilution. Schattauer, Stuttgart, pp: 115–124 (1987)
227. Landgraf H, Ehrly AM, Saeger-Lorenz K, Vogel C: Untersuchung über den Einfluß einer Infusion von mittelmolekularer Hydroxyäthylstärke (Haes-steril 10%) auf die Fließeigenschaften des Blutes gesunder Probanden. Infusionstherapie 4: 200–204 (1981)
228. Landgraf H, Ruppel C, Saeger-Lorenz K, Vogel C, Ehrly AM: Verbesserung der Fließfähigkeiten des Blutes von Patienten mit peripherer AVK durch niedermolekulare Hydroxyäthylstärke. Infusionstherapie 9: 202–206 (1982)
229. Landon J, Fawcett JK, Wynn V: Blood pyruvate concentration measured by a specific method in control subjects. J Clin Path 15: 579–584 (1962)
230. La Rue L, Alter M, Min Lai S, Friday G, Sobel E, Levitt L, Mc Coy R, Isack T: Acute stroke, hematocrit and blood pressure. Stroke 18: 565–569 (1987)
231. Laubenthal H: Anaphylaktoide/anaphylaktische Reaktionen bei Infusion kolloidaler Plasmaersatzlösungen. In: Peter K, Schimetta W, Bergmann H, Gerlach E, Meßmer K, Steinbereithner K. (eds). Hydroxyäthylstärke (HES), Aktuelle Theorie und Praxis. Beiträge zur Anaesthesiologie und Intensivmedizin 26, Verlag Wilhelm Maudrich, Vienna, pp: 63–73 (1988)
232. Laubenthal H, Peter K, Messmer K: Unverträglichkeitsreaktionen auf kolloidale Plasmaersatzlösungen. Anästh Intensivmed 23: 26–33 (1982)
233. Leonhardt H, Arntz HR: Zusammenhänge zwischen kariovaskulären Risikofaktoren und der Blutviskosität unter besonderer Berücksichtigung der Hyperlipoproteinämien. Rheol Acta 16: 368 (1977)
234. Leschke M, Motz W, Strauer BE: Hämorheologisch-therapeutische Anwendungsmöglichkeiten bei der koronaren Herzerkrankung. Wiener Med Wochenschr: 17–24 (1986)
235. Liley AW: Clinical and laboratory significance and variations in maternal plasma volume in pregnancy. Internat J Gynaec Obstet 8: 358–364 (1970)
236. Linkesch W: Physiologie und Pathophysiologie des Eisenstoffwechsels. Wiener Med Wochenschr 3/4: 59 (1984)
237. Lipowsky H: Determinations of microvascular blood flow. Physiologist 25: 357–363 (1982)
238. Lipowsky H, Firrell J: Microvascular hemodynamics during systemic hemodilution and hemoconcentration. The American Physiological Society, New York, H: 908–923 (1986)
239. List WF: Vergleichende Blutgasuntersuchungen von Kapillarblut aus Ohrläppchen und Finger mit arteriellem Blut unter Anwendung der Astrupmethode. Z Prakt Anästh Wiederbeleb 2: 345–355 (1967)
240. Littmann H: Zur Bestimmung der wahren Größe eines Objekts auf dem Hintergrund des gesunden Auges. Klin Mbl Augenheilk 180: 286–289 (1982)
241. Loew PG, Thews G: Die Altersabhängigkeit des arteriellen Sauerstoffdruckes bei der berufstätigen Bevölkerung. Klin Wochenschr 40: 1093–1100 (1962)

242. Löllgen H: Sauerstofftransport bei kritisch Kranken. Intensivmedizin im Dialog: 5–7 (1989)
243. Löllgen H, Ulmer HV: Ergometrie-Empfehlungen zur Durchführung und Bewertung ergometrischer Untersuchungen. Klin Wochenschr 63: 651–677 (1985)
244. Lowe GDO, Jaap AJ, Forbes CD: Relation of atrial fibrillation and high haematocrit to mortality in acute stroke. Lancet I: 784–786 (1983)
245. Lutz H: Plasmaersatzmittel. Thieme, Stuttgart (1986)
246. Lyden PD, Alving LI, Zivin JA, Rothrock JF: Hemodilution with low-molecular-weight hydroxyethyls starch after experimental focal cerebral ischemia in rabbits. Stroke 19: 223–227 (1988)
247. Maas AHJ, Veefkind AH, Van den Camp R, Teunissen AJ, Winckers EKA, Jansen AP: Evaluation of ampouled tonometered puffer solutions as quality control system for pH, $pCO_2$ and $pO_2$ measurements. J Clin Chem Clin Biochem 15: 174–180 (1977)
248. Macintyre E, Mackie I, HO D, Tinker J, Bullen C, Machin SJ: The haemostatic effects of hydroxyethyl starch (HES) used as a volume expander. Intensive Car Med 11: 300–303 (1985)
249. Marshall J: The role of hemodilution in the management of cerebral ischemia. In: Hartmann A, Kuschinsky W. (eds) Cerebral ischemia and hemorheology. Springer, Berlin Heidelberg, pp: 411–415 (1987)
250. Mast H, Marx P: Neurological deterioration under hemodilution in cerebral ischemia. Clin Hemorheology 9: 498 (1989)
251. Matthews WB, Oxbury JM, Graininger KMR: A. blind controlled trial of dextran 40 in the treatment of ischemic stroke. Brain 99: 193–206 (1976)
252. Mattle H, Mumenthaler M: Diagnose, Therapie und Prävention zerebrovaskulärer Erkrankungen. I. Klinik und Diagnose. Schweiz Med Wschr 119: 613–629 (1989)
253. Mattle H, Mumenthaler M: Diagnose, Therapie und Prävention zerebrovaskulärer Erkrankungen. II. Therapie und Prävention. Schweiz Med Wschr 119: 656–670 (1989)
254. Mau G: Hemoglobin changes during pregnancy and growth disturbances in the neonate. J Perinat Med 5: 172–177 (1977)
255. Meier-Baumgartner HP: Das Bobath-Konzept. Z Gerontol 20: 377–380 (1987)
256. Messinezy M, Pearson TC, Prochazka A, Wetherly-Mein G: Treatment of primary proliferative polycythaemia by venesection and low dose busulphan: retrospective study from one centre. Br J Haematol 61: 657–666 (1985)
257. Messmer K, Sunder-Plassmann L, Klövekorn WP, Holper K: Circulatory significance of hemodilution: rheological changes and limitations. Adv Microcirc 4: 1–77 (1972)
258. Messmer K, Sunder-Plassmann L, von Hesler F, Endrich B: Hemodilution in peripheral occlusive disease: a hemorheological approach. Clin Hemorheology 2: 721–731 (1982)
259. Metcalf W, Papdopoulos A, Tufaro R, Barth A: Clinical physiologic study of hydroxyethyl starch. Surgery, Gynecology, Obstetrics 131: 255 (1970)
260. Metzler de Höhmann U, Weigelin E: Fibrinolyse und Antikoagulantientherapie bei retinalen Venenverschlüssen. Medizinische Verlag, Marburg/Lahn, pp: 1–79 (1977)
261. Millar-Craig MW, Bishop CN, Raftery EB: Circadian variation of blood-pressure. Lancet 15: 795–797 (1978)
262. Mirhashemi S, Messmer K, Arfors KE, Intaglietta M: Microcirculatory effects of normovolemic hemodilution in skeletal muscle. Int J Microcirc Clin Exp 6: 359–369 (1987)
263. Mohr JP: American trial of nimodipine in acute ischemic stroke. 2nd International Symposium on Nimodipine. Acute Indications, Miami Beach, Florida: 38–42 (1990)
264. Müller N, Popov-Cenic S, Kladetzky RG, Hack G, Lang U, Safer A, Rahlfs VW: Hydroxyäthylstärke und ihr Einfluß auf die intra – sowie postoperative Haemostase. Infusionstherapie 3: 305–309 (1976)
265. Müller-Bühl U, Diehm C, Sieben U: Prävalenz und Risikofaktoren von peripherer arterieller Verschlußkrankheit und koronarer Herzkrankheit. Vasa Suppl 4, Huber, Bern (1987)
266. Müller-Bühl U, Combert HU, Diehm C: Hämodilutionstherapie der arteriellen Verschlußkrankheit mit Hydroxyäthylstärke 200/0,5. Münch Med Wschr 124: 241–243 (1982)

267. Müller-Matthesius R: Amylase-Bestimmung mit p-Nitrophenyl-maltosiden. Internist 23: 575–578 (1982)
268. Müller-Plathe O: Säure-Basen Haushalt und Blutgase. Thieme, Stuttgart (1982)
269. Murphy JF, O'Riordan J, Newcombe RG, Coles EC, Pearson JF: Relation of haemoglobin levels in first and second trimester to outcome of pregnancy. Lancet II: 992–995 (1986)
270. Naeye RL, Tafari N: Risk factors in pregnancy and diseases of the fetus and newborn. Williams and Wilkins, Baltimore (1985)
271. Nardini M, Rossi G, Martini A, Bono G, Brambilla GM, Candelise L, De Zanche, Iadecola C, Inzitari D, Mariani F, Fieschi C: Italian study of cerebral reversible ischemic attacks. Eur Neurol 22 (Supplement 1): 83–88 (1983)
272. Needergard M: Mechanisms of brain damage in focal cerebral ischemia. Acta Neurol Scand 77: 81–101 (1988)
273. Neuhof H, Wolf H: Oxygen uptake during hemodilution. Biblthca Haemat 41: 66–75 (1975)
274. Newhouse VL, Lecong PL, Furgason ES, Ho CT: On increasing the range of pulsed doppler system for blood flow measurement. Ultrasound Med Biol 6: 233–237 (1980)
275. Newhouse VL, Nathan RS, Hertzler LW: A proposed standard target for ultrasound doppler gain calibration. Ultrasound Med Biol 8: 313–316 (1982)
276. Newsholme EA, Start C: Regulation des Stoffwechsels. Verlag Chemie, Weinheim (1977)
277. Niswander KR, Gordon M: The women and their pregnancies. Saunders, Philadelphia (1972)
278. Nobbe F: Akute cerebrale Ischämie: Symptomatik, Sofortmaßnahmen, Diagnostik und Therapie. Klinikarzt 13: 941–947 (1984)
279. Noll F: In: Bergemeyer HU (ed.). Methoden der enzymatischen Analyse. Verlag Chemie, Weinheim, pp: 1521–1526 (1974)
280. Nückel M, Singer I, Kaps M, Hornig C, Dorndorf W: Wie häufig kann man mit einer Indikation zur Thrombolyse rechnen? Abstractband 7. Arbeitstreffen der Arbeitsgemeinschaft "Neurologische Intensivmedizin" München 80 (1990)
281. Olsen TS: Regional cerebral blood flow after occlusion of the middle cerebral artery. Acta Neurol Scand 73: 321–337 (1986)
282. Olsen TS: Regional cerebral blood flow after stroke. In: Haaß A (ed.). Hemodilution in stroke. Springer, Berlin Heidelberg New York, in press (1991)
283. Olsen TS, Larsen B, Herning M, Bech Skriver E, Lassen NA: Blood flow and vascular reactivity in collaterally perfused brain tissue. Evidence of an ischemic penumbra in patients with acute stroke. Stroke 14: 332–341 (1983)
284. Ostendorf P: Therapie mit Antikoagulantien und Thrombozytenaggregationshemmern bei extracraniellen Gefäßstenosen und Gefäßverschlüssen. Internist 20: 539–546 (1979)
285. Ozaita G, Calandre L, Peinado E, Rodriguez-Antigüedad A, Bermejo F: Hematocrit and clinical outcome in acute cerebral infarction. Stroke 18: 1166–1168 (1987)
286. Paulini K, Sonntag W: Veränderungen des RES der Ratte nach parenteraler Gabe von Dextran 40 und Hydroxyäthylstärke (Mw 40.000). Chemische, licht- und elektronenmikroskopische Untersuchung. Infusionstherapie 3: 294–299 (1976)
287. Pearce JMS, Chandrasekera CP, Ladusans EJ: Lacunar infarcts in polycythaemia with raised packed cell volumes. Br Med J 287: 935–936 (1983)
288. Pearson TC, Wetherley-Mein G: Vascular occlusive episodes and venous haematocrit in primary prolifertive polycythaemia. Lancet 2: 1219–1222 (1978)
289. Pentoxifylline Study Group: Pentoxifylline (PTX) in acute ischemic stroke. Stroke 18: 298 (1987)
290. Peter K, Gander HP, Lutz H, Nold W, Stosiek E: Die Beeinflussung der Blutgerinnung durch Hydroxyäthylstärke. Anästhesist 24: 219 (1975)
291. Pfeifer U, Kult J, Förster H: Aszites als Komplikation hepatischer Speicherung von Hydroxyäthylstärke (HES) bei Langzeitdialyse. Klin Woschensch 62: 862–866 (1984)

292. Pindur G, Haaß A, Treib J, Miyashita C, Köhler M, Seyfert UT, Wenzel E: Changes in haemostasis during hydroxyethyl starch (HES) treatment. J Clin Exp Hematol 58: 106 (1989)
293. Pits RF: Physiologie der Niere und der Körperflüssigkeiten. Schattauer, Stuttgart (1972)
294. Poeck K, Hacke W: Akuter ischämischer zerebraler Gefäßinsult. Voraussetzungen für Studien über die Wirksamkeit aktiver Enzyme. Dtsch Ärzteblatt 86/ 1/2: 33–34 (1989)
295. Pollock S, Tsitsopoulos P, Harrison MJG: The effect of haematocrit on cerebral perfusion and clinical status following carotid occlusion in the gerbil. Stroke 13: 167–170 (1982)
296. Popov-Cenic S, Müller N, Kladetzky RG, Hack G, Lang U, Safer A, Rahlfs VW: Durch Prämedikation, Narkose und Operation bedingte Änderungen des Gerinnungs- und Fibrinolysesystems und der Thrombozyten: Einfluß von Dextran und Hydroxyäthylstärke (HÄS) während und nach der Operation. Anaesthesit 26: 77–84 (1977)
297. Powers WJ, Raichle ME: Positron emission tomography and its application to the study of the study of cerebrovascular disease in man. Stroke 16: 361–376 (1985)
298. Ranft J, Heidrich H, Peters A, Trampisch H: Laser-Doppler examinations in persons with healthy vasculare and in patients with peripheral arterial occlusive disease. Angiology 37: 818–827 (1986)
299. Rapopori SM: Medizinische Biochemie. VEB Verlag Volk und Gesundheit, Berlin, pp: 362 (1966)
300. Reed AH, Cannon DC, Winkelman JW, Bhasin YP, Henry RJ, Pileggi VJ: Estimation of normal ranges from a controlled sample survey. I. Sex- and age-related influence on the SMA 12/60 screening group of tests. Clin Chem 18: 57–66 (1972)
301. Von Restorff W, Höfling B, Holtz J, Bassenge E: Effect of increased blood fluidity through hemodilution on general circulation at rest and during exercise in dogs. Pflügers Archiv 357: 25–34 (1975)
302. Rieger H: Induziert Blutverdünnung (Hämodilution) als neues Konzept der Therapie peripherer Durchblutungsstörungen. Internist 23: 375–382 (1982)
303. Rieger H, Reinicke B: Ergebnisse spezieller Behandlungsmethoden bei ischämischen Gewebsläsionen. Internist 25: 434 (1984)
304. Ring J, Messmer K: Anaphylaktoide Reaktionen nach Infusion kolloidaler Volumenersatzmittel. Internist Prax 16: 579 (1976)
305. Ring J, Messmer K: Incidence and severity of anaphylactoid reactions to colloid volume substitutions. Lancet I: 466 (1977)
306. Ring J, Richter W: Wirkungsmechanismus unerwünschter Reaktionen von Haes und Humanalbumin. Allergologie 3: 79 (1980)
307. Ringelstein EB, Koschorke S, Holling A, Thron A, Lambertz H, Minale C: Computed tomographic patterns of proven embolic brain infarctions. Ann Neurol 26: 759–765 (1989)
308. Ringelstein EB, Mauckner A, Schneider R, Sturm W, Doering W, Wolf S, Maurin N, Willmes K, Schlenker M, Brückmann H, Eschenfelder V: Effects of enzymatic blood defibrination in subcortical arteriosclerotic encephalopathy. J Neurol Neurosurg Psychiat 51: 1051–1057 (1988)
309. Ringelstein EB, Zeumer H, Schneider R: Der Beitrag der zerebralen Computertomographie zur Differentialtypologie und Differentialtherapie des ischämischen Großhirninfarktes. Fortschr Neurol Psychiat 53: 315–336 (1985)
310. Roggenkamp HG, Jung F, Kiesewetter H: Ein Gerät zur elektrischen Messung der Verformbarkeit von Erythrozyten. Biomed Tech 28: 100–104 (1982)
311. Rudofsky G: Postoperativer Verlauf von hämodynamischen und hämorheologischen Parametern. In: Kiesewetter H, Ehrly M, Jung F: Hämorheologische Meßmethoden. Münch Wiss Publ: 255–266 (1985)
312. Rudofsky G, Brock FE, Nobbe F: Beeinflussung der reaktiven Hyperämie durch die isovolämische Hämodilution bei Patienten mit arterieller Verschlußkrankheit. VASA 8: 320–323 (1979)
313. Rudofsky G, Meyer P, Strohmeyer HU: Effect of haemodilution on resting blood flow and reactive hyperaemia in lower limbs. Bibl Haemat No 47: 157–164 (1981)

314. Sachs L: Angewandte Statistik. Springer, Berlin Heidelberg New York (1984)
315. Sakai F, Igarashi H, Suzuki S, Tazaki Y: Cerebral blood flow and cerebral hematocrit in patients with cerebral ischemia measured by single-photon emission computed tomography. Acta Neurol Scand Suppl 127: 9–13 (1989)
316. Scandinavian Stroke Study Group: Multicenter trial of hemodilution in acute ischemic stroke. Stroke 18: 691–699 (1987)
317. Scandinavian Stroke Study Group: Multicenter trial of hemodilution in acute ischemic stroke. Results of subgroup analyses. Stroke 19: 464–471 (1988)
318. Scharf J, Von Kummer R, Back T, Reich H, Machens G, Wildemann B: Haemodilution with dextran 40 and hydroxyethyl starch and its effect on cerebral microcirculation. J Neurol 236: 164–167 (1989)
319. Scheffler P: Klinische Aussagekraft nicht-invasiver, arterieller Blutflußmessungen mit einem rechnergestützten Ultraschallverfahren. Habilitationsschrift, Universität des Saarlandes (1987)
320. Scheffler P, Hellstern P, Weiss H, Schneider A, Wenzel E: Die hämodynamische Beeinflußbarkeit der cerebralen Durchblutung bei Gefäßgesunden und bei Patienten mit Arteriosklerose. Dtsch.-Jap. Kongreß für Angiologie. Demeter Verlag, Stuttgart: 249–256 (1985)
321. Schmid-Schönbein H: Blood rheology and cardiac microcirculation: Is there a place for hemodilution in coronary insufficiency? In: Tillmanns H, Kübler W, Zebe H (eds) Microcirculation of the Heart. Springer, Berlin Heidelberg New York, p: 325 (1982)
322. Schmid-Schönbein H: Physiologie und Pathophysiologie der Mikrozirkulation aus rheologischer Sicht. In: Trübestein G: Art. Verschlußkrankheit und tiefe Venenthrombose. Thieme, Stuttgart (1984)
323. Schmid-Schönbein H, Engler RL: No-reflow in the microcirculation. The granulocyte tragedy. In: Hartmann A, Kuschinsky W (eds) Cerebral ischemia and hemorheology. Springer, Berlin Heidelberg New York, pp: 464–471 (1987)
324. Schmid-Schönbein H: Macrorheology and microrheology of blood in cerebrovascular insufficiency. Eur Neurol 22: 2–22 (1983)
325. Schmidt FH: Die enzymatische Bestimmung von Glukose und Fruktose nebeneinander. Klin Wochenschr 39: 1244–1248 (1961)
326. Schneider R: Hämodilution beim ischämischen Hirninfarkt. Deutsche Gesellschaft für Angiologie, Demeter Verlag, Stuttgart, p: 3 (1989)
327. Schneider R, Kiesewetter H: Parenterale Pentoxifyllin-Applikation beim ischämischen Insult. Dtsch Med Wochenschr 44: 1674–1677 (1982)
328. Schoop W: Bewegungstherapie bei peripheren Durchblutungsstörungen. Med Welt 10: 502–506 (1964)
329. Schröcksadel W, Gabl F: Die Diagnostik des gestörten Eisenstoffwechsels. WMW 3/4: 63 (1984)
330. Schwab J, Schramm A, Blüm A, Goller B: Therapie des apoplektischen Insults beim alten Menschen. Z Geriatrie Rehab 2: 151–152 (1989)
331. Schwab W, Tritschler W, Kessler AC, Bablok W: Neue enzymatische Lactatbestimmung: methodische Aspekte und Probengewinnung. J Clin Chem Clin Biochem 17: 65–70 (1979)
332. Scully RE, McNeely BU, Galdabini JJ: Normal reference laboratory values. New Engl J Med 302: 37–48 (1980)
333. Seaman GVF, Engel R, Swank RL, Hissen W: Circadian periodicity in some physiological parameters of circulating blood. Nature 4999: 833–835 (1965)
334. Share L: In: Greep RO, Astwood EB (eds). Handbook of physiology. Williams and Wilkins, Baltimore, pp: 25–55 (1974)
335. Siegenthaler W, Kaufmann W, Hornbostel H, Waller H-D: Lehrbuch der inneren Medizin. Thieme, Stuttgart (1987)
336. Siedel H, Schlumberger G, Klose S, Ziegenhorn J, Wahlefeld AW: Improved reagent for the enzymatic determination of serum cholesterol. J Clin Chem Biochem 19: 838 (1981)
337. Siemkowicz E: The effect of glucose upon restitution after transient cerebral ischemia. A summary. Acta Neurol Scand 71: 414–427 (1985)

338. Siggaard-Anderson 0: The acid-base status of the blood. Munksgaard, Kopenhagen, pp: 2–20 (1974)
339. Siggaard-Andersen O, Engel K, Jörgensen K, Astrup P: A micromethod for determination of pH, carbon dioxide tension, base excess and standard bicarbonate in capillary blood. Scand J Clin Lab Invest 12: 172–176 (1960)
340. Siggaard-Andersen O, Jörgensen K, Naerea N: Spectrophotometric determination of oxygen saturation in capillary blood. Scand J Clin Lab Invest 14: 298 (1962)
341. Simon J, Jung F, Holbach T, Mrowietz C, Jaschke H, Kiesewetter H: Mikrobandscheibenoperationen. Krankenhausarzt 59: 814–821 (1986)
342. Sirtl C, Jesch F: In: Peter K, Schimetta W, Bergmann H, Hübner G, Gerlach E, Meßmer K, Steinbereithner K (eds.). Hydroxyäthylstärke (HES), Aktuelle Theorie und Praxis. Beiträge zur Anaesthesiologie und Intensivmedizin 26, Verlag Wilhelm Maudrich, Vienna, pp: 74–97 (1988)
343. Sirtl C, Laubenthal H, Dietrich HJ, Hügler P, Peter K: Nebenwirkungen von künstlichen kolloidalen Plasmaersatzmitteln unter besonderer Berücksichtigung von Hydroxyäthylstärke (HES). In: Penzer H, Pauser G, Bergmann H, Schimetta W (eds): Hydroxyäthylstärke (HES) Lungen – Volumen – Flüssigkeit. Beiträge zur Anaesthesiologie und Intensivmedizin 31, Verlag Wilhelm Maudrich, Vienna, pp: 35–53 (1990)
344. Sommermayer K, Cech F, Schmidt B, Weidler B: Klinisch verwendete Hydroxyäthylstärke: Physikalisch-Chemische Charakterisierung. Krankenhauspharmazie 8: 271–278 (1987)
345. Sorlie PD, Garcia-Palmieri M, Costas R, Havlik R: Hematocrit and risk of coronary heart disease: the Puerto Rico heart health program. Am Heart J 101: 456–461 (1981)
346. Spudis EV, De La Torre E, Pikula L: Management of completed stroke with dextran 40. Stroke 4: 895–897 (1973)
347. Stacher A: Klinik und Therapie des Eisenmangels. Wiener Med Wochenschr 3/4: 76 (1984)
348. Staedt U, Schwarz M, Bayerl JR, Tornow K, Heene DL: Hämodilution bei akuter zerebraler Ischämie. Med Welt 37: 695–699 (1986)
349. Statistisches Bundesamt: Statistisches Jahrbuch 1990 für die Bundesrepublik Deutschland. Kohlhammer, Stuttgart, in press (1990)
350. Steiner TJ: Naftidrofuryl in the treatment of recent stroke. Results of a controlled clinical trial. Vasa, Suppl 24: 44–47 (1988)
351. Strand T, Asplund S, Eriksson E, Hägg E, Lithner P, Westrer P: A randomized controlled clinical trial of hemodilution therapy in acute ischemic stroke. Stroke 15: 980–989 (1984)
352. Strauer BE: Hypertensive Herzkrankheit. Therapiewoche 34: 1–14 (1984)
353. Strauss RG: Review of the effects of hydroxyethyl starch on the blood coagulation system. Transfusion 21: 299–303 (1981)
354. Strauss RG, Stansfield C, Henriksen RA, Villhauer PJ: Pentastarch may cause fewer effects of hydroxyethyl on coagulation than hetastarch. Transfusion 28: 257–260 (1988)
355. Strauss RG, Stump DC, Henriksen RA: Hydroxyethyl starch accentuates von Willebrand's disease. Transfusion 25: 235–237 (1985)
356. Stump DC, Strauss RG, Henriksen RA, Petersen RE, Saunders R: Effects of hydroxyethyl starch on the blood coagulation, particularly factor VIII. Transfusion 25: 349–354 (1985)
357. Sunder-Plassmann L, von Hesler F, Endrich B, Messmer K: Improvement of collateral circulation in chronic vascular occlusive disease of the lower extremity. Biblthca Haemat 47: 43–53 (1981)
358. Sunder-Plassmann L, Klövekorn WP, Messmer K: Blutviskosität und Hämodynamik bei Anwendung kolloidaler Volumenersatzmittel. Anaesthesit 20: 172–180 (1971)
359. Sundt JR, TM, Waltz AG: Hemodilution and anticoagulation. Effects on the microvasculare and microcirculation of the cerebral cortex after arterial occlusion. Neurol 17: 230–238 (1967)

360. Sundt JR, TM, Waltz AG, Sayre G: Experimental cerebral infarction: modification by treatment with haemodiluting. Haemo-concentration and dehydrating agents. J Neurosurg 26: 46–56 (1967)
361. Symington B: Hetastarch and bleeding complications. Ann Intern Med 105: 627–629 (1986)
362. Tauchert M: Atypische Koronarerkrankung. In: Hombach V (ed) Kardiologie. Schattauer, Stuttgart, pp: 137–148 (1984)
363. Tenland T: Laser Doppler flowmetry. Methods and microvascular applications. Linköping Studies in Science and Technology Dissertations No 83: (1982)
364. Thomas L: Eiweiß-Elektrophorese. Urban and Schwarzenberg, Munich (1981)
365. Thompson WL: Hydroxyethylstarch. In: W Hennessen (ed) Developments in Biological Standardization. Karger, Basel, pp: 259 (1981)
366. Todd MM, Tommasino C, Moore S: Cerebral effects of isovolemic hemodilution with a hypertonic saline solution. J Neurosurg 63: 944–948 (1985)
367. Toghi H, Yamanouchi H, Murakami M, Kameyama M: Importance of hematocrit as a risk factor in cerebral infarction. Stroke 9: 369–374 (1978)
368. Tozer BA: The calculation of maximum permissible exposure level for laser radiation. J Phys E Sci Instrum 12: 922–926 (1979)
369. Trampisch HJ: Statistische Basis für kontrollierte klinische Studien bei peripherer arterieller Verschlußkrankheit. Angio Archiv 13: 9–13 (1980)
370. Tranmer B, Iacobacci R, Kindt G: Colloid Volume Expansion and Brain Edema. In: Hoff J, Betz A (eds) Intracranial pressure VII. Springer, Berlin Heidelberg New York, pp: 992–994 (1989)
371. Tranmer B, Keller T, Nagata K, Kindt G, Adey G: Blood volume expansion with hetastarch in acute ischaemic stroke: the effects on local cerebral blood flow and computer mapped EEG. Neurol Res 8: 177–181 (1986)
372. Tu Y, Heros RC, Karakostas D, Liszczak T, Hyodo A, Candia G, Zervas N, Lagree K: Isovolemic hemodilution in experimental focal cerebral ischemia. J Neurosurg 69: 82–91 (1988)
373. Überla K: In: von Eichstätt KW, Gross F (eds.). Arzneimittelprüfung. Fischer, Stuttgart, pp: 137–145 (1975)
374. Vara-Thorbeck R, Guerrero-Fernandez-Marcote JA: Hemodynamic response of elderly patients undergoing major surgery under moderate normovolemic hemodilution. Eur Surg Res 17: 372–376 (1985)
375. Vass K, Tomida S, Hossmann K, Nowak JR, T, Klatzo I: Microvascular disturbances and edema formation after repetitive ischemia of gerbil brain. Acta Neuropathol 75: 288–294 (1988)
376. Vaupel P: Der gegenwärtige Stand der Milzphysiologie. Rheinl Pfälz Ärztebl 27: 735–745 (1974)
377. Vaupel P: In: Tillmann W, Ehrly AM (eds.). Hämorheologie und Hämatologie. Münch Wiss Publikationen, Munich, pp: 14–28 (1986)
378. Vossen W: Die Bestimmung des Sauerstoffgehaltes aus Sauerstoffpartialdruck und Sauerstoffsättigung für die klinische Routine. Dissertationsschrift, Universität Düsseldorf (1977)
379. Wade P: Transport of oxygen to the brain in patients with elevated haematocrit values before and after venesection. Brain 106: 513–523 (1983)
380. Wade P, Du Boulay G, Marshall J, Pearson TC, Ross-Russel R, Shirley A, Symon L, Wetherley-Mein G, Zilkha E: Cerebral blood flow, haematocrit and viscosity in subjects with a high oxygen affinity haemoglobin variant. Acta Neurol Scand 61: 210–215 (1980)
381. Wade P, Taylor D, Barnett H, Hachinsky V: Hemoglobin concentration and prognosis in symptomatic obstructive cerebrovascular disease. Stroke 18: 68–71 (1987)
382. Wagner KH, Wagner-Hering E: L (+)-Lactat im intermediären Stoffwechsel. Physikal Rehabilitation 10: 123–130 (1969)
383. Waldhausen P, Kiesewetter H, Leipnitz G, Koscielny J, Jung F, Bambauer R, von Blohn G: Durch Hydroxyäthylstärke induzierte passagere Niereninsuffizienz bei vorbestehen-

der glomerulärer Schädigung. Acta Medoca Austriaca (AMA), Jg. 18/1991, Sonderheft 1, 52–55 (1991)
384. Walker AE, Robins M, Weinfeld FD: Clinical findings. Stroke 12 (Suppl I: I/13–I/24): 13 (1981)
385. Wallenfels K, Földi H, Niermann H, Bender H, Linder D: The enzymic synthesis, by transglucosylation of a homologous series of glycosidically substituted maltooligosaccharides, and their use as amylase substrates. Carbohydr Res 61: 359–368 (1978)
386. Weichselbaum TE: An accurate and rapid method for the determination of proteins in small-amounts of blood serum and plasma. Am J Clin Pathol 16: 40–45 (1946)
387. Weidinger P, Bach N: 5 Jahre Wiener Erfahrungen mit ambulanten Claudicatio-Gruppen. In: Kiesewetter H, Jung F (eds) Konservative Therapie peripherer und zerebraler arterieller Durchblutungsstörungen, Ermer Verlag, pp: 21–36 (1987)
388. Weidinger P, Becsi C, Wehofer D: Hämodilution bei peripherer AVK: Vergleich hypervolämische Hämodilution und isovolämische Beutelplasmapherese. Haemostaseologie 8: 53 (1988)
389. Weidinger P, Becsi C, Wehofer D: Die Hämodilution als neuer Weg in der konservativen Therapie bei der peripheren arteriellen Verschlußkrankheit – Vergleich zwischen Beutelplasmapherese und hypervolämischer Hämodilution. Med Welt, in press (1990)
390. Weisskopf V, Mueller C, Weidler B, Balzer K, Fanoulas G, Fidora K: Erfahrungen mit der conjunktivalen Sauerstoffpartialdruckmessung im Rahmen rekonstruktiver Operationen an den extrakraniellen Hirngefäßen. Angio 9: 237–246 (1987)
391. Weth G: Kann eine Acutbehandlung des Schlaganfalls Paresen sofort zurückbilden? Z Geriatrie Rehab 2: 310–314 (1989)
392. Wilhelm HJ, Jung F, Kiesewetter H, Recktenwald C: On haemodilution therapy for patients with sudden loss of hearing. Klin Wochenschr 64: 1058 (1986)
393. Willison J, Du Boulay G, Paul E, Russell R, Thomas D, Marshall J, Pearson T, Symon L, Wetherley-Mein G: Effect of high haematocrit on alertness. Lancet: 846–848 (1980)
394. Wintrobe MM: Clinical hematology. Lea and Febiger, Philadelphia (1981)
395. Wise R, Bernardi S, Frackowiak R, Legg N, Jones T: Serial observations on the pathophysiology of acute stroke. Brain 106: 197–222 (1983)
396. Wolf S, Arend O, Bertram B, Schulte K, Kaufhold F, Teping C, Reim M: Hämodilution bei Patienten mit Zentralvenenthrombose der Retina: Eine placebokontrollierte randomisierte Studie. Fortsch Ophthal, in press (1990)
397. Wolf S, Hoberg A, Bertram B, Jung F, Kiesewetter H, Reim M: Videofluoreszenzangiographische Verlaufsbeobachtung bei Patienten mit retinalen Arterienverschlüssen. Klin Mbl Augenhlk 195: 154–160 (1989)
398. Wolf S, Hoberg A, Bertram B, Teping C, Reim M: Haemodilution therapy in retinal artery occlusion. In: Ferraz LN, Oliveira D (eds) Ophthalmology today. Elsevier, Amsterdam, pp: 531–533 (1988)
399. Wolf S, Jung F, Kiesewetter K, Körber N, Reim M: Videofluorescein angiographie: method and clinical application. Graefes Arch Clin Exp Ophthalmol 227: 145–151 (1989)
400. Wood JH, Fleischer A: Observations during hypervolemic hemodilution of patients with acute focal cerebral ischemia. JAMA 248: 2999–3014 (1982)
401. Wood JH, Simeone F, Fink E, Golden M: Hypervolemic hemodilution in experimental focal cerebral ischemia. J Neurosurg 59: 500–505 (1983)
402. Wood JH, Simeone F, Reuben E, Snyder L: Experimental hypervolemic hemodilution: physiological correlations of cortical blood flow, cardiac output and intracranial pressure with fresh blood viscosity and plasma volume. J Neurosurg 14: 709–723 (1984)
403. World Health Organisation: Who Expert Committee on arterial Hypertension, Technical Report Series, No 628, Genf (1978)
404. Wu KK, Hoak JC: A new method for the quantitative detection of platelet aggregates in patients with arterial insufficiency. Lancet: 924 (1974 II)
405. Yates CJP, Berrent PA, Andrews V, Dormandy JA: Increase in leg blood flow by normovolemic hemodilution in intermittent Claudication. Lancet I: 166 (1979)
406. Yett H, Skillman J, Salzman E: The hazards of aspirin plus heparin. N Engl J Med: 1092 (1978)

407. Yoshida M, Yamashita T, Matsuo J, Kishikawa T: Enzymic degradation of hydroxyethyl starch. Die Stärke 25: 373–378 (1973)
408. Zander R: Sauerstofftransportvermögen von Blutersatzflüssigkeiten im Vergleich mit anderen Infusionslösungen. Klin Wochenschr 56: 567–573 (1978)
409. Zander R: Zur Beteiligung potentieller Blutersatzlösungen mit Sauerstoffträgereigenschaften und deren Einsatzmöglichkeiten. Infusionstherapie 8: 274–286 (1981)
410. Zeumer H: Fibrinolyse hirnversorgender Arterien beim akuten ischämischen Insult. Vortrag auf dem Kongreß "Neue Strategien in der Behandlung des akuten ischämischen Insultes", Homburg-Saar (1987)
411. Zondervan HA: Blood viscosity in complicated pregnancy. Thesis, Amsterdam (1988)
412. Zumkley H: Klinik des Wasser-, Elektrolyt- und Säure-Basen-Haushaltes. Thieme, Stuttgart, pp: 102–105 (1977)

# Subject Index